Oral Mucosal Drug Delivery

DRUGS AND THE PHARMACEUTICAL SCIENCES

DRUGS AND THE PHARMACEUTICAL SCIENCES

A Series of Textbooks and Monographs

edited by

James Swarbrick
AAI, Inc.
Wilmington, North Carolina

1. Pharmacokinetics, *Milo Gibaldi and Donald Perrier*
2. Good Manufacturing Practices for Pharmaceuticals: A Plan for Total Quality Control, *Sidney H. Willig, Murray M. Tuckerman, and William S. Hitchings IV*
3. Microencapsulation, *edited by J. R. Nixon*
4. Drug Metabolism: Chemical and Biochemical Aspects, *Bernard Testa and Peter Jenner*
5. New Drugs: Discovery and Development, *edited by Alan A. Rubin*
6. Sustained and Controlled Release Drug Delivery Systems, *edited by Joseph R. Robinson*
7. Modern Pharmaceutics, *edited by Gilbert S. Banker and Christopher T. Rhodes*
8. Prescription Drugs in Short Supply: Case Histories, *Michael A. Schwartz*
9. Activated Charcoal: Antidotal and Other Medical Uses, *David O. Cooney*
10. Concepts in Drug Metabolism (in two parts), *edited by Peter Jenner and Bernard Testa*
11. Pharmaceutical Analysis: Modern Methods (in two parts), *edited by James W. Munson*
12. Techniques of Solubilization of Drugs, *edited by Samuel H. Yalkowsky*
13. Orphan Drugs, *edited by Fred E. Karch*
14. Novel Drug Delivery Systems: Fundamentals, Developmental Concepts, Biomedical Assessments, *Yie W. Chien*
15. Pharmacokinetics: Second Edition, Revised and Expanded, *Milo Gibaldi and Donald Perrier*
16. Good Manufacturing Practices for Pharmaceuticals: A Plan for Total Quality Control, Second Edition, Revised and Expanded, *Sidney H. Willig, Murray M. Tuckerman, and William S. Hitchings IV*
17. Formulation of Veterinary Dosage Forms, *edited by Jack Blodinger*

18. Dermatological Formulations: Percutaneous Absorption, *Brian W. Barry*
19. The Clinical Research Process in the Pharmaceutical Industry, *edited by Gary M. Matoren*
20. Microencapsulation and Related Drug Processes, *Patrick B. Deasy*
21. Drugs and Nutrients: The Interactive Effects, *edited by Daphne A. Roe and T. Colin Campbell*
22. Biotechnology of Industrial Antibiotics, *Erick J. Vandamme*
23. Pharmaceutical Process Validation, *edited by Bernard T. Loftus and Robert A. Nash*
24. Anticancer and Interferon Agents: Synthesis and Properties, *edited by Raphael M. Ottenbrite and George B. Butler*
25. Pharmaceutical Statistics: Practical and Clinical Applications, *Sanford Bolton*
26. Drug Dynamics for Analytical, Clinical, and Biological Chemists, *Benjamin J. Gudzinowicz, Burrows T. Younkin, Jr., and Michael J. Gudzinowicz*
27. Modern Analysis of Antibiotics, *edited by Adjoran Aszalos*
28. Solubility and Related Properties, *Kenneth C. James*
29. Controlled Drug Delivery: Fundamentals and Applications, Second Edition, Revised and Expanded, *edited by Joseph R. Robinson and Vincent H. Lee*
30. New Drug Approval Process: Clinical and Regulatory Management, *edited by Richard A. Guarino*
31. Transdermal Controlled Systemic Medications, *edited by Yie W. Chien*
32. Drug Delivery Devices: Fundamentals and Applications, *edited by Praveen Tyle*
33. Pharmacokinetics: Regulatory • Industrial • Academic Perspectives, *edited by Peter G. Welling and Francis L. S. Tse*
34. Clinical Drug Trials and Tribulations, *edited by Allen E. Cato*
35. Transdermal Drug Delivery: Developmental Issues and Research Initiatives, *edited by Jonathan Hadgraft and Richard H. Guy*
36. Aqueous Polymeric Coatings for Pharmaceutical Dosage Forms, *edited by James W. McGinity*
37. Pharmaceutical Pelletization Technology, *edited by Isaac Ghebre-Sellassie*
38. Good Laboratory Practice Regulations, *edited by Allen F. Hirsch*
39. Nasal Systemic Drug Delivery, *Yie W. Chien, Kenneth S. E. Su, and Shyi-Feu Chang*
40. Modern Pharmaceutics: Second Edition, Revised and Expanded, *edited by Gilbert S. Banker and Christopher T. Rhodes*
41. Specialized Drug Delivery Systems: Manufacturing and Production Technology, *edited by Praveen Tyle*
42. Topical Drug Delivery Formulations, *edited by David W. Osborne and Anton H. Amann*
43. Drug Stability: Principles and Practices, *Jens T. Carstensen*

44. Pharmaceutical Statistics: Practical and Clinical Applications, Second Edition, Revised and Expanded, *Sanford Bolton*
45. Biodegradable Polymers as Drug Delivery Systems, *edited by Mark Chasin and Robert Langer*
46. Preclinical Drug Disposition: A Laboratory Handbook, *Francis L. S. Tse and James J. Jaffe*
47. HPLC in the Pharmaceutical Industry, *edited by Godwin W. Fong and Stanley K. Lam*
48. Pharmaceutical Bioequivalence, *edited by Peter G. Welling, Francis L. S. Tse, and Shrikant V. Dinghe*
49. Pharmaceutical Dissolution Testing, *Umesh V. Banakar*
50. Novel Drug Delivery Systems: Second Edition, Revised and Expanded, *Yie W. Chien*
51. Managing the Clinical Drug Development Process, *David M. Cocchetto and Ronald V. Nardi*
52. Good Manufacturing Practices for Pharmaceuticals: A Plan for Total Quality Control, Third Edition, *edited by Sidney H. Willig and James R. Stoker*
53. Prodrugs: Topical and Ocular Drug Delivery, *edited by Kenneth B. Sloan*
54. Pharmaceutical Inhalation Aerosol Technology, *edited by Anthony J. Hickey*
55. Radiopharmaceuticals: Chemistry and Pharmacology, *edited by Adrian D. Nunn*
56. New Drug Approval Process: Second Edition, Revised and Expanded, *edited by Richard A. Guarino*
57. Pharmaceutical Process Validation: Second Edition, Revised and Expanded, *edited by Ira R. Berry and Robert A. Nash*
58. Ophthalmic Drug Delivery Systems, *edited by Ashim K. Mitra*
59. Pharmaceutical Skin Penetration Enhancement, *edited by Kenneth A. Walters and Jonathan Hadgraft*
60. Colonic Drug Absorption and Metabolism, *edited by Peter R. Bieck*
61. Pharmaceutical Particulate Carriers: Therapeutic Applications, *edited by Alain Rolland*
62. Drug Permeation Enhancement: Theory and Applications, *edited by Dean S. Hsieh*
63. Glycopeptide Antibiotics, *edited by Ramakrishnan Nagarajan*
64. Achieving Sterility in Medical and Pharmaceutical Products, *Nigel A. Halls*
65. Multiparticulate Oral Drug Delivery, *edited by Isaac Ghebre-Sellassie*
66. Colloidal Drug Delivery Systems, *edited by Jörg Kreuter*
67. Pharmacokinetics: Regulatory • Industrial • Academic Perspectives, Second Edition, *edited by Peter G. Welling and Francis L. S. Tse*
68. Drug Stability: Principles and Practices, Second Edition, Revised and Expanded, *Jens T. Carstensen*

69. Good Laboratory Practice Regulations: Second Edition, Revised and Expanded, *edited by Sandy Weinberg*
70. Physical Characterization of Pharmaceutical Solids, *edited by Harry G. Brittain*
71. Pharmaceutical Powder Compaction Technology, *edited by Göran Alderborn and Christer Nyström*
72. Modern Pharmaceutics: Third Edition, Revised and Expanded, *edited by Gilbert S. Banker and Christopher T. Rhodes*
73. Microencapsulation: Methods and Industrial Applications, *edited by Simon Benita*
74. Oral Mucosal Drug Delivery, *edited by Michael J. Rathbone*
75. Clinical Research in Pharmaceutical Development, *edited by Barry Bleidt and Michael Montagne*

ADDITIONAL VOLUMES IN PREPARATION

The Drug Development Process: Increasing Efficiency and Cost-Effectiveness, *edited by Peter G. Welling, Louis Lasagna, and Umesh V. Banakar*

Microparticulate Systems for the Delivery of Proteins and Vaccines, *edited by Smadar Cohen and Howard Bernstein*

Good Manufacturing Practices for Pharmaceuticals: A Plan for Total Quality Control, Fourth Edition, Revised and Expanded, *Sidney H. Willig and James R. Stoker*

Aqueous Polymeric Coatings for Pharmaceutical Dosage Forms: Second Edition, *edited by James W. McGinity*

Oral Mucosal Drug Delivery

edited by

Michael J. Rathbone
InterAg
Hamilton, New Zealand

Marcel Dekker, Inc. **New York • Basel • Hong Kong**

Library of Congress Cataloging-in-Publication Data

Oral mucosal drug delivery / edited by Michael J. Rathbone.
p. cm. — (Drugs and the pharmaceutical sciences ; 74)
Includes indexes.
ISBN 0-8247-9744-2 (hardcover : alk. paper)
1. Oral medication. 2. Oral mucosa. I. Rathbone, Michael J. II. Series.
[DNLM: 1. Administration, Oral. 2. Mouth Mucosa—metabolism. 3. Cell Membrane Permeability—physiology. 4. Drug Delivery Systems.
W1 DR893B v.74 1996 / WB 350 063 1996]
RM162.073 1996
615'.6—dc20
DNLM/DLC
for Library of Congress 96-14719
CIP

The publisher offers discounts on this book when ordered in bulk quantities. For more information, write to Special Sales/Professional Marketing at the address below.

This book is printed on acid-free paper.

MARCEL DEKKER, INC.
270 Madison Avenue, New York, New York 10016

Current printing (last digit):
10 9 8 7 6 5 4 3 2 1

PRINTED IN THE UNITED STATES OF AMERICA

To my son Camryn

Preface

The administration of drugs to or via the oral cavity is a difficult problem that offers many challenges to the pharmaceutical scientist. A good understanding of the anatomy and physiology of the oral cavity, a detailed consideration and understanding of the problems and limitations of the oral cavity as a site for drug delivery, the role of saliva in the distribution and clearance of drugs in the oral cavity, and knowledge of the mechanisms, pathways, and barriers to drug permeation are all required to successfully formulate an optimized oral mucosal drug delivery system.

Recent years have seen rapid developments in the field of oral mucosal drug delivery: new approaches to overcoming the problems associated with the oral cavity as a site for drug delivery, more detailed insights into the structure and organization of oral mucosa, novel in vitro and in vivo methods for assessing the permeability of oral mucosa, and innovative, rationally designed delivery systems that overcome the problems that have previously frustrated the formulation scientist.

Although the pharmaceutical and dental literature contains many publications on the general topic of oral mucosal drug delivery, there have thus far been few efforts to present the whole subject methodically in a single reference.

The purpose of this book is fourfold. The first is to review the unique aspects of the oral cavity that make it a distinctive site for drug delivery, e.g., anatomy and physiology of the oral cavity, structure and organization of the oral mucosa, routes of drug transport through oral mucosa, salivary mucins, and saliva kinetics. The second purpose is to detail the current approaches that formulation scientists adopt to overcome the problems associated with drug delivery to or via this site, e.g., permeation enhancement and retention. The third is to review current in vitro and in vivo methodologies that allow an investigator to establish the suitability of a drug candidate. Finally, the book outlines the currently available and emerging oral mucosal drug delivery systems.

The term "oral mucosal drug delivery" is used in this book in its general sense to cover the delivery of drugs both locally to, and systemically via, the oral cavity. Local delivery to the oral cavity can encompass delivery into the membranes that line the oral cavity; delivery to the dental tissues found in the oral cavity, e.g., teeth; delivery to microenvironments that exist within the mouth, e.g., the periodontal pocket; and delivery to the saliva. Each chapter is intended to be a complete treatise on a particular topic. The chapters are designed to complement one another and provide the reader with a better understanding of the oral cavity as a site for drug delivery, the problems that await the formulator, how such problems can be overcome, the methods available to assist the formulator in preformulation studies, and the delivery systems that are currently available or emerging, so that a rational approach to the formulation of an oral mucosal drug delivery system, be it for local or systemic use, can be adopted.

Although the aims of local and systemic oral mucosal drug delivery are very different, because of the inherent characteristics of the oral cavity, there is considerable overlap in the problems associated with these modes of delivery and in the design of delivery systems that achieve these different aims. It has proven very difficult to establish a definitive dividing line between those systems designed for local use and those intended for systemic delivery. This is reflected in the book. Although some chapters are devoted exclusively to systemic or local delivery, many provide a generalized overview applicable to both systemic and local drug delivery system design.

The 15 chapters are contributions from established or emerging researchers around the world who have been working in this field. The book is designed for individuals from diverse backgrounds who are interested in the problems, limitations, and advantages of the oral cavity as a site for drug delivery, and in the design, fabrication, optimization, and assessment of oral mucosal drug delivery systems. The chapters offer a good introduction to the uninitiated scientist, and an in-depth analysis of some fundamental considerations.

The anatomy and physiology of the oral cavity and its implications for oral mucosal drug delivery are reviewed by Squier and Wertz in Chapter 1. These authors expand on this subject in Chapter 2 and look closely at the structure and organization of the oral mucosal membranes and the potential barriers to a penetrant. Based on this knowledge, Zhang and Robinson in Chapter 3 discuss the potential routes for drug transport through oral mucosa. The route of drug delivery having been identified, Aungst (Chapter 4) discusses the possibilities and limitations of enhancing the permeation of a drug through oral mucosa.

Having an appreciation of the relevant anatomy and physiology of the oral cavity, the formulator must next assess the suitability of the drug for delivery. In this respect the permeability of the oral mucosa to the drug is an important consideration and the following three chapters (5, 6 and 7) discuss in vitro and in vivo methods for measuring the permeability of oral mucosa. Chapter 8 deals with a major problem that is encountered in oral mucosal drug delivery: saliva. This chapter discusses the location of the sites of secretion, identifies the flow patterns associated with saliva in the oral cavity, and discusses the possible implications of these flow patterns with respect to oral mucosal drug delivery. The oral cavity membranes are lined with a mucin layer, which may have implications in the barrier function of the oral cavity and play a role in drug delivery. Such possibilities are discussed by Schenkels et al in Chapter 9. The presence of salivary mucins in the oral cavity provides the formulator with a handle with which to overcome a major problem associated with the oral cavity as a site for drug delivery: retention of the delivery system, a particular problem when attempting to delivery drugs for extended periods of time. Kellaway and Warren discuss this aspect in Chapter 10 and provide us with our first insight into the range of delivery systems that are available for local and/or systemic use in the oral cavity.

The remaining chapters of the book focus on delivery systems used in the oral cavity. An overview of systemic drug delivery and delivery systems is presented by Rathbone et al in Chapter 11, while Chapter 12 is devoted to a recent innovation: patch design, manufacture, and assessment. Chewing gum as an oral mucosal drug delivery system is considered by Rassing in Chapter 13. This delivery system has the potential for both local and systemic oral mucosal drug delivery, and both of these aspects are considered. Chapters 14 and 15 consider local delivery to specialized areas of the mouth—the periodontal pocket and the teeth. Much research time and effort have been focused on these areas in recent years, and numerous innovative and highly specialized delivery systems have evolved from this research.

I am indebted to all of the authors who prepared chapters. It has been my pleasure to collaborate with these knowledgeable and cooperative individuals whose efforts have been essential to the completion of this work. Special appreciation is extended to Professor Christopher Squier for his valuable and constructive comments during its conception and production. To all of the reviewers of the chapters I send thanks for the time they devoted to this task. A very special thanks goes to James Townshend, who reviewed the entire manuscript and made many helpful comments. Finally, I wish to thank my wife, Judith, for her endless patience, kindness, and love.

Michael J. Rathbone

Contents

Preface *v*
Contributors *xi*

1. Structure and Function of the Oral Mucosa and Implications for Drug Delivery 1
Christopher A. Squier and Philip W. Wertz

2. Biochemical Basis of the Permeability Barrier in Skin and Oral Mucosa 27
Philip W. Wertz, A. Janet Hoogstraate, and Christopher A. Squier

3. Routes of Drug Transport Across Oral Mucosa 51
Hao Zhang and Joseph R. Robinson

4. Oral Mucosal Permeation Enhancement: Possibilities and Limitations 65
Bruce J. Aungst

5. In Vitro Methods for Measuring Permeability of the Oral Mucosa 85
Hao Zhang and Joseph R. Robinson

6. Buccal Epithelial Cell Cultures as a Model to Study Oral Mucosal Drug Transport and Metabolism 101
Kenneth L. Audus

7. In Vivo Techniques for Studying the Oral Mucosal Absorption Characteristics of Drugs in Animals and Humans 121
Michael J. Rathbone, Robert Purves, Firoz A. Ghazali, and Ping C. Ho

8. The Flow of Saliva and Its Influence on the Movement, Deposition and Removal of Drugs Administered to the Oral Cavity 157
John A. Weatherell, Colin Robinson, and Michael J. Rathbone

9. Salivary Mucins: Their Role in Oral Mucosal Barrier Function and Drug Delivery 191
Leon C. P. M. Schenkels, Tarikere L. Gururaja, and Michael J. Levine

10. Mucoadhesive Hydrogels for Buccal Delivery 221
Ian W. Kellaway and Simon J. Warren

11. Systemic Oral Mucosal Drug Delivery and Delivery Systems 241
Michael J. Rathbone, Gilles Ponchel, and Firoz A. Ghazali

12. Specialized Oral Mucosal Drug Delivery Systems: Patches 285
Gary DeGrande, Luce Benes, Françoise Horrière, Herve Karsenty, Claire Lacoste, Roy McQuinn, Jian-Hwa Guo, and Robert Scherrer

13. Specialized Oral Mucosal Drug Delivery Systems: Chewing Gum 319
Margrethe Rømer Rassing

14. Intra-periodontal Pocket Drug Delivery Systems 359
W. Aubrey Soskolone and Michael Freidman

15. The Intraoral Delivery of Fluoride 381
Bernadette K. Drummond and John C. Rodda

Author Index *407*
Subject Index *437*

Contributors

Kenneth L. Audus, Ph.D. School of Pharmacy, Department of Pharmaceutical Chemistry, The University of Kansas, 3006 Malott Hall, Lawrence, Kansas 66045, USA.

Bruce J. Aungst, Ph.D. The DuPont Merck Pharmaceutical Company, Pharmaceutical Research and Development, Experimental Station, PO Box 80400, Wilmington, Delaware 19880, USA.

Luce Benes, Ph.D. Laboratoires 3M Santé, Avenue du 11 Novembre - 45312, Pithiviers Cedex, France.

Gary DeGrande, Ph.D. Directeur Technique, Laboratoires 3M Santé, Avenue du 11 Novembre - 45312, Pithiviers Cedex, France.

Bernadette K. Drummond, Head of Department of Community Dental Health, School of Dentistry, University of Otago, Dunedin, New Zealand.

Michael Friedman, Ph.D. Department of Pharmacy, Hebrew University Faculty of Medicine, Jerusalem, Israel.

Firoz A. Ghazali, M.Pharm. School of Pharmacy, University of Otago, Dunedin, New Zealand.

Jian-Hwa Guo, Ph.D. 3M Pharmaceuticals, 3M Center, Building 270-2S-06, St. Paul, Minnesota 55144, USA.

Tarikere L. Gururaja, Ph.D. Department of Oral Biology and Dental Research Institute, State University of New York at Buffalo, 109 Foster Hall, 3435 Main Street, Buffalo, New York 14214, USA.

Ping C. Ho, M.Sc. School of Pharmacy, University of Otago, Dunedin, New Zealand.

A. Janet Hoogstraate, Ph.D. Leiden/Amsterdam Center for Drug Research, Division of Pharmaceutical Technology, Center for Bio-Pharmaceutical Sciences, Gorlaeus Laboratories, Einsteinweg 55, 2300 RA Leiden, The Netherlands.

Françoise Horrière, Ph.D. Laboratories 3M Santé, Avenue du 11 Novembre - 45312, Pithiviers Cedex, France.

Herve Karsenty, Ph.D. Laboratories 3M Santé, Avenue du 11 Novembre - 45312, Pithiviers Cedex, France.

Ian W. Kellaway, D.Sc. Professor, The Welsh School of Pharmacy, University of Wales College of Cardiff, Redwood Building, King Edward VII Avenue, Cardiff, CF1 3XF, Wales.

Claire Lacoste, Ph.D. Laboratoires 3M Santé, Avenue du 11 Novembre - 45312, Pithiviers Cedex, France.

Michael J. Levine, Ph.D. Professor, Department of Oral Biology and Dental Research Institute, State University of New York at Buffalo, 109 Foster Hall, 3435 Main Street, Buffalo, New York 14214, USA.

Roy McQuinn, Ph.D. 3M Pharmaceuticals, 3M Center, Building 270-2S-06, St. Paul, Minnesota 55144, USA.

Gilles Ponchel, Ph.D. Laboratoire de Pharmacotechnie et de Biopharmacie, URA CNRS 1218, Faculté de Pharmacie, University of Paris XI, 5 rue Jean-Babtiste Clément, 92296 Châtenay-Malabry Cedex, France.

Robert Purves, Ph.D. Department of Pharmacology, University of Otago, Dunedin, New Zealand.

Margrethe Rømer Rassing, Ph.D. Associate Professor, Royal Danish School of Pharmacy, Department of Pharmaceutics, 2 Univeritetsparken, DK - 2100, Copenhagen 0, Denmark.

Michael J. Rathbone, Ph.D. Manager, Research and Development, InterAg, 558 Te Rapa Road, Hamilton, New Zealand.

Colin Robinson, Ph.D. Division of Oral Biology, Leeds Dental Institute, Clarendon Way, Leeds, LS2 9LU, England.

Joseph R. Robinson, Ph.D. Professor, University of Wisconsin-Madison, School of Pharmacy, 425 North Charter Street, Madison, Wisconsin 53706, USA.

John C. Rodda, Associate Professor, Head of Department of Restorative Dentistry, School of Dentistry, University of Otago, Dunedin, New Zealand.

Leon C. P. M. Schenkels, Ph.D. Department of Oral Biology and Dental Research Institute, State University of New York at Buffalo, 109 Foster Hall, 3435 Main Street, Buffalo, New York 14214, USA.

Robert Scherrer, Ph.D. 3M Pharmaceuticals, 3M Center, Building 270-2S-06, St. Paul, Minnesota 55144, USA

W. Aubrey Soskolone, Ph.D. Department of Periodontics, Hebrew University-Hadassah Faculty of Dental Medicine, Jerusalem, Israel.

Christopher A. Squier, Ph.D. Assistant Dean for Research, Dows Institute for Dental Research, College of Dentistry, The University of Iowa, Iowa City, Iowa 52242, USA.

Simon J. Warren, Ph.D. Cardiff Scintigraphics Limited, Tower Block, Park Place, Cardiff, CF1 3XR, Wales

John Weatherell, Ph.D. Division of Oral Biology, Leeds Dental Institute, Clarendon Way, Leeds, LS2 9LU, England.

Philip W. Wertz, Ph.D. Department of Oral Pathology, Radiology and Medicine, The University of Iowa, Iowa City, Iowa 52242, USA.

Hao Zhang, Ph.D. Anesta Corporation, 350 West 800 North, Suite 320, Salt Lake City, Utah 84103, USA.

Oral Mucosal Drug Delivery

1

Structure and Function of the Oral Mucosa and Implications for Drug Delivery

Christopher A. Squier
The University of Iowa, USA

Philip W. Wertz
The University of Iowa, USA

I. INTRODUCTION

To the pharmacologist interested in oral drug delivery, the mucosa of the mouth may appear to differ little from the rest of the moist lining of the gastrointestinal tract. In fact, with the notable exceptions of the esophagus and uterine cervix, this tissue is remarkably different from all other mucosae of the body, and probably has more in common with skin, with which it is forms a junction at the lips, than with the intestinal mucosa. The use of the oral mucosa for drug delivery has led to the tendency, at least in the dermatological literature, to regard oral mucosa as a highly permeable tissue [1, 2]. Such an assumption is not borne out by clinical experience. For example, despite an abundant oral flora containing many opportunistic organisms, inflammatory lesions with a microbial etiology are relatively infrequent in the oral mucosa except around the teeth. A permeable mucosa might also be expected to permit transudation of tissue fluid so as to maintain a moist oral lining, even in individuals with salivary insufficiency. That dry mouth (xerostomia) is common under conditions of hyposalivation is evidence of the relative impermeability of the oral mucosa. Clearly, the permeability of oral mucosa is a complex topic and will reflect the structure and pathological status of the tissue as well as the nature of the penetrants.

This Chapter will first describe the organization of the oral mucosa, pointing out the functional implications of structure for permeability. It will then examine the effects that pathological changes in this tissue may have on permeability and, finally, will compare the structure of oral mucosa in several animal species that are traditionally used as models for human.

II. STRUCTURE AND BARRIER FUNCTION OF ORAL MUCOSA

All covering and lining tissues of the body consist of a surface epithelium supported by a fibrous connective tissue. Epithelium, by virtue of the close packing and constant turnover of cells, is well adapted to protect underlying tissues and organs against mechanical and chemical insult whereas the connective tissue, consisting of relatively few cells in an extensive matrix, provides mechanical support and nutrients for the epithelium. In comparing the structure of skin and oral mucosa to the gastrointestinal tract, a major difference emerges in the organization of the epithelium, which reflects the different functions of these regions. The lining of the stomach and the small and large intestine consist of a simple epithelium (Figure 1a) composed of only a single layer of cells which facilitates absorption across the tissue. Skin, oral mucosa and esophagus are covered by a stratified epithelium (Figure 1b) composed of multiple layers of cells which show various patterns of differentiation (or maturation) between the deepest cell layer and the surface. The type of differentiation tends to reflect the functional demands placed on the tissue, such as a requirement for flexibility or rigidity and resistance to mechanical damage. This variation will be described in the next section.

A. Regional Variation in the Oral Mucosa

The lining mucosa of the oral cavity is covered by a stratified, squamous epithelium and three different types of oral mucosa are recognized (Figure 2). *Masticatory mucosa* covers the gingiva and hard palate, regions that are subject to the mechanical forces of mastication, such as abrasion and shearing. It consists of a cornified, or keratinized, epithelium that closely resembles the epidermis of the skin in its pattern of maturation [3, 4] and is usually tightly attached to underlying structures by a collagenous connective tissue. *Lining*

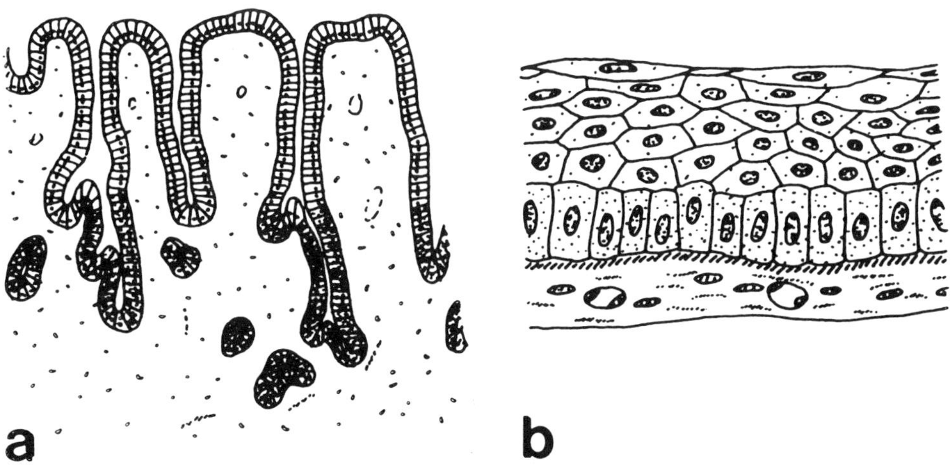

Figure 1. (a) simple (single layered) epithelium that makes up the lining of the gastrointestinal tract and (b) stratified (multilayered) epithelium that lines the esophagus and oral cavity.

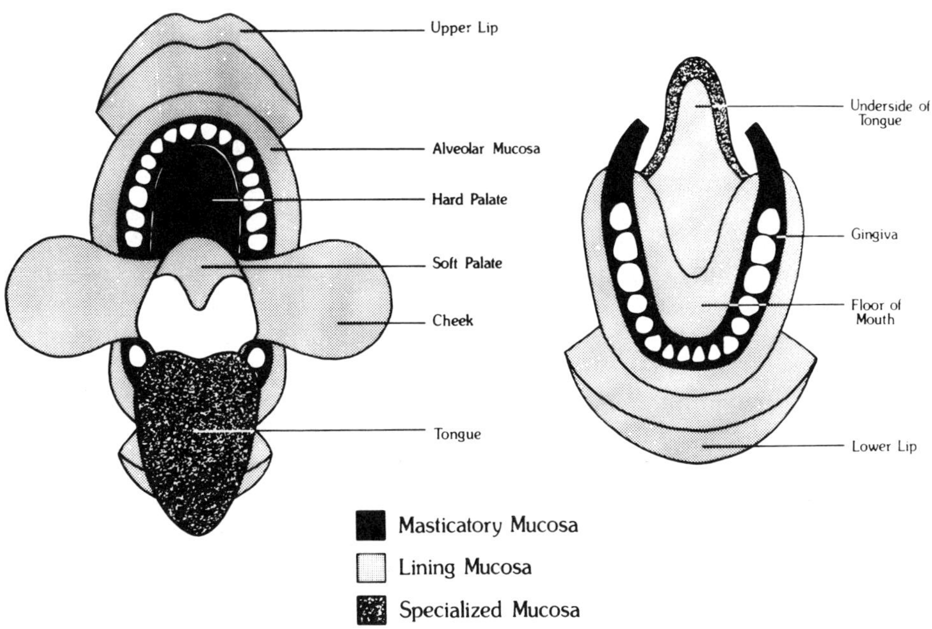

Figure 2. Diagram showing the location in the oral cavity of the three major types of oral mucosa; masticatory mucosa, lining mucosa and specialized mucosa.

Table 1. Thickness and Turnover Time for Human Oral Epithelium and Epidermis.

	Mean thickness[a] (μm)	Median turnover time[b] (days)
Epidermis	120	27
Hard palate	310	24
Buccal mucosa	580	13
Floor of mouth mucosa	190	20

[a]values from reference 27, [b]values from reference 8.

mucosa covers the remaining regions, except for the dorsal surface of the tongue, and provides an elastic, deformable surface, capable of stretching with movements such as mastication and speech. It is covered with an epithelium that does not have a cornified or keratinized surface layer and so is termed nonkeratinized. This epithelium can vary considerably in thickness in different oral regions (Table 1) and is more permeable than the keratinized masticatory regions or skin [5]. Lining mucosa is attached by a loose, elastic connective tissue to underlying structures. A similar nonkeratinized tissue lines the human esophagus [6] and uterine cervix [7]. *Specialized mucosa*, with characteristics of both masticatory and lining mucosa, is found on the dorsum of the tongue. It has a surface consisting of areas of both keratinized and nonkeratinized epithelium [8] which is tightly bound to the underlying muscle of the tongue. The various types of oral mucosa differ in their relative surface area in the oral cavity; from measurements made by Collins and Dawes [9] it can be calculated that the masticatory mucosa represents approximately 25%, the specialized mucosa (dorsum of tongue) approximately 15%, and the lining mucosa approximately 60% of the total surface area of the oral lining. Both the structure and the relative area of the different types of mucosa will influence the delivery of substances across the oral lining. Regional differences in oral epithelium arise during the process of differentiation as the epithelial cells (termed keratinocytes) move from the deeper, basal region to the surface. Basal keratinocytes are cuboidal or columnar cells with a bounding plasma membrane and a full complement of the normal intracellular organelles (Figure 3). These cells are capable of division so as to maintain a constant epithelial population as cells are shed from the surface. Tissue homeostasis requires differentiation and desquamation at the epithelial surface to be matched by cell division. Many factors, including aging and disease, can alter this balance so that an epithelium may become thicker (hyperplastic) or thinner (atrophic) than normal. The possible influence of these factors on permeability is discussed later (Section III). Tissue turnover (i.e., the time taken for the entire thickness of an epithelium to be replaced) varies considerably between regions and tends

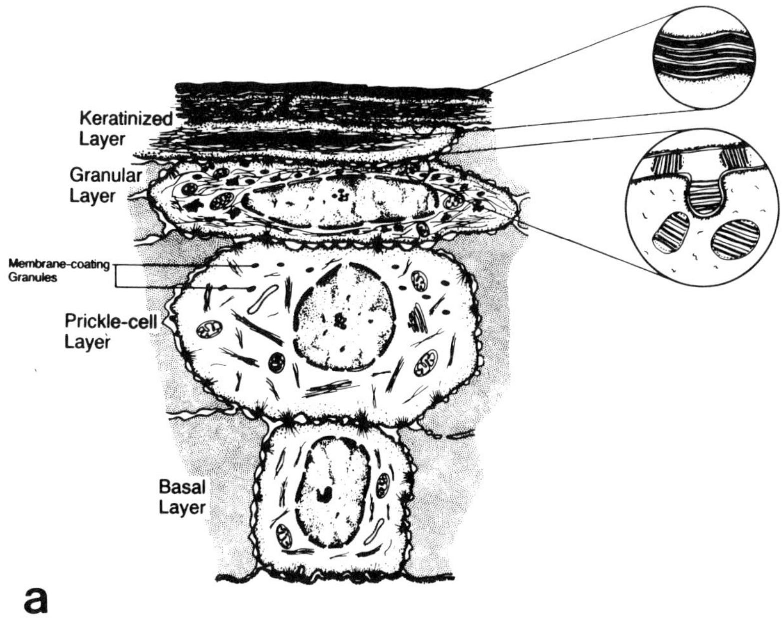

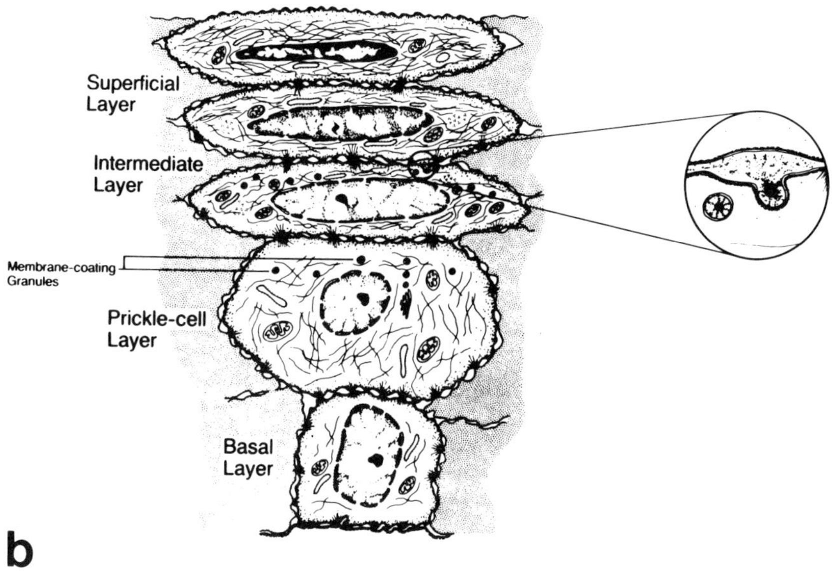

Figure 3. Diagrams to show the major structural changes during maturation in (a) keratinized epithelium and (b) nonkeratinized epithelium. (Modified from reference 111).

to be related to the pattern of epithelial differentiation and thickness. The rate of turnover in oral epithelium is, in general, slower than that occurring in the gastrointestinal epithelium but faster than in epidermis. There are regional differences within the oral cavity (Table 1) so that the keratinized epithelium of the oral mucosa has a slower turnover time than the nonkeratinized oral regions. Such differences can have important implications for healing and the rate of recovery of the tissue from damage.

The principal patterns of differentiation are represented by keratinized and nonkeratinized epithelium. Differentiation in keratinized epithelia (Figure 3a) leads to production of the stratum corneum [10]. The cornified cells making up this layer are flat and hexagonal in shape [11], filled with a compact array of condensed cytokeratin filaments [12], bounded by a thickened cell envelope [10, 13, 14] and surrounded by an external lipid matrix [15-17]. As will be described in this, and other chapters of this book, it is this extracellular lipid which determines the diffusional resistance (permeability) of the tissue to many substances.

As cells leave the basal layer and enter into differentiation, they become larger and begin to flatten and to accumulate lipids and cytoplasmic protein filaments, representing the cytokeratins. A portion of the accumulating lipid is packaged in small organelles known as membrane-coating granules or lamellar granules that become evident in the prickle cell layer (Figure 3a) [18, 19]. In addition to the accumulation of lipids and keratins [10, 12], the differentiating keratinocytes synthesize and retain a number of specific proteins including profillagrin [20, 21], involucrin [22, 23] and other precursors required for the thickening of the cell envelope [24]. At the boundary between the granular and cornified layers, the membrane-coating granules migrate to the superficial (apical) aspect of the keratinocyte, where the bounding membrane of the organelle fuses with the cell plasma membrane so that the lipid lamellae are extruded into the extracellular spaces of the surface layer [10, 15, 18, 25]. Thus the membrane coating granules are believed to be responsible for the formation of the superficial permeability barrier in stratified squamous epithelium; the evidence for this is presented in a subsequent section (Section II C). After the granules are extruded, the interior of the cell becomes filled with aggregated cytokeratin filaments, and involucrin and other proteins are deposited on the inner aspect of the plasma membrane as a thick band of protein which becomes covalently cross-linked.

In epidermis, the short stacks of lipid lamellae that are extruded from the membrane-coating granules fuse at the edges [26] to produce multiple broad lipid sheets which fill most of the extracellular spaces of the stratum corneum. Remnants of the cell attachment apparatus (desmosomes) are sparse and are found mainly near the ends of the cornified cells. In keratinized oral epithelium about 50% of the intercellular space of the stratum corneum is occupied by desmosomes [27], and the interdesmosomal regions are frequently dilated. Although the extruded membrane-coating granule contents fuse to form multiple broad lipid sheets in the intercellular spaces of the stratum corneum of this tissue, the number of individual lamellae in oral tissue is less than that observed in epidermis. These differences are discussed more fully in Chapter 2.

In nonkeratinizing epithelia (Figure 3b), the accumulation of lipids and of cytokeratins in the keratinocytes is less evident and the change in morphology is far less marked than in keratinizing epithelia. The mature cells in the outer portion of nonkeratinized epithelia become large and flat and possess a cross-linked protein envelope, but they retain nuclei and other organelles, and the cytokeratins do not aggregate to form bundles of filaments as seen in keratinizing epithelia. As cells reach the upper one-third to one-quarter of the epithelium, membrane coating granules become evident at the superficial aspect of the cells and appear to fuse with the plasma membrane so as to extrude their contents into the intercellular space. The membrane-coating granules found in nonkeratinizing epithelia are spherical in shape, membrane-bounded and measure about 0.2 micron in diameter [28]. They have often been referred to as cored granules because of their appearance in transmission electron micrographs of conventional, osmium tetroxide fixed, tissue. Such granules have been observed in a variety of human nonkeratinized epithelia, including oral mucosa [29-31] uterine cervix [32] and esophagus [6]. Recent studies employing ruthenium tetroxide as a post-fixative indicate that a small proportion of the granules in nonkeratinized epithelium do contain lamellae, which may be the source of short stacks of lamellar lipid scattered throughout the intercellular spaces in the outer portion of the epithelium [33]. In contrast to the appearance of the intercellular spaces of the surface layer of keratinized epithelia, those of the superficial layer of nonkeratinizing epithelia contain electron lucent material, which may represent nonlamellar phase lipid, with only occasional short stacks of lipid lamellae. It is the absence of organized lipid lamellae in the intercellular spaces that accounts for the greater permeability of this tissue (see Chapter 2).

B. The Interface Between Oral Mucosa and Tooth (The Dento-gingival Junction)

The region where the oral mucous membrane is penetrated by the erupted tooth is a unique junction between two dissimilar tissues. At the dento-gingival junction (Figure 4), the keratinized gingival (or oral) epithelium (OE) which covers the jawbone, becomes continuous with a region of non-keratinized epithelium which lines a shallow sulcus around the tooth (the oral sulcular epithelium, OSE). This, in turn, is attached to the surface of the tooth enamel by a stratified epithelium called the junctional epithelium (JE). This epithelium is unusual in lacking morphological and biochemical evidence of differentiation, such as a characteristic pattern of cytokeratins, membrane

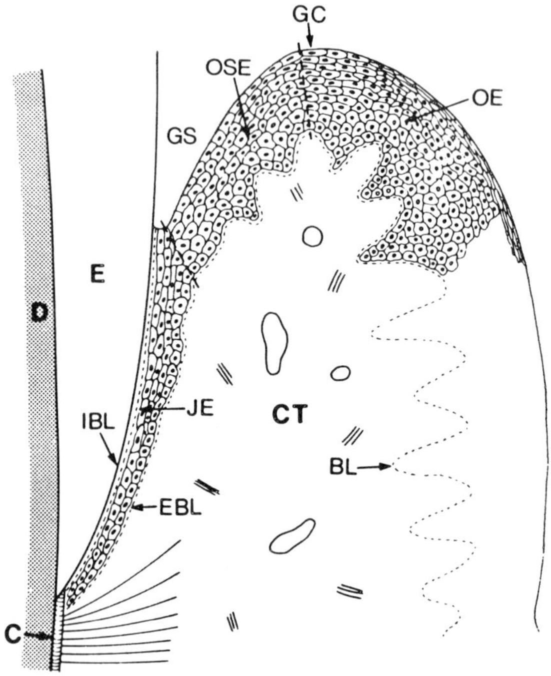

Figure 4. Diagram of the interface between oral mucosa and tooth: C = cementum of tooth, D = dentine of the tooth, E = tooth enamel, JE = junctional epithelia, IBL = inner basal lamina, EBL = external basal lamina, GS = gingival sulcus, OSE = oral subcular epithelium, GC = gingival crest, OE = oral epithelium, CT = connective tissue, BLG = basal lamina of gingiva. (From reference 8).

thickening or cell surface markers [34]. It also lacks membrane-coating granules [27]. The junctional epithelium of the tooth thus represents a unique example of an undifferentiated tissue persisting until maturity and even old age [35]. The absence of differentiation in junctional epithelium may be an adaptation to attachment at the enamel surface [36] or it may serve to limit apical migration of the adjacent oral epithelium [34]. Regardless of the reason, the result is a tissue that lacks a superficial permeability barrier and which has been shown to be permeable to a variety of materials ranging from carbon particles [37] to proteins [38]. When a tracer protein molecule, such as horseradish peroxidase, is introduced into the gingival sulcus in vivo it is able to penetrate the intercellular regions of the junctional epithelium and enter the underlying connective tissue. However, the tracer does not enter the adjacent sulcular epithelium, where membrane-coating granules are present [39]. The junctional epithelium is therefore a route by which toxins, antigens and enzymes derived from bacterial plaque, which forms at the tooth surface, can penetrate the epithelium and enter the subepithelial connective tissue. This sets up a cycle of inflammation and tissue damage that will facilitate entry of irritants from the dental sulcus and so exacerbate damage. Eventually the tissue destruction (periodontal disease) will involve the tooth-supporting structures and lead to tooth loss.

From the point of view of periodontal therapy, attempts to remove bacterial plaque by mechanical and chemical means will reduce the potential for injurious substances to penetrate into the gingival tissues and so tend to promote clinical health. Nevertheless, the intrinsic permeability of the junctional epithelium will always provide access to some exogenous materials, which probably accounts for the invariable subclinical inflammation observed in this region [40]. On the other hand, the permeability of this region may also facilitate the local delivery of antimicrobial and anti-inflammatory agents to suppress the disease cycle.

C. Membrane-coating Granules and the Location of a Permeability Barrier in Oral Mucosa

In 1969, Schreiner and Wolff [41] used the protein horseradish peroxidase (MW 40 kDa) as a tracer to demonstrate the location of a permeability barrier in human epidermis. After being injected intradermally, the peroxidase molecule was seen to have crossed the basal lamina and penetrated the intercellular spaces of the epidermis as far as the boundary of the granular and layers; no tracer was seen in the intercellular region of the stratum corneum. The level at which the penetration of peroxidase ceased corresponded with the site at which membrane-coating granules extruded their lamellate contents into the intercellular space. In a series of studies, Squier and coworkers [42-45] used horseradish peroxidase or lanthanum to demonstrate the location of the permeability barrier in oral mucosa. In keratinized mucosa, the limit of penetration of the tracers was at the boundary of the granular and keratinized layers, as in epidermis [42, 43]. When the procedure was carried out using nonkeratinized oral mucosa, the tracers failed to penetrate the outer one-third to one-quarter of the epithelium [42, 43]. This coincided with the level at which the membrane coating granules of this tissue appear to fuse with the superficial cell membrane and extrude their contents into the intercellular space. Although these granules differ morphologically from those of keratinized epithelium, they appear to be homologous with the granules of keratinized epithelia in their location and behavior [28].

If the presence of membrane-coating granules in a stratified squamous epithelium is a pre-requisite for the formation of a permeability barrier, then tissues from which they are absent might be expected to lack such a barrier. Epithelial cells from skin and keratinizing oral mucosa maintained in a submerged culture system show poor differentiation, and membrane-coating granules have rarely been described in ultrastructural studies. When such cultures are treated topically with horseradish peroxidase it readily penetrates between the cells of the superficial layer, indicating that a permeability barrier is not present [46]. The use of raised (interface) cultures has been found to facilitate epithelial differentiation, including the development of membrane coating granules in epidermis [47, 48] and oral epithelium [49]. The permeability of such a system tends to be slightly higher than that of skin in vivo [50, 51] although equivalence has been reported [52]. Thus, in the junctional epithelium of the tooth, and in tissue culture systems, the presence or absence of membrane-coating granules can be related to the permeability properties of the tissue.

D. Other Permeability Barriers in Oral Mucosa

Although the superficial layers of the oral epithelium represent the primary barrier to the entry of substances from the exterior, it is evident that the basement membrane also plays a role in limiting the passage of materials across the junction between epithelium and connective tissue [53]. Thus intravenously injected horseradish peroxidase can enter the intercellular spaces of the epidermis, but the passage of the larger molecules of the protein, thorotrast, is restricted [54]. A similar mechanism appears to operate in the opposite direction. When labeled albumin is applied to the surface of the oral mucosa of animals sensitized to this protein, immune complexes that are formed in the epithelium are trapped above the basement membrane, suggesting that whereas immunoglobulins can traverse this region, the larger immunocomplexes do not [55]. It has recently been proposed that the basal region of pig buccal epithelium may represent the site of a barrier to small substances such as β-blocking agents [56]. Measurements of the permeability of different strata of buccal epithelium isolated by enzymatic separation or horizontal (en-face) sectioning suggest that the barrier to water is confined to the superficial layers of the epithelium [57]. The accumulation of materials in the basal region may represent the nonspecific binding of charged molecules to components of the basal lamina.

E. The Role of the Connective Tissue

The epithelium of the oral mucosa is supported on a dense irregular connective tissue, termed the lamina propria, from which it is separated by a basement membrane. Although these two regions may limit the movement of

Table 2. Blood Flow in Different Regions of Oral Mucosa and Skin from Rhesus Monkey (Values from reference 58).

Region	Mean blood flow (mL per minute per 100 g tissue)
Dorsum of tongue	100.6
Vermilion border of lip	49.9
Labial mucosa	28.3
Buccal mucosa	20.3
Attached gingival[a]	19.5
Ventral surface of tongue	13.9
Floor of mouth	12.2
Skin[a]	9.4
Soft palate	9.2
Hard palate[a]	7.0

[a]Keratinized region

macromolecules and complexes they are unlikely to affect the diffusion of most compounds of pharmacological interest. Epithelium is an avascular tissue and it is the presence of small vessels and capillaries in the lamina propria that provides access to the vascular system for compounds traversing the mucosa. Blood flow in the oral mucosa varies in different regions (Table 2), but is generally greater than that in the skin [58]. Factors that might affect the clearance of drugs from the connective tissue include inflammatory and vascular changes associated with disease, and these will be discussed later (Section III A).

The vascular drainage from the oral mucosa is principally via the lingual, facial and retromandibular veins which open into the internal jugular vein. This avoids hepatic first pass clearance, a limiting factor in oral (intestinal) drug absorption. Anastomoses between intracranial and extracranial veins and the infrequency of valves to prevent backflow in the facial veins provide a route between the oral mucosa and the brain that might be exploited for the delivery of therapeutic compounds such as neuropeptides.

III. PATHOPHYSIOLOGY OF ORAL MUCOSA AND PERMEABILITY

The oral cavity has sometimes been described as a mirror that reflects the health of the individual. Changes indicative of disease may be seen clinically as alterations in the oral mucosa that can reveal systemic conditions such as diabetes or vitamin deficiency, or the local effects of chronic tobacco or alcohol use. Such conditions may result in an alteration in permeability and are discussed in this section.

A. Aging and the Permeability of Oral Mucosa

Skin shows well documented changes in structure and function with age, most of which arise from chronic exposure to ultraviolet radiation (i.e., photoaging). The oral mucosa, being protected from such environmental effects, shows few changes that can be unambiguously ascribed to aging. In some regions there is a slight thinning of the epithelium with a concomitant flattening of the epithelial-connective tissue interface [59]. Despite claims of a reduction in the rate of cell proliferation with age there is no clear data to support this for human tissue, although there may be some increase in turnover time [60].

The limited information available on the permeability of oral mucosa indicates that there is a trend towards decreased permeability to water with age which is statistically significant for floor of mouth mucosa from females [61]. It is of interest to note that in skin, where the morphological changes with age are more marked than in oral mucosa, there have been a number of reports which demonstrate a significant decrease in permeability with age; the reasons for this have been discussed by Squier et al [61].

The age changes evident in the lamina propria that could have an influence on drug delivery are those affecting the vascular system. Although there is some evidence for a reduction in the number of individual vessels with active flow [62] it is not known whether these affect overall blood flow and perfusion. Systemic conditions encountered in the elderly which can affect the oral vasculature include diabetes and atherosclerosis [63, 64]; in a study of blood flow in atheroscerotic monkeys, Goodman and Squier [65] reported a 50% reduction of flow in the oral mucosa. However, given the ample blood supply to the oral tissues (Table 2) it is likely that perfusion is still sufficient to maintain drug clearance even in the presence of these vascular alterations [66].

B. Reactive Changes in the Oral Mucosa

1. *Inflammation*

The most common mucosal reaction to insult or disease is inflammation. The abundant vasculature ensures rapid infiltration of the tissue with inflammatory cells in response to mechanical or chemical insult. A mild degree of inflammation stimulates epithelial proliferation, leading to hyperplastic changes, whereas severe inflammation suppresses proliferation [67] so that the epithelium may become thinner or even be lost (i.e., ulcerated). As already mentioned, the accumulation of bacteria in plaque around the teeth gives rise to toxins and antigens that produce chronic inflammation in the periodontal tissues of many individuals. Similarly, infection of the mucosal surface with the fungus Candida is widespread, particularly in individuals who are immunocompromized or taking antibiotics, and if untreated will lead to chronic inflammation.

A common site for mucosal inflammation is under dentures. Riber and Kaaber [68] found inflammatory changes of the palatal mucosa after 12 months in one-third of a group of denture wearers. Permeability measurements on the inflamed tissue under the dentures revealed a threefold increase in permeability as compared to values for normal palate [69]. This effect seemed to be associated with a shift in epithelial differentiation in the presence of chronic inflammation towards that of nonkeratinization with a concomitant increase in permeability. Inflammation in denture wearers is almost invariably associated with the presence of Candidal infection, and Martin, et al [70] have demonstrated that the permeability barrier in rat palate is compromized when a plate infected with Candida is applied to the surface. The evidence thus seems to suggest that chronic inflammation leads to increased mucosal permeability associated with an alteration in epithelial differentiation.

2. *Extrinsic factors*

A variety of extrinsic factors can bring about changes in the oral mucosa that have a potential for altering permeability. The most frequent of these is irritation from physical damage, such as cheek biting, rough dental fillings or toothbrushing, or from chemical irritants such as tobacco and tobacco smoke, alcohol, toothpastes and mouthrinses. Assuming that inflammation is not severe (see previous section) oral epithelium responds to irritation by an increase in cell proliferation that results in a thickening of the tissue; keratinized regions tend to show a thickening of the keratinized layer (hyperkeratinization) and nonkeratinized regions frequently develop a keratinized layer in these circumstances. The most dramatic hyperkeratotic changes in the oral mucosa are seen in the palate of smokers and at sites in the mouth such as the cheek, inner lip and gums, where users of snuff or chewing tobacco place the product. These reactive changes presumably offer greater mechanical protection to the tissue but do not appear to improve its barrier properties. Indeed, hyperkeratotic hamster cheek pouch, induced by chemical or mechanical means, shows permeability values that are either no different from, or are greater than, normal tissue [71]. Such findings are consistent with data from skin, where the thickened epidermis of the palmar and plantar regions has a higher permeability than thin skin [11] and where the pathological thickening that is evident in conditions such as psoriasis and in various ichthyoses, results in an increased permeability to water [72]. The reduced barrier function in conditions of epithelial thickening is probably a reflection of the increased cell proliferation and faster epithelial transit time characteristic of hyperplasia; this reduces the opportunity for membrane granule extrusion and adequate formation of the intercellular barrier material (see Chapter 2).

Apart from tobacco, one of the most common agents to be introduced into the oral cavity is alcohol, either in the form of alcoholic beverages or in mouthrinses. There is little consistent data to suggest that alcohol has a direct effect on the human oral mucosa [73, 74] but there is no doubt that the use of both tobacco and alcohol significantly increases the relative risk of oral cancer [75, 76]. The effect may be due to ethanol acting as an effective vehicle for enhancing the penetration of compounds, including tobacco carcinogens, across the oral epithelium [77-79]. Such a mechanism would also explain epidemiological data suggesting a significantly increased relative risk of oral cancer among individuals who frequently use mouthrinse containing alcohol [80, 81]. However, this effect also offers possibilities for enhancing drug delivery across the oral epithelium.

One of the changes sometimes seen in individuals using mouthrinses or toothpaste is a sloughing of the epithelial surface [82]. This is usually due to the presence of surface active agents that are added to improve solubility or increase foaming of the products [83]. Siegel and Gordon [84, 85] have demonstrated that these agents increase the permeability of oral epithelium in animals and that this effect is related to the extent of tissue destruction; ionic surfactants such as sodium lauryl sulfate cause more damage than non-ionic agents such as Tween-80. Given the vulnerability of damaged oral tissue to infection, these compounds are not likely to be of much value in facilitating oral drug delivery.

C. Specific Mucosal Disease

Apart from the reactive lesions that appear as a thickening, the majority of mucosal diseases result in thinning (atrophy) or breakdown (ulceration) of the oral epithelium. The most common of these is aphthous ulceration (aphthous stomatitis), affecting 20-60% of the population, and typically occurring on the nonkeratinized regions of the mucosa such as the floor of mouth, cheek, and inside lip. A less common condition, found in 2-4% of the population, is lichen planus, that can manifest as an atrophic form on the cheek and palate. The etiology of both conditions is obscure but it has been suggested that they may represent immunologically mediated lesions as a result of a local tissue reaction to food or bacterial derived antigens that have penetrated the epithelium [86]. In this regard, it is interesting to note that the diseases are most frequently found on the more permeable, lining mucosa. Less common of all are the so-called blistering conditions (vesiculo-bullous lesions) with a viral or autoimmune etiology. In all the above lesions atrophy or ulceration of the epithelium will result in impairment of the barrier layer and an increase in permeability.

D. Iatrogenic Disease

Modern anti-cancer therapy represents a significant challenge to the integrity of covering and lining tissues, including the oral mucosa. Both chemotherapeutic agents and radiation limit the proliferative ability of the epithelium so that it becomes thinner or ulcerated. This is first seen in the more rapidly proliferating tissues such as intestinal and oral lining mucosa. Such changes are likely to impair barrier function and increase permeability. There may also be indirect effects, such as damage to the salivary glands, which will reduce salivary production and impair barrier efficiency, and a reduction in immunocompetence as a result of myeloablative therapy. This will increase the risk of local infection from oral organisms.

E. Mucosal Disease and Drug Delivery

Although the overall effects of disease processes on the oral mucosa are to impair the integrity of the tissue, this will tend to facilitate local delivery of agents that might be used to treat mucosal conditions. However, it will complicate the use of more sophisticated delivery devices which involve the use of mucoadhesives for retention and controlled release of drugs, because of the marked changes at the mucosal surface that may include increased desquamation or sloughing. On the other hand, the oral mucosa is thicker than epidermis or intestinal epithelium, is rarely involved in hypersensitivity reactions common in the skin and heals rapidly. These characteristics confer robustness and permit rapid recovery when adhesives and occlusive dressings are applied topically.

IV. STRUCTURE OF ORAL MUCOSA IN EXPERIMENTAL ANIMALS

The benefit of using human oral mucosa for drug delivery is that it offers an area of nonkeratinized, lining mucosa which is more permeable than the keratinized oral regions or the skin. However, there are considerable limitations to experimental studies of oral mucosal drug delivery in humans. Non-invasive approaches such as the buccal absorption test have limited value and there are ethical constraints on the size and number of surgical biopsies that can be removed for in vitro studies. As a consequence, many investigators have chosen to use animal models to study oral mucosal permeability and drug delivery (see Chapters 5, 6 and 7).

There are numerous reports of the use of small laboratory animals for permeability studies, including rats [87-91] hamsters [92-94] and guinea pigs [38, 55]. Unfortunately, such choices seriously limit the value of the data obtained for, unlike human, most laboratory animals have an oral lining that is totally keratinized. For example, the rat has a buccal mucosa with a very thick, keratinized, surface layer (Figure 5d). The hamster has an extensive cheek pouch that can be easily everted so as to provide access to a large area of mucosa. However, this is a thin, keratinized tissue (Figure 5e) more closely resembling skin than oral mucosa. Functioning as a site for storage of food, the hamster cheek pouch is a static environment that is not flushed with saliva in the same way as the lining of the oral cavity proper. Although it may be reasonable to use this tissue for comparative studies, such as the relative effectiveness of permeabilizers in facilitating drug penetration, results cannot be directly extrapolated to human mucosa. The rabbit represents the only laboratory rodent that has nonkeratinized lining mucosa resembling human tissue (Figure 5c) and has been extensively utilized in experimental studies [85, 95-98]. Rabbit buccal mucosa has been well characterized morphologically [99] but the difficulty of access, the small area of nonkeratinized tissue and the abrupt transition to keratinized tissue at the margins limit its value for in vivo studies.

The oral mucosa of larger experimental animals that has been used for permeability and drug delivery studies include monkeys [100], dogs [101-104] and pigs [5, 38, 105, 106]. The monkey, being a primate, has a very similar oral mucosa to that of human, although in the common laboratory species (for example, the Macaque or Rhesus) the oral cavity is smaller and the epithelium generally thinner (Table 3). There have been few comparative studies of the

Table 3. Epithelial Thickness and Permeability Constants (K_p) for Buccal Mucosa from Different Species for Tritiated Water.

Species	$K_p \times 10^{-7}$ cm/minute (± SD)	Thickness μm (± SD)
Human	579 ± 122[a]	580 ± 90[d]
Pig	634 ± 60[a]	772 ± 150[e]
Monkey	1025 ± 154[b]	271 ± 50[c]
Dog	1045 ± 37[c]	126 ± 20[c]

[a]Lesch et al [5], [b]Mehta et al [100], [c]Kramer and Squier [unpublished results], [d]Schroeder [27], [e]Squier and Hall [106].

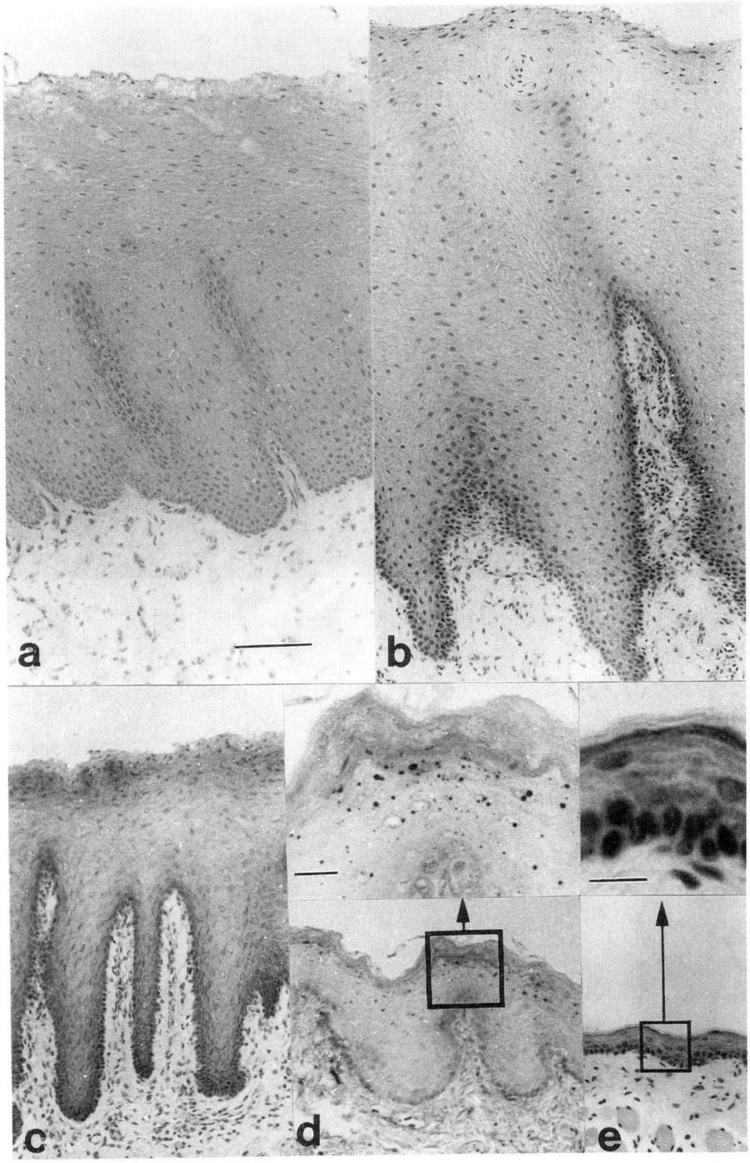

Figure 5. Histological sections through the buccal mucosa of different species. All are reproduced at the same magnification (bar represents 100 μm); note the extreme differences in epithelial thickness between species. Where, a = human, b = pig, c = rabbit, d = rat, e = hamster cheek pouch. The inserts in d and e are at higher magnifications (bar represents 20 μm) to show the keratinized surface of the epithelia in these species.

permeability of monkey oral mucosa but Mehta et al [100] reported permeability coefficient values for water for buccal mucosa that appear to be higher than those obtained for human and pig (Table 3). The high costs of purchasing and maintaining monkeys, and the difficulties of handling them, including the risks of infection, make these animals impractical in vivo models in most laboratories.

Dogs are less expensive and easier to handle than monkeys and have an oral mucosa very similar to that of human although the epithelium is somewhat thinner. However, comparative studies indicate that the tissue is more permeable than that of human (Table 3).

The considerable similarities between pig and human in terms of anatomy, metabolism, disease and wound healing make this a very attractive animal model [107]. The oral mucosa probably resembles that of the human more closely than any other animal in terms of structure [108, 109] and composition [110] although the epithelium tends to be thicker than in human (Figures 5a and b). Measurements of permeability reveal no significant differences from human oral mucosa for water (Table 3). For use in in vivo studies pigs are relatively inexpensive to maintain although they grow rapidly and thus become more difficult to handle. Miniature breeds have been used to overcome this problem [105] but are extremely expensive and a more practical solution for short term projects is to work with young (weanling) domestic breeds. For in vitro studies it is relatively easy to obtain large amounts of pig oral mucosa from a slaughterhouse.

The use of inappropriate animal species represents one of the weaknesses of research into oral mucosal drug delivery. Characterization of the structure and permeability of oral mucosa so as to identify a suitable model remains a priority.

V. ACKNOWLEDGMENTS

This work was supported in part by grants R01 DE07930, R01 DE10516 and P30 DE10126 from the National Institutes of Health. We thank Sherrie Sheldon for typing the manuscript.

REFERENCES

1. F. D. Malkinson, Permeability of the stratum corneum, *The Epidermis* (W. Montagna, and W. C. Lobitz, eds.), Academic Press, New York, 1964, p. 435.
2. R. K. J. Winkelmann, The relationship of the structure of the epidermis to percutaneous absorption, *Br. J. Derm. 81*:12 (1969).

3. O. F. Alvares, and J. Meyer, Variable features and regional differences in oral epithelium, *Current Concepts of the Histology of Oral Mucosa* (C. A. Squier, and J. Meyer, eds.), Charles C. Thomas, Springfield, IL, 1971, p. 97.
4. S -Y. Chen, and C. A. Squier, The ultrastructure of the oral epithelium, *The Structure and Function of Oral Mucosa* (J. Meyer, C. A. Squier, and S. J. Gerson, eds.), Pergamon Press, Oxford, 1984, Chapter 7.
5. C. Lesch, C. A. Squier, A. H. Cruchley, D. M. Williams, and P. M. Speight, The permeability of human oral mucosa and skin to water, *J. Dent. Res. 68*:1345 (1989).
6. D. Hopwood, K. R. Logan, and I. A. D. Bouchier, The electron microscopy of normal human esophageal epithelium, *Virchows Arch. B. Cell Path. 26*:345 (1978).
7. M. Hackemann, C. Grubb, and K. R. Hill, The ultrastructure of normal squamous epithelia of the human cervix utero. *J. Ultrastruct. Res. 22*:443 (1968).
8. C. A. Squier, N. W. Johnson, and R. M. Hopps, *Human Oral Mucosa; Development, Structure and Function*, Blackwell Scientific, Oxford, 1976.
9. L. M. C. Collins, and C. Dawes, The surface area of the adult human mouth and the thickness of the salivary film covering the teeth and oral mucosa, *J. Dent. Res. 66*:1300 (1987).
10. A. G. Matoltsy, Keratinization, *J. Invest. Dermatol. 67*:20 (1976).
11. A. M. Kligman, The biology of the stratum corneum, *The Epidermis* (W. Montagna, and W. C. Lobity, eds.), Academic Press, New York 1964, p. 387.
12. P. M. Steinert, and J. S. Cantieri, Epidermal keratins, *Biochemistry and Physiology of the Skin* (L. A. Goldsmith, ed.) Volume I, Oxford University Press, New York, 1983, p. 169.
13. R. H. Rice, and H. Green, Presence in human epidermal cells of a soluble protein precursor of the cross-linked envelope: activation of the cross-linking by calcium ions, *Cell 18*:681 (1979).
14. D. C. Swartzendruber, P. W. Wertz, K. C. Madison, and D. T. Downing, Evidence that the corneocyte has a chemically bound lipid envelope, *J. Invest. Dermatol. 88*:709 (1987).
15. P. M. Elias, and D. S. Friend, The permeability barrier in mammalian epidermis, *J. Cell Biol. 65*:180 (1975).
16. A. S. Breathnach, T. Goodman, C. Stolinski, and M. Gross, Freeze-fracture replication of cells of stratum corneum of human epidermis, *J. Anat. 114*:65 (1973).

17. K. C. Madison, D. C. Swartzendruber, P. W. Wertz, and D. T. Downing, Presence of intact intercellular lipid lamellae in the upper layers of the stratum corneum, *J. Invest. Dermatol. 88*:714 (1987).
18. L. Landmann, The epidermal permeability barrier, *Anat. Embryol. 178*:1 (1988).
19. I. R. Martinez, and A. Peters, Membrane-coating granules and membrane modifications in keratinizing epithelia, *Am. J. Anat. 130*:93 (1971).
20. B. A. Dale, and S. Y. Ling, Evidence of a precursor form of stratum corneum basic protein in rat epidermis, *Biochemistry 18*:3539 (1979).
21. B. A. Dale, K. A. Holbrook, and P. M. Steinert, Assembly of stratum corneum basic protein and keratin filaments in macrofibrils, *Nature 276*:729 (1978).
22. R. H. Rice, and H. Green, The cornified envelope of terminally differentiated human epidermal keratinocytes consists of cross-linked protein, *Cell 11*:417 (1979).
23. F. M. Watt, and H. Green, Involucrin synthesis is correlated with cell size in human cultures, *J. Cell Biol. 90*:738 (1981).
24. M. Simon, and H. Green, Participation of membrane-associated proteins in the formation of the cross-linked envelope of the keratinocyte, *Cell 36*:327 (1984).
25. R. M. Lavker, Membrane coating granules: the fate of the discharged lamellae, *J. Ultrastruc. Res. 55*:79 (1976).
26. L. Landmann, Epidermal permeability barrier: transformation of lamellar granule-disks into intercellular sheets by a membrane fusion process, *J. Invest. Dermatol. 87*:202 (1986).
27. H. E. Schroeder, *Differentiation of Human Oral Stratified Epithelium,* S. Karger, Basel, 1981, p. 33.
28. C. A. Squier, Membrane coating granules in nonkeratinized oral epithelium, *J. Ultrastruc. Res. 60*:212 (1977).
29. K. Hashimoto, R. J. Dibella, and G. Shklar, Electron microscopic studies of the normal human buccal mucosa, *J. Invest. Dermatol. 47*:512 (1966).
30. P. Schenk, and J. Wersall, The ultrastructure of papillae-filliformes of human tongue, *Arch. Dermatol. Forsch. 252*:91 (1975).
31. A. F. Hayward, Membrane coating granules, *Int. Rev. Cytol. 59*:97 (1979).
32. C. Grubb, M. Hackemann, and K. R. Hill, Small granules and plasma membrane thickening in human cervical squamous epithelium, *J. Ultrastruct. Res. 22*:258 (1968).
33. P. W. Wertz, D. C. Swartzendruber, and C. A. Squier, Regional variation in the structure and permeability of oral mucosa and skin, *Adv. Drug Del. Rev. 12*:1 1993.

34. I. C. Mackenzie, Nature and mechanisms of regeneration of the junctional epithelial phenotype, *J. Periodontol. Res.* *22*:243 (1987).
35. H. E. Schroeder, and M. A. Listgarten, *Fine Structure of the Developing Epithelial Attachment of Human Teeth*, 2nd Edition, S. Karger, Basel, 1977.
36. C. A. Squier, Keratinization of the sulcular epithelium - a pointless pursuit?, *J. Periodontol.* *52*:426 (1981).
37. D. H. Fine, J. L. Pechersky, and D. H. McKibben, The penetration of human gingival sulcular tissue by carbon particles, *Arch. Oral Biol.* *14*:1117 (1969).
38. K. J. Tolo, A study of permeability of gingival pocket epithelium to albumin in guinea pigs and Norwegian pigs, *Arch. Oral Biol.* *16*:881 (1971).
39. A. R. Romanowski, C. A. Squier, and C. A. Lesch, Permeability of rodent junctional epithelium to exogenous protein, *J. Periodont. Res.* *23*:81 (1988).
40. H. E. Schroeder, Transmigration and infiltration of leucocytes in human junctional epithelium, *Helv. Odonto. Acta.* *17*:6 (1973).
41. E. Schreiner, and K. Wolff, Die permeabilitat des epidermalen intercellularraumes fur kleinmolekulares protein, *Arch. Klin. Dermatol.* *235*:78 (1969).
42. C. A. Squier, The permeability of keratinized and non-keratinized oral epithelium to horseradish peroxidase, *J. Ultrastruct. Res.* *43*:160 (1973).
43. C. A. Squier, and L. Rooney, The permeability of keratinized and nonkeratinized oral epithelium to lanthanum in vivo, *J. Ultrastruct. Res.* *54*:286 (1976).
44. C. A. Squier, and R. M. Hopps, A study of the permeability barrier in epidermis and oral epithelium using horseradish peroxidase as a tracer in vitro, *Br. J. Dermatol.* *95*:123 (1976).
45. C. A. Squier, and J. Edie, Localization of lanthanum tracer in oral epithelium using transmission electron microscopy and the electron microprobe, *Histochem. J.* *15*:1123 (1983).
46. C. A. Squier, O. Fejerskov, and A. Jepsen, The permeability of a keratinizing squamous epithelium in culture, *J. Anat.* *126*:103 (1978).
47. M. Prunerias, M. Regnier, and D. Woodley, Methods for culture of keratinocytes with an air-liquid interface, *J. Invest. Dermatol.* *82*:285. (1989).
48. K. C. Madison, D. C. Swartzendruber, P. W. Wertz, and D. T. Downing, Lamellar granule extrusion and stratum corneum intercellular lamellae in murine keratinocytes, *J. Invest. Dermatol.* *90*:110 (1988).
49. J. H. Lillie, D. K. MacCullum, and A. Jepsen, Growth of stratified squamous epithelium on reconstituted extracellular matrices: long-term culture, *J. Invest. Dermatol.* *90*:100 (1988).

50. D. B. Guzek, A. H. Kennedy, S. C. McNeill, E. Wakshull, and R. O. Potts, Transdermal drug transport and metabolism, Comparison of in vitro and in vivo results, *Pharmacol. Res. 6*:33 (1989).
51. N. B. Cumpstone, A. H. Kennedy, C. S. Hannon, and R. O. Potts, The water permeability of primary mouse keratinocyte cultures grown at the air-liquid interface, *J. Invest. Dermatol. 92*:598 (1989).
52. C. L. Cannon, P. J. Neal, J. Kubilus, M. Klausner, D. C. Swartzendruber, C. A. Squier, M. J. Kremer, and P. W. Wertz, Lipid and ultrastructural characterization of a new epidermal model shows good correspondence to normal human epidermis, *J. Invest. Dermatol. 102*:600 (1994).
53. M. C. Alfano, A. E. Chasen, and C. W. J. Masi, Autoradiographic study of the penetration of radiolabeled dextrans and inulin through non-keratinized oral mucosa in vitro, *J. Periodont. Res. 12*:368 (1977).
54. K. Wolff, and H. Honigsmann, Permeability of the epidermis and the phagocytic activity of keratinocytes. Ultrastructural studies with thorotrast as a marker, *J. Ultrastruct. Res. 36*:176 (1971).
55. K. J. Tolo, Penetration of human albumin through oral mucosa of guinea pigs immunized to this protein, *Arch. Oral Biol. 19*:259 (1974).
56. M. E. de Vries, H. E. Boddé, H. E. Junginger, The in-vitro penetration of β-blocking agents through porcine buccal epithelium, *Proc. of Int. Symp. Control. Rel. Bioact. Mater. 17*:295 (1990).
57. M. J. Kremer, W. B. Shade, N. S. Holbrook, P. W. Wertz, and C. A. Squier, Morphologic location of the buccal permeability barrier, *J. Dent. Res. 71*:213 (1992).
58. C. A. Squier, and D. Nanny, Measurement of blood flow in the oral mucosa and skin of the Rhesus monkey using radiolabeled microspheres, *Arch. Oral Biol. 30*:313 (1985).
59. D. M. Williams, and A. R. Cruchley, Structural aspects of aging in the oral mucosa, *The Effect of Aging in Oral Mucosa and Skin*, (C. A. Squier, and M. W. Hill, eds.), CRC Press, Boca Raton, 1994, p. 65.
60. M. W. Hill, Epithelial proliferation and turnover in oral epithelia and epidermis with age, *The Effect of Aging in Oral Mucosa and Skin*, (C. A. Squier and M. W. Hill eds.), CRC Press, Boca Raton, 1994, p. 75.
61. C. A. Squier, P. W. Wertz, D. M. Williams, and A. T. Cruchley, Permeability of oral mucosa and skin with age, *The Effect of Aging in Oral Mucosa and Skin* (C. A. Squier, and M. W. Hill, eds.), CRC Press, Boca Raton, 1994, p. 91.
62. D. Johnson, G. Roth, D. Richardson, and J. Matheny, Effect of age on the dynamics of human gingival microcirculation, *J. Dent. Res. 72*:1780 (1992).
63. A. Murrah, Diabetics Mellitus and associated oral manifestations: A review, *J. Oral Pathol. 14*:271 (1985).
64. I. Semba, A histometrical analysis of age changes in the human lingual artery, *Arch. Oral Biol. 34*:483 (1989).

65. C. H. Goodman, and C. A. Squier, Blood flow in the oral mucosa of normal and atherosclerotic rhesus monkeys, *J. Oral Pathol. 17*:34 (1988).
66. G. K. Johnson, Effects of aging on the microvasculature and microcirculation in skin and oral mucosa, *The Effect of Aging in Oral Mucosa and Skin*, (M. W. Hill, and C. A. Squier, eds.), CRC Press, Boca Raton, 1994, p. 99.
67. R. M. Hopps, and N. W. Johnson, Relationship between histological degree of inflammation and epithelial proliferation in macaque gingiva, *J. Periodont. Res. 9*:273 (1974).
68. E. Riber, and S. Kaaber, A 12-month study on changes in the barrier properties of denture-loaded palatal mucosa in immediate denture wearers, *Scand. J. Dent. Res. 88*:250 (1980).
69. E. Riber, and S. J. Kaaber, Barrier properties of inflamed denture-loaded palatal mucosa to water, *Scand. J. Dent. Res. 86*:386 (1978).
70. M. V. Martin, J. Appleton, J. Chesters, and J. W. Smalley, The effect of Candida albicans on the permeability of rat palatal epithelia; an ultrastructural and biochemical study, *J. Med. Vet. Mycol. 25*:19 (1987).
71. C. A. Squier, and B. K. Hall, The permeability of hyperplastic oral epithelium, *J. Oral Pathol. 14*:357 (1985).
72. R. A. Grice, Transepidermal water loss in pathological skin, *The Physiology and Pathophysiology of the Skin* (A. Jarrett, ed.), Academic Press, London, 1980.
73. C. Mascres, and P. Franchebois, Observations histochimiques de la muqueuse buccale chez le patient cirrhotique non fumeur, *Path. Biol. 29*:203 (1981).
74. R. W. Hillman, and B. Kissin, Oral cytological patterns and nutritional status; some relationships in alcoholic subjects, *Oral Surg. Oral Med. Oral Pathol. 49*:34 (1980).
75. G. D. McCoy, S. A. Hecht, and E. L. Wynder, The roles of tobacco, alcohol and diet in the etiology of upper alimentary and respiratory tract cancers, *Prev. Med. 9*:622 (1980).
76. W. J. Blot, J. K. McLaughlin, D. M. Winn, D. F. Austin, R. S. Greenberg, S. Preston-Martin, L. Bernstein, J. B. Schoenberg, A. Sternhagen, and J. F. Fraumeni, Smoking and drinking in relation to oral pharyngeal cancer, *Canc. Res. 48*:3282 (1988).
77. C. S. Lieber, H. K. Seitz, A. J. Garro, and T. M. Wamer, Alcohol-related diseases and carcinogenesis, *Canc. Res. 89*:2844 (1979).
78. A. J. Tuyns, Alcohol, *Cancer Epidemiology and Prevention* (D. Schottenfeld, and J. F. Fraumeni, eds.), W. B. Saunders, Philadelphia, 1982, p. 293.

79. C. A. Squier, P. Cox, and B. K. Hall, Enhanced penetration of nitrosonornicotine across oral mucosa in the presence of ethanol, *J. Oral Pathol. 15*:276 (1986).
80. W. Weaver, S. M. Fleming, and D. C. Smith, Mouthwash and oral cancer: carcinogen or coincidence?, *J. Oral Surg. 37*:250 (1979).
81. W. J. Blot, D. M. Winn, and J. F. Fraumeni, Oral cancer and mouthwash, *J. Natl. Cancer Inst. 70*:251 (1983).
82. W. C. Rubright, J. A. Walker, U. L. Karlsson, and D. L. Diehl, Oral slough caused by dentifrice detergents and aggravated by drugs with antisialic activity, *J. Am. Dent. Assoc. 97*:215 (1978).
83. P. Barkvoll, and G. Rolla, Possible effects of sodium lauryl sulfate (SLS) on the oral mucosa, *J. Dent. Res. 58*:991 (1989).
84. I. A. Siegel, and H. P. Gordon, Effects of surfactants on the permeability of canine oral mucosa in vitro, *Tox. Lett. 26*:153 (1985).
85. I. A. Siegel, and H. P. Gordon, Surfactant-induced alterations of permeability of rabbit oral mucosa in vitro, *Exp. Mol. Pathol. 44*:132 (1986).
86. S. J. Challacombe, Oral manifestations of food allergy and intolerance, *Food Allergy and Intolerance* (J. Brestoff, and S. J. Challacombe, eds.), Bailliere Tindall, London, 1987, p. 511.
87. B. J. Aungst, N. J. Rogers, and E. Shefter, Comparison of nasal, rectal, buccal, sublingual, and intramuscular insulin efficacy and the effects of a bile salt absorption promoter, *J. Pharmacol. Exp. Ther. 244*:23 (1988).
88. B. J. Aungst, and N. J. Rogers, Comparison of the effects of various transmucosal absorption promoters on buccal insulin delivery, *Int. J. Pharm. 53*:227 (1989).
89. I. A. Siegel, and H. P. Gordon, Surfactant-induced increases of permeability of rat oral mucosa to non-electrolytes in vivo, *Arch. Oral Biol. 30*:43 (1985).
90. S. A. Simon, R. Robb, and S. S. Schiffman, Transport pathways in rat lingual epithelium, *Pharm. Biochem. Behav. 29*:257 (1988).
91. O. Lhote, A. Decoodt, A. Moulin, and A. Dufoir, In vivo approach to determine the route of optimal drug absorption in rats, *Eur. J. Drug Metab. Pharmacokin., Special No. 3*:43 (1991).
92. M. Tanaka, N. Yanagibashi, H. Fukuda, and T. Nagai, Absorption of salicylic acid through the oral mucous membrane of hamster cheek pouch, *Chem. Pharm. Bull. 28*:1056 (1980).
93. Y. Kurosaki, S-I Hisaichi, L-Z Hong, T. Nakayama, and T. Kimura, Enhanced permeability of keratinized oral mucosa to salicylic acid with 1-dodecylazacycloheptan-2-one (Azone): In Vitro studies in hamster cheek pouch, *Int. J. Pharm. 49*:47 (1989).

94. Y. Kurosaki, S. I. Hisaichi, C. Hamada, T. Nakayama, and T. Kumura, Effects of surfactants on the absorption of salicylic acid from hamster cheek pouch as a model of keratinized oral mucosa, *Int. J. Pharm. 47*:13 (1988).
95. I. A. Siegel, and K. T. J. Izutsu, Permeability of oral mucosa to organic compounds, *J. Dent. Res. 59*:1604 (1980).
96. I. A. Siegel, Effect of chemical structure on non-electrolyte penetration of oral mucosa, *J. Invest. Dermatol. 76*:137 (1981).
97. C. K. Oh, and W. A. Ritschel, Absorption characteristics of insulin through the buccal mucosa, *Meth. Find. Exp. Clin. Pharmacol. 12*:275 (1990).
98. M. E. Dowty, K. E. Knuth, B. K. Irons, and J. R. Robinson, Transport of thyrotropin releasing hormone in rabbit buccal mucosa in vitro, *Pharm. Res. 9*:1113 (1992).
99. S -Y Chen, Comparison of the fine structure of the mucosa of cheek and hard palate in the rabbit, M.Sc. Thesis, University of Illinois, Chicago (1970).
100. M. Mehta, B. W. Kemppainen, and R. G. Stafford, In vitro penetration of tritium-labelled water (THO) and (3H)PbTx-3 (a red tide toxin) through monkey buccal mucosa and skin, *Toxicology Letters 55*:185 (1991).
101. M. M. Veillard, M. A. Longer, T. W. Martens, and J. R. Robinson, Preliminary studies of oral mucosal delivery of peptide drugs, *J. Control. Rel. 6:*123 (1987).
102. M. Ishida, Y. Machida, N. Nambu, and T. Nagai, New mucosal dosage form of insulin, *Chem. Pharm. Bull. 29*:810 (1981).
103. T. Nagai, Adhesive topical drug delivery system, *J. Control. Rel. 2*:121 (1985).
104. C. L. Barsuhn, L. S. Olanoff, D. Gleason, E. L. Adkins, and N. F. H. Ho, Human buccal absorption of flurbiprofen, *Clin. Pharmacol. Ther. 44*:225 (1988).
105. E. Quadros, J. Cassidy, J. Gniecko, and S. LeRoy, Buccal and colonic absorption of CGS 16617, a novel ACE inhibitor, *J. Control. Rel. 19*:77 (1991).
106. C. A. Squier, and B. K. Hall, The permeability of skin and oral mucosa to water and horseradish peroxidase as related to the thickness of permeability barrier, *J. Invest. Dermatol. 84*:176 (1985).
107. L. E. Mount, and D. L. Ingram, *The Pig as a Laboratory Animal*, Academic Press, London, 1991, p. 175.
108. T. G. Heaney and R. S. Jones, Histological investigation of the influence of adult porcine alveolar mucosal connective tissue on epithelial differentiation, *Arch. Oral Biol. 23*:713 (1978).
109. P. Collins, J. Laffoon, and C. A. Squier, Comparative structure of porcine oral epithelia, *J. Dent. Res. 60*:543 (1981).

110. C. A. Squier, P. Cox, and P. W. Wertz, Lipid content and water permeability of skin and oral mucosa, *J. Invest. Dermatol. 96*:123 (1991).

111. C. A. Squier, and M. W. Hill, Oral mucosa, *Oral Histology; Development Structure and Function*, (A. R. Ten Cate, ed.), Mosby, St. Louis, 1994, p. 389.

2

Biochemical Basis of the Permeability Barrier in Skin and Oral Mucosa

Philip W. Wertz
The University of Iowa, USA

A. Janet Hoogstraate
Leiden/Amsterdam Center for Drug Research, The Netherlands

Christopher A. Squier
The Univeristy of Iowa, USA

I. INTRODUCTION

The purpose of the present chapter is to provide an introduction to the biochemistry underlying the epithelial permeability barriers of the skin and oral mucosa. Some aspects of the physiology, function and ultrastructure of permeability barriers will also be included.

For collections of recent review articles on related topics the reader is referred to volume 8, issue 3 of *Critical Reviews in Therapeutic Drug Carrier Systems* (1991) and volume 12, issues 1 and 2 of *Advanced Drug Delivery Reviews* (1993). Other excellent review articles and chapters have discussed the epidermal permeability barrier [1, 2], percutaneous absorption [3] and the oral mucosal permeability barrier [4, 5].

II. HISTORICAL OVERVIEW

A. Localization of the Epidermal Permeability Barrier to the Stratum Corneum

Historically, our concept of the permeability barrier was developed to explain the water-proof nature of the skin and was applied only later to the oral mucosa. The development of a water-impermeable skin was an essential step in the evolution of terrestrial life [6], and speculation on the location of the epidermal water barrier in man appeared in the literature as early as 1853 [7]. However, most of the early investigators who considered this problem were misled by the artefactual appearance of skin in routine histology preparations [8]. Specifically, in routine histological cross-sections of tissue, the epidermal stratum corneum has a loosely woven basket weave appearance, and it is difficult to imagine that such a grossly open porous structure composed of dead cells could provide any kind of barrier. Active transport processes or electrochemical mechanisms based in the living cells of the epidermis were postulated to account for the barrier [9, 10].

In 1944, Winsor and Burch [11] performed a classic experiment that conclusively demonstrated that the stratum corneum does provide the water barrier. These investigators monitored water flux through the abdominal skin of anesthetized surgery patients while using sandpaper to progressively remove epidermal cells. They observed that there was no large increase in water flux until the very lowest layers of the stratum corneum were breached, and it was concluded that the stratum corneum provides the epidermal barrier. Subsequently, Blank [12] performed a refined variation of this experiment in which cells were removed by stripping with cellophane tape. Again, it was observed that water flux did not increase much until the innermost layers of cornified cells were removed. Although it was initially concluded that the innermost portion of the stratum corneum provided the barrier, it was subsequently shown that this type of experiment cannot distinguish between a barrier localized to the inner cell layers of the stratum corneum and one in which all layers of the stratum corneum contribute equally [13, 14]. Nevertheless, the experiments of Winsor and Burch [11] and of Blank [12] convincingly localized the barrier to the stratum corneum. Several other studies confirmed this conclusion by directly demonstrating that isolated stratum corneum alone provides a barrier equivalent to that of the intact skin [15, 16].

Only in the early 1960's with the introduction of alkali expansion of frozen sections was it conclusively demonstrated that the stratum corneum from most regions of the skin is in fact a highly ordered structure consisting of stacks of flattened, hexagonal cells with a narrow zone of interdigitation at the edges of adjacent stacks [17-19]. Such a structure is consistent with the provision of a passive physical barrier to diffusion. That the barriers of the skin and oral mucosa are passive was proven by demonstrations that rates of diffusion are nondirectional and are not altered by metabolic inhibitors such as cyanide [20].

B. Tracer and Freeze Fracture Studies of Epithelial Barriers

Although Kligman argued as early as 1964 [8] that all cell layers within the stratum corneum contribute to its barrier function, this view was not immediately accepted. Not until the tracer experiments were performed [21-23] was there direct experimental support for this view. Schreiner and Wolff [21] were the first investigators to use the protein, horseradish peroxidase, as a water soluble tracer in skin. Using electron microscopy, these investigators observed that when peroxidase was injected intradermally, it could cross the basement lamina and diffuse outward through the intercellular spaces, but its outward movement stopped at the boundary between the stratum granulosum and stratum corneum, where the lamellar granule contents have been extruded. Squier [22] subsequently confirmed this observation on horseradish peroxidase penetration through the dermis and viable portion of the epidermis, and in addition, demonstrated that when applied topically, this tracer penetrated only the most superficial cell layers that were in the process of desquamation. These observations are in accord with Kligman's [8] suggestion that all layers of the stratum corneum contribute to its barrier function. Similar observations were made for keratinized oral epithelium from the hard palate and gingiva [22]. With the nonkeratinized oral epithelia, it was demonstrated that the superficial cell layers corresponding to approximately the outer one-quarter to one-third of the epithelium provide a barrier [22].

Objections that horseradish peroxidase, with a molecular weight of 44,000 daltons, is too large to be a good indicator of the movement of water were overcome by the subsequent use of lanthanum salts [23-25]. With this smaller electron dense tracer, all of the conclusions based on experiments employing horseradish peroxidase were confirmed.

There has been much debate about the pathway or pathways by which substances traverse the barrier. In simple epithelia such as that lining the gut, materials penetrate by a transcellular route, and their uptake is generally by either active or facilitated transport. With skin and mucosa, these mechanisms do not appear to be involved and most evidence supports a paracellular pathway with little or no contribution from transcellular or appendageal routes [4, 26]. The paracellular pathway through epidermal stratum corneum was first convincingly demonstrated by Elias and Nemanic [27], who allowed n-butanol to diffuse across skin and then reacted the tissue with osmium tetroxide. When the reaction product was visualized by transmission electron microscopy, it was found exclusively in the intercellular spaces of the stratum corneum, indicating that the paracellular route is followed by this penetrant. More recently, Squier and Lesch [28] have shown by autoradiography that radiolabeled water, ethanol and cholesterol all follow a paracellular route through the barriers of the epidermis, keratinized oral epithelium and nonkeratinized oral epithelium. Several investigators have presented theoretical considerations supporting the paracellular route in both skin and oral mucosa [29, 30]. Perhaps the most elegant and most convincing demonstration of the paracellular pathway has been achieved through the application of laser confocal microscopy to visualize the distribution of fluorescent probes in intact vital tissue [31]. The distribution of fluorescein isothiocyanate labeled dextran 4000 in buccal epithelium as revealed by confocal microscopy is shown in Figure 1. This method employs fresh tissue and involves less manipulation of the sample than any other available method, and therefore, is less subject to artefact.

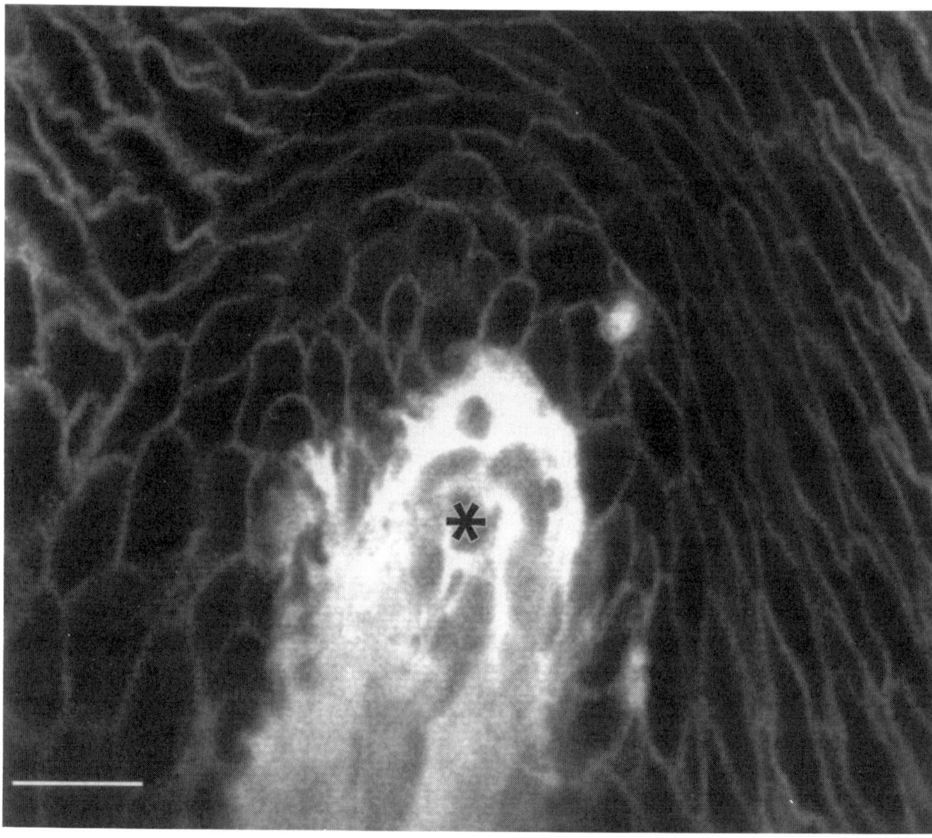

Figure 1. Distribution of fluorescein isothiocyanate labeled dextran 4000 from the floor of the mouth as revealed by laser confocal microscopy. Bar = 25 μm. Connective tissue denoted by asterisk (*).

III. LIPID NATURE OF THE PERMEABILITY BARRIER

A. Modulation of Lipid Composition with Differentiation

Following the demonstration by Winsor and Burch [11] that the epidermal stratum corneum provides the permeability barrier of the skin, numerous studies were conducted to determine the relative roles of stratum corneum proteins versus lipids. In a series of studies employing skin in vitro [32-36], it was shown that lipid removal could produce a large increase in permeability; however, it was not possible to directly correlate the extent of lipid removal with increased permeability. One of the complicating factors in this series of experiments was the recovery from the skin surface of sebaceous lipids, which do not contribute to barrier function. Another problem in some studies was contamination of samples with subcutaneous triglycerides when excised skin was used in vitro. Dimethylsulfoxide used in some of these studies extracts only small amounts of lipid, but partitions into the stratum corneum and increases permeability by acting as a permeability enhancer, and there is no solvent capable of complete removal of one class of barrier lipid without removing other lipid classes. In one more recent study [37], the extent of lipid removal from hairless mouse skin by acetone or hexane was shown to be directly proportional to the increase in permeability, and it was suggested that sphingolipids and sterols are more important for barrier function than other nonpolar lipids. However, in another recent study of human skin [38], it was found that neither hexane nor acetone removed significant amounts of lipids other than sebaceous lipids, and neither of these solvents produced significant impairment of barrier function. In general, organic solvents that remove stratum corneum lipids increase permeability. However, some solvents may influence permeability independently of lipid removal, and it is likely that all stratum corneum lipids are important for barrier function.

As epidermal or oral epithelial cells undergo maturation, they accumulate lipids, the composition of which alters dramatically as a function of differentiation [39, 40]. A number of investigators have studied this modulation of lipid composition with differentiation in epidermis [41-46] and more recently in oral epithelium [47, 48].

In epidermis, basal keratinocytes contain mainly phospholipids, the most abundant of which are sphingomyelin, phosphatidylcholine and phosphatidylethanolamine [39, 44]. Serine and inositol phosphatides are present in lesser amounts. Phosphatidyl-N-acylethanolamine, once thought to be a major epidermal lipid [49], is now known to be produced only in response to tissue damage and necrosis [50]. As epidermal cells migrate outward from the basal layer they become larger, flatter and accumulate additional phospholipids of the same types. They also accumulate cholesterol, glucosylceramides and ceramides. In the final stages of the differentiation process, the phospholipids are completely broken down and the glucosylceramides are deglycosylated to produce a mixture of ceramides, cholesterol and fatty acids as the principal lipids in the stratum corneum [39, 40]. In keratinized oral epithelium, essentially the same lipid transformations occur, except the phospholipid breakdown and glycolipid deglycosylation are incomplete, so that small proportions of phospholipids and glycosylceramides persist in oral stratum corneum [48]. In nonkeratinizing oral epithelia there is a general accumulation of phospholipids and cholesterol with cell maturation with little change in the proportions of the different lipid classes, except for a dramatic accumulation of glycosylceramides [47].

B. Lipid Synthesis

The epidermal lipids, and presumably those of the oral epithelia, are mainly synthesized in the epithelium from acetate [51], which is present in substantial concentrations (0.17 mM) in human blood [52]. Following intradermal injection of ^{14}C-acetate [51], the radioactivity is rapidly incorporated into the epidermal phospholipids followed by glucosylceramides. After several days the specific activity of the glucosylceramides begins to decrease as that of the ceramides increases. In similar experiments, radiolabeled glucose is rapidly converted to the glycerol portion of the phosphoglycerides and is incorporated into glycolipids but does not appear to be a carbon source for synthesis of the fatty chains or cholesterol.

In epidermis and all regions of oral epithelium, sphingolipids are major products of differentiation [40, 47]. Sphingosine is synthesized from palmitoyl-CoA and serine [53-55]. In the initial, rate limiting step 3-ketodihydrosphinganine is produced in a reaction catalyzed by palmitoyl-CoA serine palmitoyl transferase. This intermediate is rapidly reduced to produce dihydrosphingosine, which can then be dehydrated to produce sphingosine or hydroxylated to produce phytosphingosine. The free long-chain bases are efficiently acylated to produce ceramides, which may be glycosylated by means of a glycosyl transferase to produce a glycosylceramide or converted to sphingomyelin by transfer of a phosphoryl-choline from CDP-choline.

Cholesterol is another major lipid in epidermis and in oral epithelium [56]. Basal keratinocytes in epidermis, and presumably oral epithelium, have cell surface lipoprotein receptors and are able to derive cholesterol from the circulation; however, as cells move outward from the basal layer, these receptors are internalized and degraded [57]. The cholesterol that accumulates from this point onward is synthesized in the epithelial cell from acetate [51]. Hydroxymethylglutaryl-CoA (HMG-CoA) reductase catalyzes the rate-limiting step in this pathway [58], and it has been demonstrated that this enzyme is regulated by phosphorylation [59, 60]: the dephosphorylated enzyme is active, whereas the phosphorylated counterpart is not. The state of phosphorylation of this as well as other regulatory enzymes is determined by the relative activities of protein kinase C and by protein phosphatases, which are in turn influenced by diacylglycerol [61], lysosphingolipids [62], calcium [63] and by other less well defined factors.

C. Essential Fatty Acids

Linoleic acid is required in the mammalian diet [64, 65]. If omitted, one of the first symptoms of essential fatty acid deficiency to be noted is rough scaly skin and impaired permeability barrier function manifest by increased water consumption to compensate for increased water loss through the skin [66]. Subsequently, growth, reproductive capability and kidney function become impaired and death may result. The scaly skin symptom is coupled to hyperproliferation and reflects the inability to produce eicosanoids [67]. In normal epidermis and keratinizing oral epithelium prostaglandin E_2 and 12-HETE are the most abundant eicosanoids [68, 69]. Liver and a number of other tissues convert linoleate to arachidonate by means of desaturation and chain extension [70]. However, epidermis does not have the required Δ6-desaturase to mediate this conversion [71], and so must obtain both linoleate and arachidonate from the circulation. Retroconversion of arachidonate to linoleate by epidermis has been reported [72].

The impaired barrier function in essential fatty acid deficiency is specifically related to the need for linoleate in an unusual acylglucosylceramide [73-76], shown in Figure 2, and a related acylceramide [77] which have been implicated in assembly of the barrier. It has been proposed [78] that the very long ω-hydroxyacyl chain in this molecule completely spans one bilayer while the linoleate inserts into an adjacent bilayer, thus riveting the two together. This molecular rivet action could result in the aggregation and flattening of small membrane vesicles to produce the contents of the lamellar granules. In essential fatty acid deficiency the acylglucosylceramide is synthesized but contains oleate instead of linoleate [76, 79]. In this condition water loss through the skin may be increased as much as 10-fold, but the provision of linoleate, either in the diet [75] or topically [67], rapidly restores both the sphingolipid molecules and the permeability barrier function to normal.

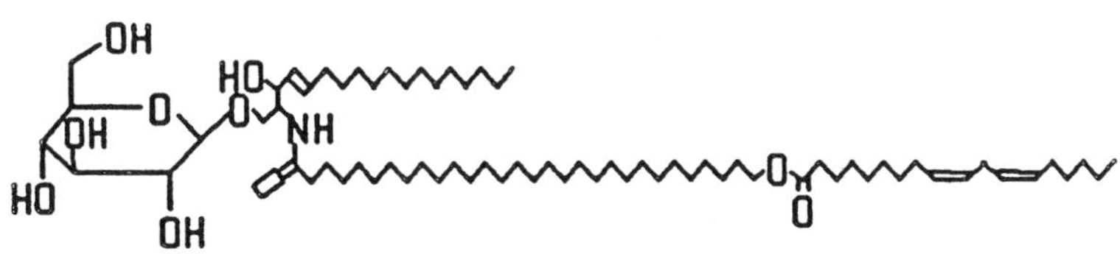

Figure 2. Structure of the linoleate-containing acylglucosylceramide from keratinizing epithelia. (From references 73 and 74).

D. Lipid Degradation

In the final stages of differentiation in keratinizing epithelia, a variety of hydrolases are involved in lipid modification and maturation of the barrier [39]. A number of hydrolytic enzymes have been associated with lamellar granules [80, 81] and are presumed to be delivered to the intercellular spaces via this organelle. Sphingomyelinase, which has been shown to be much more abundant in epidermis and keratinizing oral epithelium than in nonkeratinized oral epithelium [82], converts sphingomyelin to ceramides. Accordingly, sphingomyelin is abundant in the viable cells of epidermis, palatal epithelium and gingival epithelium, but is completely absent or present in only trace amounts in stratum corneum from these epithelia [47, 48]. Likewise, β-glucocerebrosidase is most abundant in the keratinizing epithelia [83], especially in the upper granular layer [84], and converts glucocerebrosides to ceramides in the vicinity of the boundary between the granular and cornified layers. A variety of phospholipases degrade the phosphoglycerides [85]. Linoleic acid, released from acylglucosylceramide, appears to be recycled [86], whereas monounsaturated fatty acids selectively become esterified to cholesterol [87]. The fatty acids that survive as such into the stratum corneum are entirely saturated, straight-chained and mainly 20 through 24 carbons in length [87]. In the nonkeratinizing epithelia, the levels of hydrolytic enzymes are appreciably lower [82, 83], and accordingly, phospholipids and glycosylceramides survive into the superficial cell layers [47].

E. Membrane-coating Granules

In keratinizing epithelia, the lipids that accumulate with maturation are largely packaged in small organelles known as membrane-coating granules or lamellar granules [2]. These organelles are formed in the region of the Golgi [2, 88, 89]. They are membrane-bounded and contain one or several tightly packed stacks of flattened lipid vesicles. Direct chemical analysis [80, 90, 91] of isolated membrane coating granules from epidermis have demonstrated that these organelles contain phospholipids, cholesterol, fatty acids, cholesterol esters, ceramides and glycolipids, mainly monohexosylceramides, the proportions of which are summarized in Table 1. The most unusual of these lipids is the linoleate-rich acylglucosylceramide discussed above and depicted in Figure 2 [73, 74, 92, 93]. A number of hydrolytic enzyme activities have also been demonstrated in isolated lamellar granules [80, 91]. In the final stages of differentiation, lamellar granule contents are extruded into the extracellular space at the boundary between the uppermost nucleated cells and the stratum corneum [23, 94], where they are transformed into multilamellar sheets [95], which fill most of the extracellular spaces of the stratum corneum and comprise

Table 1. Compositions (Weight Percent) of Lipids from Epidermal Lamellar Granules and from Epithelial Barriers. (From References 48, 129 and Unpublished Observations by P. W. Wertz and C. A. Squier).

	Lamellar granules	Epidermal stratum corneum	Palatal stratum corneum	Buccal barrier
Phospholipids	35.9	0.0	12.1	34.6
Cholesterol sulfate	0.0	2.0	9.8	0.9
Glycosylceramides	10.1	0.7	2.6	19.0
Acylglucosylceramide	10.8	0.0	0.0	0.0
Ceramides 2-6	13.8	34.9	23.0	8.3
Acylceramide	1.9	6.0	0.9	0.0
Cholesterol	17.4	28.4	22.5	16.6
Fatty acid	9.0	13.9	7.6	11.0
Triglyceride trace	1.3	21.1	5.2	
Cholesterol ester	1.1	12.8	1.3	3.6

the water barrier. The hydrolytic enzymes associated with the lamellar granules are thought to participate in this final biochemical and physical transformation of the lipids to form the multilamellar sheets.

In epidermis, roughly one-fifth to one-third of the linoleate-containing acylglucosylceramide is thought to be involved in the assembly of the internal lamellae of the lamellar granules [51]. However, two-thirds of the acylglucosylceramide is thought to be located in the bounding membrane of the epidermal lamellar granule [96] resulting in the introduction of this unusual lipid to the cell periphery when the bounding membrane of the granule fuses into the cell plasma membrane. At about this same time, the glucose and the linoleate are cleaved from the ceramide to produce an ω-hydroxyceramide. The glucose is used for energy production by anaerobic glycolysis [97], and the linoleate may be recycled, as noted above [86]. A thick band of protein is deposited beneath the hydroxyceramide layer [98], and the protein becomes cross-linked via both disulfide linkages [99] and isopeptide linkages [100] introduced through the action of a transglutaminase on glutamate and lysine residues [101]. The hydroxyceramide becomes ester-linked to acidic residues on the outer surface of the cross-linked protein envelope [102, 103]. This covalently linked lipid envelope may provide a template upon which the intercellular lamellae of epidermal stratum corneum form, and it appears that this ω-hydroxyceramide layer has a profound influence on the organization of the free lipids in the intercellular space [104, 105]. Recent studies have revealed that oral stratum corneum does not have this biochemical and anatomical feature, and this is reflected in differences at the ultrastructural level [105].

Membrane coating granules, similar in size and behavior to the lamellar granules in keratinized epithelia are produced in nonkeratinizing oral epithelium, but they contain a central amorphous core, rather than lamellae [106, 107]. Histochemical studies have indicated that these membrane-coating granules contain glycoconjugates [108], presumably glycolipids, which are abundant in nonkeratinizing oral epithelia [47, 109]. Although similar granules have been described in the nonkeratinized stratified squamous epithelium of uterine cervix [106] and esophagus [110] there have been no accounts of their isolation and biochemical characterization apart from a single abstract [111]. At the intermediate layer [107] within nonkeratinized epithelium, the membrane coating granules migrate to the apical aspect of the cell, and their contents are expelled into the extracellular space [107]. The location at which this occurs corresponds to the position at which the permeability barrier is formed [22].

F. Stratum Corneum Lipids

The principal lipids found in stratum corneum are the ceramides, cholesterol and fatty acids, representative structures of which are shown in Figure 3. The lipid compositions of epidermal and palatal stratum corneum are given in Table 1. In epidermal and oral stratum corneum the ceramides comprise approximately 40% and 20% of the total lipid, respectively. In both tissues cholesterol represents approximately 25% of the total [48], and fatty acid accounts for about 10% of the total. Both epidermal and oral stratum corneum contain small amounts of cholesterol sulfate, cholesterol esters and triglycerides; however, small amounts of phospholipids are found in oral stratum corneum only.

Ceramide 1 is thought to be derived from the linoleate-containing acylglucosylceramide associated with the internal lamellae of the lamellar granules. It is thought that the acylceramide may act as a molecular rivet, as discussed for the acylglucosylceramide, and may help to hold together and stabilize the multilamellar lipid arrays found in the intercellular spaces of the stratum corneum. Ceramide 2 consists of mainly 24-, 26- and 28-carbon saturated fatty acids amide-linked to sphingosine and dihydrosphingosine bases [77, 112]. The long chain base component in this ceramide includes 16- through 22-carbon sphingosines and dihydrosphingosines, but the 18- and 20-carbon species are the most abundant. Ceramide 3 contains the same range of fatty acids as found in ceramide 2, but contains mainly 18- through 22-carbon phytosphingosines instead of sphingosines. Ceramides 4 and 5 both consist of α-hydroxyacids amide linked to sphingosines. They differ in that ceramide 4

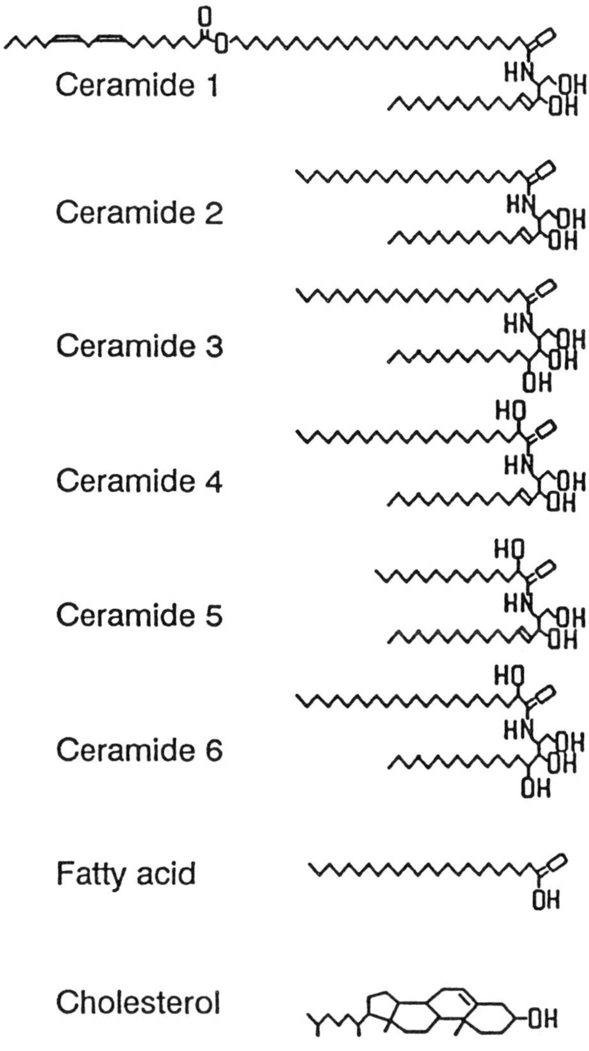

Figure 3. Representative structures of the major lipids from stratum corneum. (From references 77, 87 and 112).

contains 24- through 28-carbon hydroxyacids whereas ceramide 5 contains α-hydroxypalmitic acid. The most polar ceramide fraction, ceramide 6, contains α-hydroxyacids amide-linked to phytosphingosines.

With the exception of the linoleate chain in ceramide 1, all of the aliphatic chains in the ceramides and fatty acids are straight and saturated. This should permit the formation of highly ordered, and thereby less permeable, membrane domains. In contrast, the phospholipids that survive into the stratum corneum in keratinized oral epithelium contain unsaturated fatty acids which may cause disordering of chain packing and increased permeability.

G. Lipids in Nonkeratinized Barriers

The barrier layers of the epithelium from the floor of the mouth and the buccal regions contain mainly phospholipids, cholesterol and glycosylceramides [47], as summarized in Table 1. The phospholipids found here include sphingomyelin and the phosphatides of choline, ethanolamine, serine and inositol. There are moderate levels of triglycerides and cholesterol esters, which may be present as intracellular lipid droplets, and small proportions of fatty acids and ceramide 2 are present in these nonkeratinized epithelia. In general, the major barrier lipids in the nonkeratinizing epithelia should be capable of forming fluid liquid crystalline membranes.

H. Ultrastructures of Epithelial Permeability Barriers

At about the same time as the tracer studies were being carried out, the freeze fracture technique was introduced to study the ultrastructure of the epidermis [25, 113]. Using this method, Breathnach and coworkers [113] discovered that the intercellular spaces of epidermal stratum corneum are filled with multiple membranous structures.

Although the existence of the multiple broad lipid sheets in epidermal stratum corneum was demonstrated by the freeze-fracture technique [113], this method yields only limited information, and many of the details of organization of the intercellular lamellae remained uncertain. However, the relatively recent introduction of ruthenium tetroxide as a fixative for transmission electron microscopy [114] has permitted a more direct visualization of the intercellular lamellae. With this technique, it has been demonstrated that most of the intercellular space throughout epidermal stratum corneum is filled with multiple intercellular lamellae [114], often with the lucent bands showing an alternating broad-narrow-broad spacing [104] as illustrated in Figure 4a. In oral stratum corneum, the intercellular spaces contain more desmosomes than seen in epidermal stratum corneum, and the lamellae in the interdesmosomal regions appear to be less extensive and usually paired as can be seen in Figure 4b. These intercellular lamellae are found around the periphery of the dilations which appear to contain some electron dense material, possibly desmosomal breakdown products, and short fragments of lamellar material, possibly granule-derived lamellae that failed to reorganize into broad sheets. In nonkeratinized oral epithelium from the floor of the mouth or buccal regions,

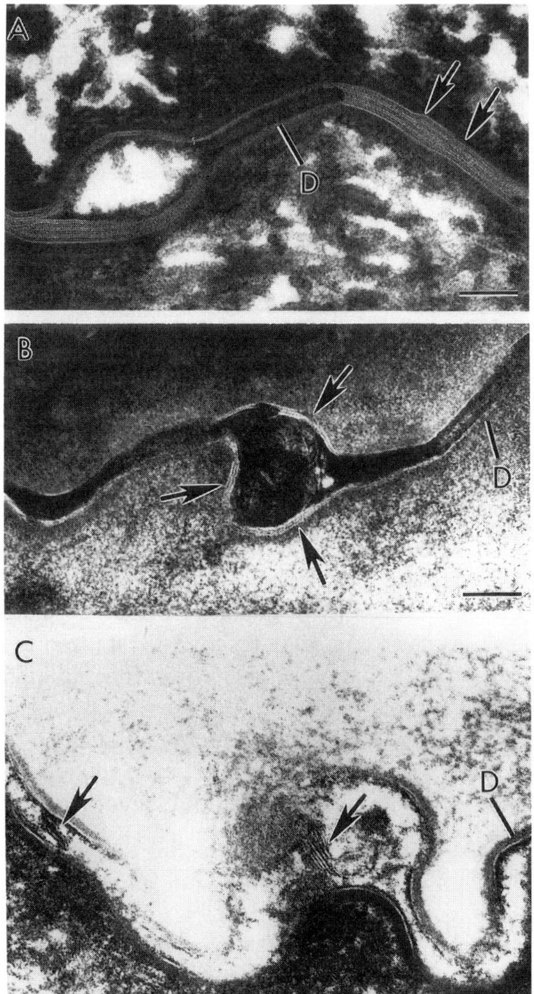

Figure 4. Organization of membrane lipids in the intercellular spaces of epidermal (A) and palatal (B) stratum corneum and in the outer cell layers of buccal epithelium (C). Lamellar lipid structures are indicated with arrows, and desmosomes are labeled D. Bars = 100 nm.

much of the intercellular space in the outer barrier layers appears empty; however, there are one or two membranous structures surrounding the cornified envelope and occasional short stacks of lipid lamellae traverse the intercellular space as shown in Figure 4c.

Table 2. Regional Variation in Permeability to Water. (From references 56 and 115).

	K_p ($\times 10^{-7}$ cm/minute)	
	Human	Pig
Skin	44	62
Palate	450	364
Buccal mucosa	579	634
Floor of mouth	973	808

IV. BARRIER FUNCTION

A. Regional Variation

Tritiated water is a commonly used indicator of permeability, and in Table 2 the permeability coefficient (K_p) values for abdominal skin and different regions of oral mucosa from pigs and humans are summarized [56, 115]. Examination of the results for human tissue reveals that there is an order of magnitude increase in permeability in going from skin to palate, and a further increase in permeability is seen in moving from keratinized to nonkeratinized oral sites. This pattern of variation is in accord with the kinds of epithelial barrier lipids found in these locations. In epidermal stratum corneum it is expected that highly ordered gel phase membrane domains will predominate, whereas in oral stratum corneum one would expect a mixture of gel and liquid crystalline domains. In nonkeratinized oral epithelium predominantly liquid crystalline domains would be expected.

B. Individual Variation

There is large variation in the permeability of skin and oral mucosa among individuals [115, 116]. With healthy tissue, it has generally been necessary to obtain ten separate measurements in order to have meaningful estimates of the mean K_p and dispersion about the mean. With skin, some of the individual variation may be an artefact resulting from contamination of the stratum corneum with subcutaneous fat, sebaceous lipids or cosmetic components. Both human and porcine subcutaneous fat is very fluid and rich in oleate, and lipases on the skin surface are capable of hydrolysing triglycerides [117]. Oleic acid could thus be liberated, and oleate is known to be a permeability enhancer [118]. Also, the amount of sebaceous lipid on the skin at different anatomical sites [119] and from different individuals [120] varies widely, and human sebum has been shown to act as a permeabilizer [121].

It has been documented that the skin becomes less permeable with increasing age [121, 122], although the effect is not large, and the barrier is known to be defective in a number of skin diseases [8, 123-126]. Changes in the permeability of oral mucosa with age have been considered in Chapter 1. Denture wearing has been reported to result in a progressive decrease in barrier function in the underlying tissue [127, 128].

V. ACKNOWLEDGEMENTS

This work was supported in part by NIH grants DEO 7930 and DE1 0516.

REFERENCES

1. P. M. Elias, Structure and function of the stratum corneum permeability barrier, *Drug Develop. Res. 13*:97 (1988).
2. L. Landmann, The epidermal permeability barrier, *Anat. Embryol. 178*:1 (1988).
3. J. E. Shaw, M. Prevo, R. Gale, and S. I. Yum, Percutaneous absorption, *Physiology, Biochemistry, and Molecular Biology of the Skin* (L. A. Goldsmith, ed.), Oxford University Press, New York, 1991, p. 1447.
4. I. A. Siegel, Permeability of the oral mucosa, *The Structure and Function of Oral Mucosa* (J. Meyer, C. A. Squier and S. J. Gerson, eds.), Pergamon Press, New York, 1984, p. 95.
5. C. A. Squier, The permeability of oral mucosa, *Crit. Rev. Oral. Biol. Med. 2*:13 (1991).
6. D. Attenborough, *Life on Earth*, Little, Brown & Co., Boston, 1980.
7. A. Homalle, Experiences physiologiques sur l'absorption par le tegument externe chez l'homme dans le bain, *Union Med. 7*:462 (1853).
8. A. M. Kligman, The biology of the stratum corneum, *The Epidermis* (W. Montagna, and W. C. Lobitz Jr., eds.), Academic Press, New York, 1964, p. 387.
9. H. Rein, Experimentelle Studien über electroendosmose an überlebender menschlicher haut, *Z. Biol. 81*:125 (1924).
10. S. Rothman, The principles of percutaneous absorption, *J. Lab. Clin. Med. 28*:1305 (1943).
11. T. Winsor, and G. E. Burch, Differential roles of layers of human epigastric skin on diffusion rate of water, *Arch. Int. Med. 74*:428 (1944).
12. I. H. Blank, Further observations on factors which influence the water content of the stratum corneum, *J. Invest. Dermatol. 21*:159 (1953).
13. I. H. Blank, Cutaneous barriers, *J. Invest. Dermatol. 45*:249 (1965).
14. R. J. Scheuplein, Percutaneous absorption after twenty-five years: Or "old wine in new wineskins", *J. Invest. Dermatol. 67*:31 (1976).

15. F. N. Marzulli, Barriers to skin penetration, *J. Invest. Dermatol. 39*:387 (1962).
16. P. J. Frosch, and A. M. Kligman, Rapid blister formation in human skin with ammonium hydroxide, *Br. J. Dermatol. 96*:461 (1977).
17. I. C. Mackenzie, Ordered structure of the stratum corneum of mammalian skin, *Nature 222*:881 (1969).
18. I. C. Mackenzie, An examination of cellular organization within the stratum corneum by a silver staining method, *J. Invest. Dermatol. 61*:245 (1973).
19. E. Christophers, Cellular architecture of the stratum corneum of mammalian skin, *J. Invest. Dermatol. 56*:165 (1971).
20. C. A. Squier, and B. K. Hall, The permeability of skin and oral mucosa to water and horseradish peroxidase as related to the thickness of the permeability barrier, *J. Invest. Dermatol. 84*:176 (1985).
21. E. Schreiner, and K. Wolff, Permeabilitat des epidermalen intercellularraumes fur kleinmolekulares proteinen, *Arch. Klin. Exp. Dermatol. 235*:78 (1969).
22. C. A. Squier, The permeability of keratinized and nonkeratinized oral epithelium to horseradish peroxidase, *J. Ultrastruct. Res. 43*:160 (1973).
23. P. M. Elias, and D. S. Friend, The permeability barrier in mammalian epidermis, *J. Cell Biol. 65*:180 (1975).
24. C. A. Squier, and L. Rooney, The permeability of keratinized and nonkeratinized oral epithelium to lanthanum in vivo, *J. Ultrastruct. Res. 54*:286 (1976).
25. P. M. Elias, N. S. McNutt, and D. S. Friend, Membrane alterations during cornification of mammalian squamous epithelia: a freeze fracture, tracer, and thin section study, *Anat. Rec. 189*:577 (1977).
26. R. J. Scheuplein, Mechanism of percutaneous absorption. Transient diffusion and the relative importance of various routes of skin penetration, *J. Invest. Dermatol. 48*:79 (1967).
27. M. K. Nemanic, and P. M. Elias, In situ precipitation: a novel cytochemical technique for visualization of permeability pathways in mammalian stratum corneum, *J. Histochem. Cytochem. 28*:573 (1980).
28. C. A. Squier, and C. A. Lesch, Penetration pathways of different compounds through epidermis and oral epithelia, *J. Oral. Path. 17*:512 (1988).
29. A. S. Michaels, S. K. Chandrasekaran, and J. E. Shaw, Drug permeation through human skin: theory and in vivo experimental measurements, *Am. Inst. Chem. Eng. J. 21*:985 (1975).
30. W. J. Albery, and J. Hadgraft, Percutaneous absorption: theoretical description, *J. Pharm. Pharmacol. 31*:129 (1979).
31. A. J. Hoogstraate, and H. E. Boddé, Methods for assessing the buccal mucosa as a route of drug delivery, *Adv. Drug Del. Rev. 12*:99 (1993).

32. G. S. Berenson, and G. E. Burch, Studies of diffusion of water through dead human skin: The effect of different environmental states and of chemical alterations of the epidermis, *Amer. J. Trop. Med. 31*:842 (1951).
33. H. D. Onken, and C. A. Moyer, The water barrier in human epidermis. Physical and chemical nature, *Arch. Dermatol. 87*:584 (1963).
34. J. W. H. Mali, The transport of water through the human epidermis, *J. Invest. Dermatol. 27*:451 (1956).
35. R. T. Treagar, The structures which limit the permeability of the skin, *J. Soc. Cosmet. Chem. 13*:145 (1956).
36. T. M. Sweeney, and D. T. Downing, The role of lipids in the epidermal barrier to water diffusion, *J. Invest. Dermatol. 55*:135 (1970).
37. G. Grubauer, K. R. Feingold, R. M. Harris, and P. M. Elias, Lipid content and lipid type as determinants of the epidermal permeability barrier, *J. Lipid Res. 30*:89 (1980).
38. K. Abrams, J. D. Harvell, D. Shriner, P. Wertz, H. Maibach, H. I. Maibach, and S. J. Rehfeld, Effect of organic solvents on in vitro human skin water barrier function, *J. Invest. Dermatol. 101*:609 (1993).
39. H. J. Yardley, and R. Summerly, Lipid composition and metabolism in normal and diseased epidermis, *Pharmacol. Ther. 13*:357 (1981).
40. P. W. Wertz, D. C. Swartzendruber, and C. A. Squier, Regional variation in the structure and permeability of oral mucosa and skin, *Adv. Drug Del. Rev. 12*:1 (1993).
41. D. J. Kooyman, Lipids of the skin. Some changes in the lipids of the epidermis during the process of keratinization, *Arch. Dermatol. Syphilol. 25*:444 (1932).
42. R. P. Reinerston, and V. R. Wheatley, Studies on the chemical composition of human epidermal lipids, *J. Invest. Dermatol. 32*:49 (1959).
43. V. J. W. Long, Variation in lipid composition at different depths in the cow snout epidermis, *J. Invest. Dermatol. 55*:269 (1970).
44. G. M. Gray, and H. J. Yardley, Different populations of pig epidermal cells. Isolation and lipid composition, *J. Lipid Res. 16*:441 (1975).
45. M. A. Lampe, M. L. Williams, and P. M. Elias, Human epidermal lipids: characterization and modulations during differentiation, *J. Lipid Res. 24*:131 (1983).
46. P. Cox, and C. A. Squier, Variations in lipids in different layers of porcine epidermis, *J. Invest. Dermatol. 87*:741 (1986).
47. C. A. Squier, P. W. Wertz, and P. Cox, Thin-layer chromatographic analysis of lipids in different layers of porcine epidermis and oral epithelium, *Arch. Oral Biol. 36*:647 (1991).
48. P. W. Wertz, M. Kremer, and C. A. Squier, Comparison of lipids from epidermal and palatal stratum corneum, *J. Invest. Dermatol. 98*:375 (1992).

49. G. M. Gray, Phosphatidyl-(N-acyl)-ethanolamine. A lipid component of mammalian epidermis, *Biochim. Biophys. Acta 431*:1 (1976).
50. P. C. Schmid, and H. H. O. Schmid, N-acylation of ethanolamine phospholipids by acyl transfer does not involve hydrolysis, *Biochim. Biophys. Acta 922*:398 (1987).
51. C. L. Hedberg, P. W. Wertz, and D. T. Downing, The time course of lipid biosynthesis in pig epidermis, *J. Invest. Dermatol. 91*:169 (1988).
52. C. L. Skutches, C. P. Holroyde, R. N. Myers, P. Paul, and G. A. Reichard, Plasma acetate turnover and oxidation, *J. Clin. Invest. 64*:708 (1979).
53. P. E. Braun, and E. E. Snell, The biosynthesis of dihydrosphingosine in cell free preparations of Hansenula ciferri, *Proc. Nat. Acad. Sci. USA 58*:298 (1967).
54. J. N. Kanfer, and S. Bates, Sphingolipid metabolism II. The biosynthesis of 3-keto-dihydrosphingosine by a partially purified enzyme from rat brain, *Lipids 5*:718 (1970).
55. A. H. Merrill, and E. Wang, Biosynthesis of long-chain (sphingoid) bases from serine by LM cells, *J. Biol. Chem. 261*:3764 (1986).
56. C. A. Squier, P. Cox, and P. W. Wertz, Lipid content and water permeability of skin and oral mucosa, *J. Invest. Dermatol. 96*:123 (1991).
57. M. Ponec, L. Havekes, J. Kempenaar, and B. J. Vermeer, Cultured human skin fibroblasts and keratinocytes: differences in the regulation of cholesterol synthesis, *J. Invest. Dermatol. 81*:125 (1983).
58. V. W. Rodwell, J. L. Nordstrom, and J. J. Mitchelsen, Regulation of HMG CoA reductase, *Adv. Lipid Res. 14*:1 (1976).
59. D. M. Gibson, and T. S. Ingelbritsen, Reversible modulation of liver 3-hydroxy-3-methylglutarylcoenzyme A reductase, *Life Sci. 23*:2649 (1978).
60. Z. H. Beg, J. A. Shonik, and H. B. Brewer, Jr., HMG CoA reductase: regulation of enzymatic activity by phosphorylation and dephosphorylation, *Proc. Nat. Acad. Sci. USA 75*:3678 (1978).
61. R. M. Bell, Protein kinase C activation by diacylglycerol second messengers, *Cell 45*:631 (1986).
62. Y. A. Hannun, and R. M. Bell, Lysosphingolipids inhibit protein kinase C: Implications for the sphingolipidoses, *Science 235*:670 (1987).
63. Y. Nishizuka, Intracellular signaling by hydrolysis of phospholipid and activation of protein kinase C, *Science 258*:607 (1992).
64. G. O. Burr, and M. M. Burr, A new deficiency disease produced by the rigid exclusion of fat from the diet, *J. Biol. Chem. 82*:345 (1929).
65. G. O. Burr, and M. M. Burr, On the nature of the fatty acids essential in nutrition, *J. Biol. Chem. 86*:587 (1930).

66. R. T. Holman, Essential fatty acid deficiency, *Progress in the Chemistry of Fats and Other Lipids* (R. T. Holman, ed.), Pergamon Press, New York, 1968, p. 275.
67. C. Prottey, Investigations into the functions of essential fatty acids in the skin, *Br. J. Dermatol. 97*:29 (1977).
68. F. E. Dewhurst, D. E. Moss, S. Offenbacher, and J. M. Goodson, Levels of prostaglandin E_2, thromboxane and prostacyclin in periodontal tissues, *J. Periodon. Res. 18*:156 (1983).
69. S. Hammerstrom, J. A. Lindgren, C. Marcelo, E. A. Duell, T. F. Andersson, and J. J. Voorhees, Arachidonic acid transformations in normal and psoriatic skin, *J. Invest. Dermatol. 73*:180 (1979).
70. H. W. Sprecher, Biochemistry of essential fatty acids, *Prog. Lipid Res. 20*:13 (1981).
71. R. S. Chapkin, and V. A. Ziboh, Inability of skin enzyme preparations to biosynthesize arachidonic acid from linoleic acid, *Biochim. Biophys. Res. Comm. 124*:124 (1984).
72. H. S. Hansen, B. Jensen, and P. Wettstein-Knowles, Apparent in vivo retroconversion of dietary arachidonic acid to linoleic acid in essential fatty acid-deficient rats, *Biochim. Biophys. Acta 878*:284 (1986).
73. P. W. Wertz, and D. T. Downing, Acylglucosylceramides of pig epidermis: structure determination, *J. Lipid Res. 24*:753 (1983).
74. W. Abraham, P. W. Wertz, and D. T. Downing, Linoleate rich acylglucosylceramides from pig epidermis: structure determination by proton magnetic resonance, *J. Lipid Res. 26*:761 (1985).
75. H. S. Hansen, and B. Jensen, Essential function of linoleic acid esterified in acylglucosylceramide and acylceramide in maintaining the epidermal water permeability barrier: Evidence from feeding studies with oleate, linoleate, arachidonate, columbinate and linolenate, *Biochim. Biophys. Acta 834*:357 (1985).
76. J. L. Melton, P. W. Wertz, D. C. Swartzendruber, and D. T. Downing, Effects of essential fatty acid deficiency on epidermal O-acylsphingolipids and transepidermal water loss in young pigs, *Biochim. Biophys. Acta 921*:191 (1987).
77. P. W. Wertz, and D. T. Downing, Ceramides of pig epidermis: structure determination, *J. Lipid Res. 24*:759 (1983).
78. P. W. Wertz, and D. T. Downing, Glycolipids in mammalian epidermis: structure and function in the water barrier, *Science 217*:1261 (1982).
79. P. W. Wertz, E. S. Cho, and D. T. Downing, Effect of essential fatty acid deficiency on the epidermal sphingolipids of the rat, *Biochim. Biophys. Acta 753*:350 (1983).
80. R. K. Freinkel, and T. N. Traczyk, Lipid composition and acid hydrolase content of lamellar granules of fetal rat epidermis, *J. Invest. Dermatol. 85*:295 (1985).

81. S. Grayson, A. D. Johnson-Winegar, and P. M. Elias, Isolation of lamellar bodies from neonatal mouse epidermis by selective sequential filtration, *Science 221*:962 (1983).
82. J. Quinn, P. Cox, C. A. Squier, and P. W. Wertz, Epithelial sphingomyelin and sphingomyelinase, *J. Dent. Res. 73*:108 (1994).
83. F. Chang, P. W. Wertz, and C. A. Squier, Comparison of glycosidase activities in epidermis, palatal epithelium and buccal epithelium, *Comp. Biochem. Physiol. 100B*:137 (1991).
84. F. Chang, P. W. Wertz, and C. A. Squier, Localization of β-glucosidase activity within keratinizing epithelia, *Comp. Biochem. Physiol. 105A*:251 (1993).
85. P. M. Elias, G. K. Menon, S. Grayson, and B. E. Brown, Membrane structural alteration in murine stratum corneum: Relationship to the localization of polar lipids and phospholipases, *J. Invest. Dermatol. 91*:3 (1988).
86. K. C. Madison, D. C. Swartzendruber, P. W. Wertz, and D. T. Downing, Murine keratinocyte cultures grown at the air/medium interface synthesize stratum corneum lipids and "recycle" linoleate during differentiation, *J. Invest. Dermatol. 93*:10 (1989).
87. P. W. Wertz, D. C. Swartzendruber, K. C. Madison, and D. T. Downing, Composition and morphology of epidermal cyst lipids, *J. Invest. Dermatol. 89*:419 (1987).
88. K. Wolff, and K. Holubar, Odland-Korper (Membrane-coating granules, keratinosomen) als epidermale lysosomen, *Arch. Klin. Exp. Dermatol. 231*:1 (1967).
89. A. F. Hayward, Membrane-coating granules, *Int. Rev. Cytol. 59*:97 (1979).
90. P. W. Wertz, D. T. Downing, R. K. Freinkel, and T. N. Traczyk, Sphingolipids of the stratum corneum and lamellar granules of fetal rat epidermis, *J. Invest. Dermatol. 83*:193 (1984).
91. S. Grayson, A. G. Johnson-Winegar, B. U. Wintraub, R. R. Isseroff, E. H. Epstein, and P. M. Elias, Lamellar body-enriched fractions from neonatal mice: Preparative techniques and partial characterization, *J. Invest. Dermatol. 85*:289 (1985).
92. G. M. Gray, R. J. White, and J. R. Majer, 1 (3' O acyl) β-glucosyl-N-dihydroxypentatriacontadienoyl-sphingosine, a major component of the glucosylceramides of pig and human epidermis, *Biochim. Biophys. Acta 528*:127 (1978).
93. P. A. Bowser, D. H. Nugteren, R. J. White, U. M. T. Houtsmuller, and C. Prottey, Identification, isolation and characterization of epidermal lipids containing linoleic acid, *Biochim. Biophys. Acta 834*:419 (1985).
94. R. M. Lavker, Membrane coating granules: the fate of the discharged lamellae, *J. Ultrastruc. Res. 55*:79 (1976).

95. L. Landmann, Epidermal permeability barrier: transformation of lamellar granule disks into intercellular sheets by a membrane fusion process, *J. Invest. Dermatol. 87*:202 (1986).
96. P. W. Wertz, and C. A. Squier, Cellular and molecular basis of barrier function in oral epithelium, *Crit. Rev. Ther. Drug Carr. Sys. 8*:237 (1991).
97. M. W. Hill, and J. Karthigasan, Glucose metabolism and protein synthesis in stratified squamous epithelia from young and old mice, *Exp. Gerontol. 24*:331 (1989).
98. R. H. Rice, and H. Green, The cornified envelope of terminally differentiated human epidermal keratinocytes consists of cross-linked protein, *Cell 11*:417 (1977).
99. A. G. Matoltsy, Keratinization, *J. Invest. Dermatol. 67*:20 (1976).
100. J. L. Abernathy, R. L. Hill, and L. A. Goldsmith, (Glutamyl)lysine cross-links in human stratum corneum, *J. Biol. Chem. 252*:1837 (1977).
101. L. A. Goldsmith, and C. M. Martin, Human epidermal transamidase, *J. Invest. Dermatol. 64*:316 (1975).
102. P. W. Wertz, and D. T. Downing, Covalently bound hydroxyacylsphingosine in the stratum corneum, *Biochim. Biophys. Acta 917*:108 (1987).
103. D. C. Swartzendruber, P. W. Wertz, K. C. Madison, and D. T. Downing, Evidence that the corneocyte has a chemically bound lipid envelope, *J. Invest. Dermatol. 88*:709 (1987).
104. D. C. Swartzendruber, P. W. Wertz, D. J. Kitko, K. C. Madison, and D. T. Downing, Molecular models of the intercellular lipid lamellae in mammalian stratum corneum, *J. Invest. Dermatol. 92*:251 (1989).
105. F. Chang, D. C. Swartzendruber, P. W. Wertz, and C. A. Squier, Covalently bound lipids in keratinizing epithelia, *Biochim. Biophys. Acta 1150*:98 (1993).
106. C. Grubb, M. Hackemann, and K. R. Hill, Small granules and plasma membrane thickening in human cervical squamous epithelium, *J. Ultrastruc. Res. 22*:458 (1968).
107. C. A. Squier, Membrane-coating granules in nonkeratinizing oral epithelium, *J. Ultrastruct. Res. 60*:212 (1977).
108. P. B. Innes, The nature of granules within sulcular epithelial cells, *J. Periodont. Res. 8*:252 (1973).
109. P. W. Wertz, P. Cox, C. A. Squier, and D. T. Downing, Lipids of epidermis and keratinized and nonkeratinized oral epithelia, *Comp. Biochem. Physiol. 83B*:529 (1986).
110. D. Hopwood, K. R. Logan, and I. A. D. Bouchier, The electron microscopy of normal human esophageal epithelium, *Virchows Arch. B Cell Pathol. 12*:187 (1978).
111. S. Y. Chen, Growth inhibitor in membrane-coating granules of oral epithelium, *J. Dent. Res. 62*:240 (1983).

112. P. W. Wertz, M. C. Miethke, S. A. Long, J. S. Strauss, and D. T. Downing, The composition of the ceramides from human stratum corneum and from comedones, *J. Invest. Dermatol. 84*:410 (1985).
113. A. S. Breathnach, T. Goodman, C. Stolinski, and M. Gross, Freeze fracture replication of cells of stratum corneum of human epidermis, *J. Anat. 114*:65 (1973).
114. K. C. Madison, D. C. Swartzendruber, P. W. Wertz, and D. T. Downing, Presence of intact intercellular lamellae in the upper layers of the stratum corneum, *J. Invest. Dermatol. 88*:714 (1987).
115. C. A. Lesch, C. A. Squier, A. Cruchley, D. M. Williams, and P. Speight, The permeability of human oral mucosa and skin to water, *J. Dent. Res. 68*:1345 (1989).
116. T. J. Franz, Percutaneous absorption. On the relevance of in vitro data, *J. Invest. Dermatol. 64*:190 (1975).
117. D. T. Downing, Lipolysis by human skin surface debris in organic solvents, *J. Invest. Dermatol. 54*:395 (1970).
118. G. M. Golden, J. E. McKie, and R. O. Potts, The role of stratum corneum lipid fluidity in transdermal drug flux, *J. Pharm. Sci. 76*:25 (1986).
119. R. S. Green, D. T. Downing, P. E. Pochi, and J. S. Strauss, Anatomical variation in the amount and composition of human skin surface lipid, *J. Invest. Dermatol. 54*:240 (1970).
120. D. T. Downing, J. S. Strauss, and P. E. Pochi, Variability in the chemical composition of human skin surface lipids, *J. Invest. Dermatol. 53*:322 (1969).
121. C. A. Squier, P. W. Wertz, D. M Williams, and A. T. Cruchley, Permeability of oral mucosa and skin with age, *The Effect of Aging in Oral Mucosa and Skin* (C. A. Squier and M. W. Hill, eds.), CRC Press, Boca Raton, 1994, p. 91.
122. A. M. Kligman, Perspectives and problems in cutaneous gerontology, *J. Invest. Dermatol. 73*:39 (1979).
123. P. Frost, G. D. Weinstein, J. W. Bothwell, and R. Wildnauer, Ichthyosiform dermatoses, *Arch. Dermatol. 98*:230 (1968).
124. P. J. Hartop, C. F. Allenby, and C. Prottey, Comparison of barrier function and lipids in psoriasis and essential fatty acid deficient rats, *Clin. Exp. Dermatol. 3*:259 (1978).
125. R. Ghadially, M. L. Williams, S, Y. E. Hou, and P. M. Elias, Membrane structural abnormalities in the stratum corneum of the autosomal recessive ichthyoses, *J. Invest. Dermatol 99*:755 (1992).
126. D. Y. M. Leung, A. R. Rhodes, R. S. Geha, L. Schneider, and J. Ring, Atopic Dermatitis (Atopic Eczema), *Dermatology in General Medicine* (T. B. Fitzpatrick, A. Z. Eisen, K. Wolff, I. M. Freedberg, and K. F. Austin, eds.), McGraw-Hill, New York, 1993, p. 1543.

127. E. Riber, and S. Kaaber, A 12-month study on changes in the barrier properties of denture-loaded palatal mucosa in immediate denture wearers, *Scand. J. Dent. Res. 88*:250 (1980).
128. E. Riber, and S. Kaaber, Barrier properties of inflamed denture-loaded palatal mucosa to water, *Scand. J. Dent. Res. 86*:386 (1978).
129. P. W. Wertz, and D. T. Downing, Stratum corneum: biological and biochemical considerations, *Transdermal Drug Delivery* (J. Hadgraft and R. H. Guy, eds.), Marcel Dekker, Inc., New York, 1989, p. 1.

3

Routes of Drug Transport Across Oral Mucosa

Hao Zhang
Anesta Corporation, USA

Joseph R. Robinson
University of Wisconsin-Madison, USA

I. INTRODUCTION

Since the early success of delivering nitroglycerin through sublingual mucosa for the treatment of angina pectoris [1], the oral mucosa has been studied extensively as a potential route for systemic drug delivery. Substantial review articles on this subject have been published [2-6].

Early oral mucosal drug delivery work focused on the phenomena that drugs can be absorbed via the oral mucosa. This interest had diminished somewhat with the finding that only a few drugs are clinically needed and practically feasible to be delivered via the oral mucosal route. More recently, interest has been renewed with the finding that certain penetration enhancers are effective in improving the permeability of oral mucosal tissue, coupled with more appropriate ways to deliver drug to this site, e.g., buccal patches. Recent research attention is on understanding the biological and physicochemical nature of the drug absorption process and the mechanism(s) of drug penetration across this tissue at the cellular and molecular level. The long term goal is to find a way to temporarily alter the permeability of the oral mucosa for drug delivery purposes. This topic is discussed in Chapter 4.

The route of penetration has been the focus of many studies because it is fundamental to intelligent design of a penetration enhancer in order to control tissue permeability. The complexity of the oral mucosa, such as the cellular structure, cell-cell interaction and communication, biochemical compositions, etc., makes it difficult to establish a simple model that will adequately describe the diffusion process inside the oral mucosa. Therefore, it is difficult to describe the precise penetration route using indirect kinetic permeability studies, since this approach requires a suitable mathematical model. Direct determination with measurable probes also has limitations.

In general, identifying and quantifying drug penetration route(s) is not an easy task. A basic understanding of the cellular structure and the physicochemical properties of the tissue, physicochemical properties of the drug, and mechanism(s) of the diffusion process are fundamental to determine the penetration route(s) of drugs absorption via the oral mucosa.

II. RELEVANT CELLULAR STRUCTURE OF THE ORAL MUCOSA

The detailed structure and function of the oral mucosa has been discussed in Chapters 1 and 2 of this book. The cellular structure of the oral mucosa consists of a superficial layer of stratified squamous epithelium, a basal lamina (basement membrane), and underlying connective tissue [7]. From the basement membrane to the epithelial surface, the cells undergo constant differentiation to form larger, but flattened, cells. In nonkeratinized oral epithelium, the superficial cells retain normal nuclei and are less flattened than in keratinized epithelium [3]. The closely compacted epithelial cells on the top quarter to one third of the epithelium form the main penetration barrier [8-10]. It is clear that the oral epithelium is not a uniform hydrophobic barrier.

The epithelial cell membrane is essentially lipophilic. The intercellular space, on the other hand, is relatively hydrophilic although there are many lipophilic components secreted from membrane coating granules into the intercellular space [11]. The entire oral epithelium can be viewed as a mosaic of hydrophilic and lipophilic regions, where the hydrophilic region is narrow and tortuous around the lipophilic cell membrane.

III. POSSIBLE ROUTES FOR DRUG TRANSPORT ACROSS THE ORAL MUCOSA

The cellular structure of the oral mucosa suggests that there are two permeability barriers. The intercellular spaces and cytoplasm are essentially

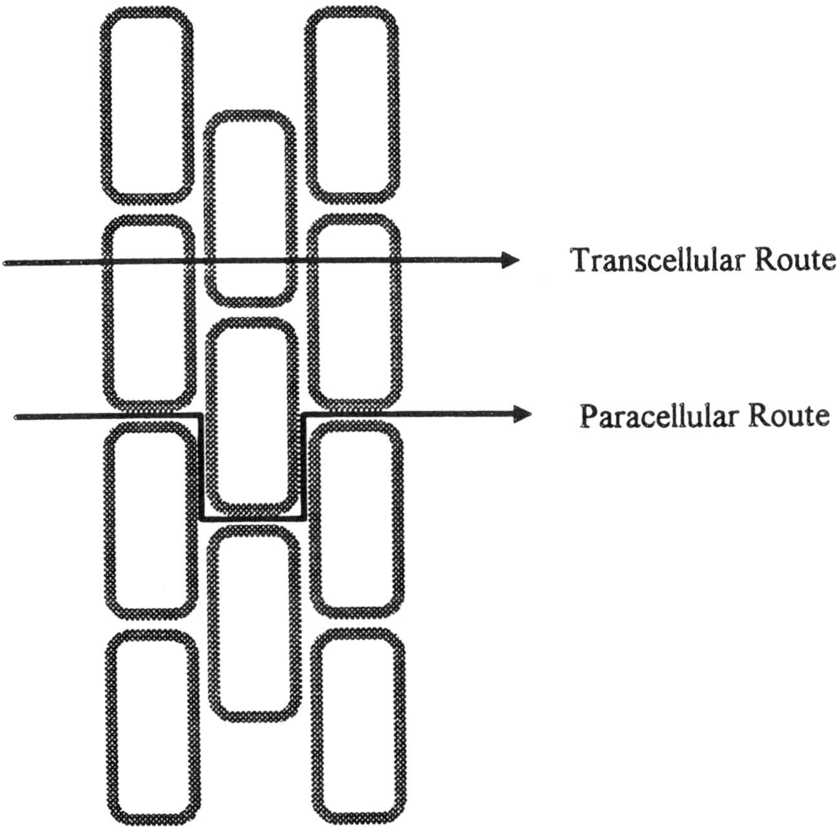

Figure 1. Schematic diagram showing that there are two possible drug transport routes, i.e., the transcellular and the paracellular routes, in the oral mucosa.

hydrophilic in character and become a transport barrier for lipophilic compounds mainly because the solubility of a lipophilic compound in this environment is low. In contrast, the cell membrane is lipophilic and the penetration of a hydrophilic compound into the cell membrane is low due to a low partition coefficient. Thus, closely compacted cell membranes become obstacles that hydrophilic compounds have to move around.

The coexistence of the hydrophilic and lipophilic regions in the oral mucosa suggests that there are two routes for drug transport, i.e., the paracellular and the transcellular routes (Figure 1). All compounds can use these two routes simultaneously, except that one route is usually preferred over the other depending on the physicochemical properties of the diffusant.

The paracellular route is the primary route for hydrophilic compounds because it is difficult for a hydrophilic compound to penetrate into the lipophilic cell membrane, and, thus, the intercellular space is the preferred route for drug transport. In this case, the limited surface area of the intercellular space and the tortuous pathways within the area are the main limitations for this route. The flux of drug movement in this route (J_H) can be written as:

$$J_H = \frac{D_H \varepsilon}{h_H} C_D \tag{1}$$

where ε is the fraction of surface area of the paracellular route, D_H is the diffusion coefficient in the intercellular spaces, h_H is the pathlength of the paracellular route, and C_D is the donor side drug concentration.

For lipophilic compounds, because the surface area for the transcellular route is large, the partition coefficients are high, and the pathlength for transcellular movement is relatively short, the permeability of lipophilic compounds across the epithelial cell membrane is typically high. In this case, drug molecules have to move across both lipophilic cell membrane and hydrophilic cytoplasm as well as the intercellular space (Figure 2). Since the main resistance of this route is the cell membrane, drug movement in the cytoplasm and intercellular space is relatively rapid and can be assumed instantaneous. Therefore, the drug flux in the transcellular route (J_L) can be expressed as:

$$J_L = \frac{(1-\varepsilon) D_L K_P}{h_L} C_D \tag{2}$$

where K_p is the partition coefficient between lipophilic region (cell membrane) and hydrophilic region (delivery solution, intercellular space and cytoplasm), h_L is the pathlength of the transcellular route.

Equation 2 shows that the permeability coefficient via the transcellular route is proportional to the partition coefficient.

The paracellular and transcellular routes depicted here are a simplified version of the oral mucosal drug absorption process. From a dynamic point of view, drug molecules will preferentially move through the route which offers the least resistance. Since the epithelium is stratified this means the movement of drug molecules may involve a mixture of these two routes, i.e., using one route in one region and the other route in the other region.

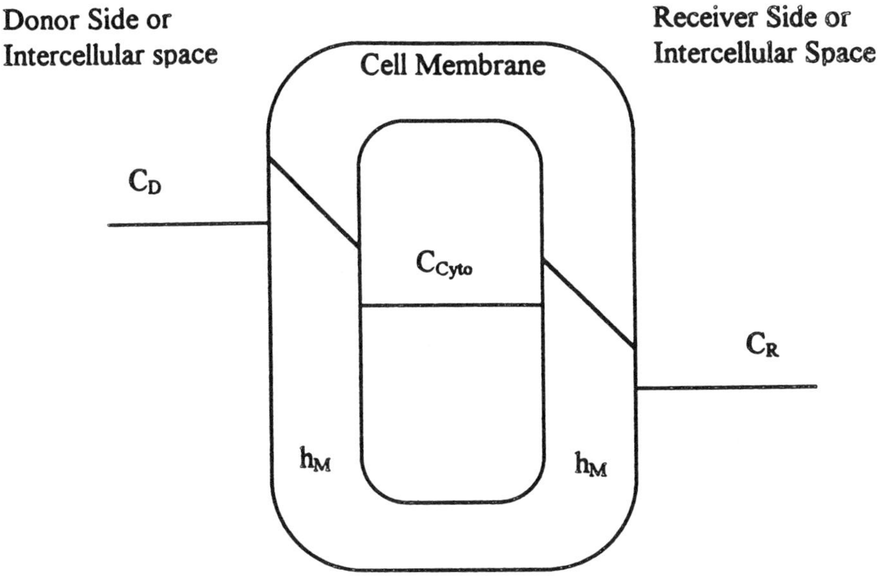

Figure 2. Schematic diagram of the transcellular route where C_D is the concentration of drug on the donor side, C_{cyto} is the concentration of drug in the cytoplasm of the cell, C_R is the concentration of drug on the receiver side and h_M is the thickness of the cell membrane. The drug has to diffuse through both the hydrophilic (cytoplasm and intercellular space) and lipophilic (cell membrane) regions. Notice that there is no concentration gradient in the hydrophilic region because the density and viscosity in the lipophilic region is much higher than that in the hydrophilic region, therefore, drug diffusion in the hydrophilic region is assumed instantaneous.

IV. EXPERIMENTAL DETERMINATION OF DRUG TRANSPORT ROUTE(S) IN THE ORAL MUCOSA

A. Direct Visualization of Probes Inside the Oral Mucosa

Drug inside oral mucosal tissue can be directly visualized. Depending on the methods of detection, direct visualization can be further classified into three categories: microscopic, autoradiographic, and confocal laser scanning microscopic.

Horseradish peroxidase was used on numerous occasions to determine the location of its movement inside human or animal oral mucosa in vivo or in vitro [8, 12-14]. As a peroxidase, horseradish peroxidase can catalyze the oxidation reaction of substrates to form a unique colored stain in an oral mucosal specimen, and thus the location of horseradish peroxidase can be detected by light microscopic examination. Other tracers have also been used to delineate the absorption pathway in oral mucosal tissue. For example, fluorescent dyes were used by Adams to study drug permeation through rat and rabbit oral mucosa [15]; lanthanum salts were used by Squier and Rooney to study the permeability of keratinized and nonkeratinized oral epithelium in vivo [9]. The location of fluorescent dyes can be easily detected by a light microscope with appropriate exciting light source and filters to reduce background fluorescence. The location of lanthanum, an electron dense substance, can be detected by electron microscopy. The same concept works for other electron dense probes, such as mercury [16]. In general, any molecule possessing special light or electron dense characteristics can be used as a tracer to show the location of the molecules inside the oral mucosa. The major limitation of using these specific tracers is that only the location of these tracers can be detected. It cannot predict the location of drugs that are physicochemically different to the tracers.

Autoradiography is another commonly used method to identify the location of a drug inside oral mucosa tissue [10, 17-19]. This method is similar to microscopic methods except that a radioactive labeled drug is used instead of tracer. The location of the radiolabeled drug can be detected by nuclear track emulsion that is sensitive to the radioactive material. This is typically a rather lengthy study. Moreover, limits on resolution can be a problem in distinguishing grains in the paracellular versus the transcellular routes.

Both microscopic and autoradiographic methods have major limitations in studying the penetration route(s), i.e., the specimen has to be fixed and embedded before examination, and the image is two dimensional. Fixing and embedding procedures have the potential of altering the location of markers or drugs in the oral mucosa. Therefore, the location detected by these methods may not represent the actual drug penetration route. In addition, with two dimensional images obtained by these methods, it is sometimes difficult to distinguish paracellular and transcellular routes.

To overcome these problems, a recently developed method, confocal laser scanning microscopy, have been employed to study the location of permeants [20-22]. The major advantages of confocal laser scanning microscopy are that an unfixed specimen can be observed directly, and a three dimensional image obtained. Direct observation without extensive sample preparation can eliminate potential artefacts often introduced by these manipulations. Meanwhile three dimensional imaging can easily detect whether the tracer is inside or outside the cell. Using confocal laser scanning microscope, Hoogstraate et al found that both 4 kDa and 10 kDa FITC-labeled dextrans were transported through porcine buccal epithelia via the paracellular route [23].

Direct visualization of diffusant inside oral mucosal tissue can tell us the distribution of diffusant in the tissue, i.e., which regions have high concentration of diffusant. However, a region with high diffusant concentration does not necessarily mean that drug transport occurs through this region. High diffusant concentration simply means that the diffusant is thermodynamically favored in this region. If the diffusant is bound to particular molecules in the region, the diffusant concentration in that region will be high, but it may not move through that region. Therefore, information provided by direct visualization measurement alone is usually inadequate to reach a conclusion about the drug transport route.

B. Indirect Examination of the Drug Transport Route

The drug transport route can be indirectly examined by permeability measurements. As discussed early, there are two possible drug transport routes in the oral mucosa, the paracellular route and the transcellular route. If the drug is transported via the paracellular route (Equation 1), the permeability of the drug is independent of its partition coefficient. Conversely, if the drug is transported via the transcellular route (Equation 2), the permeability of the drug is partition coefficient dependent.

Early oral mucosal drug absorption studies showed that oral mucosal absorption of amines and acids was proportional to their partition coefficients [24]. These results agreed with the prediction of Equation 2 that drug flux is proportional to the partition coefficient, and indicated that the transcellular route was the main drug transport pathway for these drugs. Similar partition coefficient dependencies were obtained for β-adrenoreceptor blocking drugs [25], substituted acetanilides [26], carboxylic acids [27], organic solutes [28], and other drugs [29]. All these studies suggested that the transcellular route was involved in drug transport.

The pH effect on drug absorption for ionizable compounds has been studied extensively. The pH dependency of ionizable drugs actually reflects the drug penetration route because the partition coefficient of ionizable drugs is pH dependent. Therefore, if a drug is transported via the transcellular route, the drug absorption rate is also pH dependent. However, if the drug is transported via the paracellular route where there is no partitioning involved, pH should not affect the drug absorption rate, unless it influences solubility.

Using a series of basic drugs, Beckett and Triggs found that drug loss from the oral cavity is highly dependent upon pH [30]. Similar phenomena were observed for acidic drugs except that the drug absorption rate decreased with an increase in buffer pH [31]. For other drugs, e.g., β-adrenoreceptor blocking drugs [32], morphine and its major metabolite morphine-3-

glucoronide [33], flurbiprofen [34], and fentanyl [35, 36], their absorption rates were also dependent on solution pH.

On the other hand, there are drugs whose permeability across the oral mucosa is pH independent. Dowty and Robinson studied the pH effect on thyrotropin releasing hormone (TRH) in rabbit buccal mucosa in vitro, and found that the permeability coefficients of TRH in pH 4.0 and pH 8.0 are the same [10]. Zhang et al also found that transbuccal permeability of isoproterenol, using an in vivo dog model, was independent of the donor side pH [37]. These studies suggest that the paracellular route may be used for water soluble drugs even in their unionized form.

The transport route for TRH was also examined using an osmolarity experiment [10]. In this experiment, the permeability of TRH in rabbit buccal mucosa was measured in solutions with varying osmolarity. The hypothesis was that the different buffer osmolarity can draw water in or out of the epithelial cell, therefore contracting or expanding the intercellular space, i.e., ε in Equation 1, will decrease or increase. Thus, the permeability coefficient should increase with a hypertonic solution, and decrease with a hypotonic solution, and this is exactly what was found.

The drug transport pathway can also be examined by exploring drug accumulation inside the oral mucosa. As shown in Figure 3, if an ionizable drug is transported via the transcellular route, the amount of drug accumulating inside the epithelial cell will vary depending on the pH of the buffer solution. This is because the pH of epithelial cytoplasm is closely regulated [38-41] whereas pH in the intercellular space will change with the bathing buffer pH. The pH difference across the cell membrane can cause differences in the amount of drug accumulated inside the epithelial cells. Using fentanyl as a probe, a drug accumulation study [36] revealed that fentanyl accumulation is pH dependent. This result agrees with the permeability measurement [35-36], and suggests that the transporting route for fentanyl is the transcellular route.

V. SIGNIFICANCE OF DETERMINING THE DRUG TRANSPORT ROUTES

The major problems of using the oral mucosa as a route for systemic drug delivery are its relatively low permeability to most drugs and small surface area. Therefore, using penetration enhancers to increase permeability of the oral mucosa has become the main focus of many recent studies.

A variety of enhancer types have been tested. For example, chelators can complex with calcium ion which is essential to maintain dimensions of the intercellular space. Therefore, chelators can increase the permeability of the paracellular route [42]. Some enhancers, such as oleic acid, caprylate, and mono-olein, can increase cell membrane fluidity by creating disorder in the

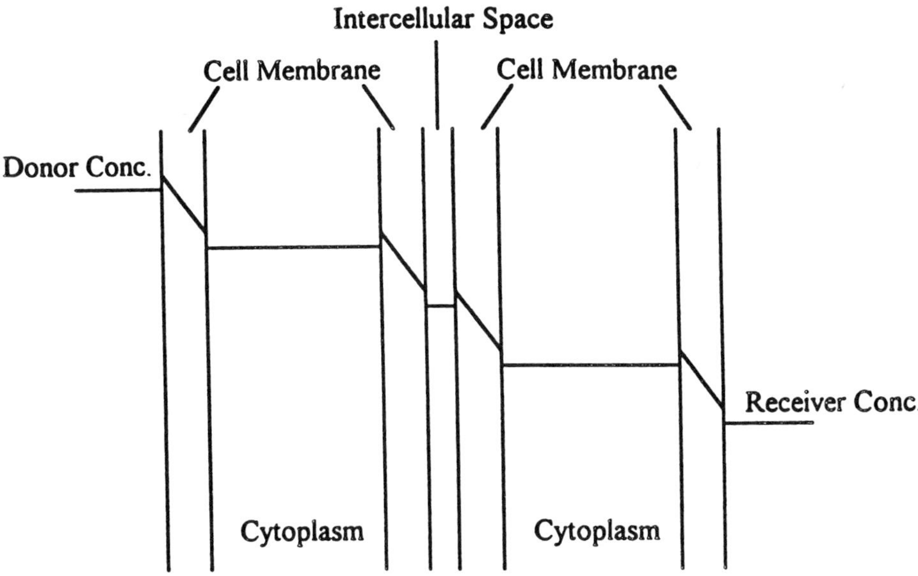

Figure 3. Transcellular drug transport across an epithelial cell layer (two cell membrane) at steady state. The diffusion inside the cytoplasm is relatively faster than inside the cell membrane, and is assumed to be instantaneous.

phospholipid domain [43-44], and thus the permeability of the transcellular route is increased.

Squier studied the effect of enzyme digestion on the permeability barrier of keratinized and nonkeratinized oral epithelium and found that there are three types of enzyme effects [45]. Phospholipases can considerably damage the cell membrane, but cannot alter the permeability barrier against horseradish peroxidase. Hyaluronidase and neuraminidase caused less structural damage and also did not impair the barrier function. Chondroitinase ABC, on the other hand, was able to effectively alter the permeability of the oral mucosa to horseradish peroxidase with minimal cellular damage.

Dowty [46] also used chondroitinase ABC in rabbit buccal mucosa and found that this enzyme can cause different permeability responses to different drugs, e.g., the permeability of salicylic acid increased 1.54 times, the permeability of choline remained the same, and the permeability of glycerol actually decreased.

Site specific enhancers that are rapidly reversible is the goal of studying the drug transport route in oral mucosa; a goal that has not yet been achieved. However, research has shown that the primary transport route of a drug can be altered by penetration enhancers. As mentioned earlier, a drug will use the route which offers the lowest diffusional resistance. Therefore, a drug that primarily uses one penetration route may switch to the other route if the properties of that route are substantially changed by a penetration enhancer. Thus a thorough understanding of the transport routes, at the cellular and molecular level, is a prerequisite for designing and selecting effective penetration enhancers.

REFERENCES

1. W. Murrell, Nitroglycerin as a remedy for angina pectoris, *Lancet 1*:80-81, 113-115, 151-152, 225-227 (1879).
2. M. Gibaldi, and J. L. Kanig, Absorption of drugs through the oral mucosa, *J. Oral Ther. Pharmacol. 1*:440 (1965).
3. C. A. Squier, N. W. Johnson, and M. Hackemann, Structure and function of normal human oral mucosa, *Oral Mucosa in Health and Disease* (A. E. Dolby, ed.), Blackwell Scientific Publications, Oxford, 1975, p. 1.
4. D. Harris, and J. R. Robinson, Drug delivery via the oral mucous membranes of the oral cavity, *J. Pharm. Sci. 81*:1 (1992).
5. M. E. de Vries, H. E. Boddé, J. C. Verhoef, and H. E. Junginger, Developments in buccal drug delivery, *Crit. Rev. Ther. Drug Carr. Syst. 8*:271 (1991).
6. P. W. Wertz, and C. A. Squier, Cellular and molecular basis of barrier function in oral epithelium, *Crit. Rev. Ther. Drug Carr. Syst. 8*:237 (1991).
7. C. A. Squier, N. W. Johnson, and R. M. Hopps, *Human Oral Mucosa; Development, Structure and Function*, Blackwell Scientific, Oxford, 1976.
8. C. A. Squier, The permeability of keratinized and nonkeratinized oral epithelium to horseradish peroxidase, *J. Ultrastruct. Res. 43*:160 (1973).
9. C. A. Squier, and L. Rooney, The permeability of keratinized and nonkeratinized oral epithelium to lanthanum in vivo, *J. Ultrastruct Res. 54*:286 (1976).
10. M. E. Dowty, K. E. Knuth, B. K. Irons, and J. R. Robinson, Transport of thyrotropin releasing hormone in rabbit buccal mucosa in vitro, *Pharm. Res. 9*:1113 (1992).
11. C. A. Squier, Membrane coating granules in nonkeratinizing oral epithelium, *J. Ultrastruct. Res. 60*:212 (1977).
12. C. A. Squier, and R. M. Hopps, A study of the permeability barrier in epidermis and oral epithelium using horseradish peroxidase as a tracer in vitro, *Br. J. Derm. 95*:123 (1976).

13. M. W. Hill, C. A. Squier, and J. E. Linder, A histological method for the visualization of the intercellular permeability barrier in mammalian stratified squamous epithelia, *Histochem. J. 14*:641 (1982).
14. C. A. Squier, and B. K. Hall, The permeability of mammalian nonkeratinized oral epithelia to horseradish peroxidase applied in vivo and in vitro, *Archs. Oral Biol. 29*:45 (1984).
15. D. Adams, The effect of saliva on the penetration of fluorescent dyes into the oral mucosa of the rat and rabbit, *Archs. Oral Biol. 19*:505 (1974).
16. H. E. Boddé, I. van den Brink, H. K. Koerten, and F. H. N. de Haan, Visualization of in vitro percutaneous penetration of mercuric chloride; transport through intercellular space versus cellular uptake through desmosomes, *J. Control. Rel. 15*:226 (1991).
17. M. C. Alfano, J. F. Drummond, and S. A. Miller, Localization of rate-limiting barrier to penetration of endotoxin through nonkeratinized oral mucosa in vitro, *J. Dent. Res. 54*:1143 (1975).
18. K. Tolo, A study of permeability of gingival pocket epithelium to albumin in guinea pigs and Norwegian pigs, *Archs. Oral Biol. 16*:881 (1971).
19. E. Haugen, and J. R. Johansen, Penetration of the oral mucosa by radiolabeled chlorhexidine in guinea pigs, *Acta Odont. Scand. 33*:365 (1975).
20. D. M. Shotton, Confocal scanning optical microscopy and its application for biological specimens, *J. Cell Sci. 94*:175 (1989).
21. S. Inové, Foundations of confocal scanned imaging in light microscopy, *Handbook of Biological Confocal Microscopy* (J. B. Pawley, ed.), Plenum Press, New York, 1990, p. 1.
22. S. Senel, A. J. Hoogstraate, F. Spies, J. C. Verhoef, H. E. Junginger, and H. E. Boddé, Visualization of enhancing effects of bile salts on buccal penetration, *Eur. J. Morph. 31*:35 (1993).
23. A. J. Hoogstraate, H. E. Boddé, C. Cullander, and H. E. Junginger, Diffusion rates and transport pathways of FITC-labelled model compounds through buccal epithelium, *Pharm. Res. 9*:S-188 (1992).
24. A. H. Beckett, and A. C. Moffat, Correlation of partition coefficients in n-heptane-aqueous systems with buccal absorption data for a series of amines and acids, *J. Pharm. Pharmacol. 21*:144S (1969).
25. P. P. H. Le Brun, P. L. A. Fox, M. E. de Vries, and H. E. Boddé, In vitro penetration of some β-adrenoreceptor blocking drugs through porcine buccal mucosa, *Int. J. Pharm. 49*:141 (1989).
26. K. W. Garren, and A. J. Repta, Buccal drug absorption II: In vitro diffusion across the hamster cheek pouch, *J. Pharm. Sci. 78*:160 (1989).
27. A. H. Beckett, and A. C. Moffat, Kinetics of buccal absorption of some carboxylic acids and the correlation of the rate constants and n-

heptane:aqueous phase partition coefficients, *J. Pharm. Pharmacol.* *22*:15 (1970).
28. I. A. Siegel, Permeability of the rat oral mucosa to organic solutes measured in vivo, *Archs. Oral Biol.* *29*:13 (1984).
29. I. A. Siegel, K. T. Izutsu, and E. Watson, Mechanisms of non-electrolyte penetration across dog and rabbit oral mucosa in vitro, *Archs. Oral Biol.* *26*:357 (1981).
30. A. H. Beckett, and E. J. Triggs, Buccal absorption of basic drugs and its application as an in vivo model of passive drug transfer through lipid membranes, *J. Pharm. Pharmacol.* *19*:31S (1967).
31. A. H. Beckett and A. C. Moffat, The influence of substitution in phenylacetic acids on their performance in the buccal absorption test, *J. Pharm. Pharmacol.* *21*:139S (1969).
32. D. C. Hicks, The buccal absorption of some β-adrenoceptor blocking drugs, *Br. J. Pharmacol.* *47*:680P (1973).
33. O. Al-Sayed-Omar, A. Johnston, and P. Turner, Influence of pH on the buccal absorption of morphine sulphate and its major metabolite, morphine-3-glucuronide, *J. Pharm. Pharmacol.* *39*:934 (1987).
34. C. L. Barsuhn, L. S. Olanoff, D. D. Gleason, E. L. Adkins, and N. F. H. Ho, Human buccal absorption of flurbiprofen, *Clin. Pharmacol. Ther.* *44*:225 (1988).
35. J. Zhang, J. Streisand, S. Niu, S. McJames, V. Freimann, B. Hague, L. Maland, R. Natte, and T. H. Stanley, Estimation of buccal fentanyl absorption bioavailability by measuring drug depletion from vehicle solutions: validation of the method in dogs, *Pharm. Res.* *9*:S-177 (1992).
36. H. Zhang, Drug transport pathways in rabbit oral mucosa, PhD Thesis, University of Wisconsin, Madison, 1994.
37. J. Zhang, C. D. Ebert, S. McJames, H. Gijsman, and T. H. Stanley, Transbuccal permeability of isoproterenol in the dog model, *Pharm. Res.* *6*:S-135 (1989).
38. M. E. Dowty, and P. Braquet, Effect of extracellular pH on cytoplasmic pH and mechanism of pH regulation in cultured bovine corneal endothelium: possible importance in drug transport studies, *Int. J. Pharm.* *68*:231 (1991).
39. C. Frelin, P. Vigne, A. Ladoux, and M. Lazdunski, The regulation of the intracellular pH in cells from vertebrates, *Eur. J. Biochem.* *174*:3 (1988).
40. W. H. Moolenaar, Regulation of cytoplasmic pH by Na^+/H^+ exchange, *Trends Biochem. Sci.* *11*:141 (1986).
41. P. S. Aronson, Kinetic properties of the plasma membrane Na^+-H^+ exchanger, *Ann. Rev. Physiol.* *45*:545 (1985).
42. V. H. L. Lee, and A. Yamamoto, Penetration and enzymatic barriers to peptide and protein absorption, *Adv. Drug Del. Rev.* *4*:171 (1991).

43. H. Kajii, T. Horie, M. Hayashi, and S. Awazu, Fluorescence study of the membrane-perturbing action of sodium caprylate as related to promotion of drug absorption, *J. Pharm. Sci. 77*:390 (1988).
44. N. Muranushi, Y. Nakajima, M. Kinugawa, S. Muranishi, and H. Sezaki, Mechanism for the inducement of intestinal absorption of poorly absorbed drugs by mixed micelles. II. Effect of the incorporation of various lipids on the permeability of liposomal membranes, *Int. J. Pharm. 4*:281 (1980).
45. C. A. Squier, Effect of enzyme digestion on the permeability barrier in keratinizing and non-keratinizing epithelia, *Br. J. Derm. 111*:253 (1984).
46. M. E. Dowty, Transport of thyrotropin releasing hormone in rabbit buccal mucosa in vitro, PhD Thesis, University of Wisconsin, Madison, 1991.

4

Oral Mucosal Permeation Enhancement: Possibilities and Limitations

Bruce J. Aungst
The DuPont Merck Pharmaceutical Company, USA

I. INTRODUCTION

Permeation enhancers are substances added to a pharmaceutical formulation in order to increase the membrane permeation rate or absorption rate of a coadministered drug. They are used to increase the bioavailability of drugs with normally poor membrane permeation properties. For permeation enhancers to be clinically acceptable they must increase bioavailability or increase membrane permeability without damaging the membrane and causing toxicity. Toxicity is probably the major concern when considering the use of excipients that are permeation enhancers for any route of administration.

This chapter reviews the literature on the use of permeation enhancers, also often referred to as absorption enhancers, for oral mucosal drug delivery. It summarizes the types of drugs for which permeation enhancement is most useful and gives examples of the extent of bioavailability enhancement that is possible. Some properties of the substances used as permeation enhancers are presented and compared, and the possible mechanisms of enhancing membrane permeation are discussed. The problems of using membrane permeation enhancers are also considered.

II. WHEN ARE PERMEATION ENHANCERS USEFUL?

When drugs are absorbed from the oral cavity they are able to bypass gastrointestinal and hepatic drug metabolizing enzymes. This is the most important advantage afforded by delivering drugs via the buccal or sublingual routes. Presystemic metabolism of drugs, which is not an unusual occurrence after intestinal absorption, results in incomplete bioavailability. Maximization of bioavailability is always desirable, because it is generally associated with minimization of the variability of blood levels and improved control of pharmacological and toxic effects. In addition, since drug that is not bioavailable is essentially wasted, the cost of drug therapy is directly influenced by the extent of bioavailability. For drugs subject to intestinal or hepatic presystemic metabolism, buccal or sublingual administration can result in an improvement in bioavailability relative to oral dosing. For example, nitroglycerin and isosorbide dinitrate have low oral bioavailabilities because of extensive presystemic metabolism, but their bioavailabilities are much improved when they are administered sublingually. Indeed, this route is used for these compounds in clinical practice.

Nitroglycerin and isosorbide dinitrate are successfully administered via this route because they are well absorbed through the oral mucosa. However, many compounds do not rapidly penetrate the oral mucosal membranes. In 1935 Walton and Lacey [1] published results of a study comparing the efficacy in dogs and humans of sublingual and subcutaneous doses of various compounds. The ratio of sublingual/subcutaneous doses producing approximately equal efficacy was 8 for atropine, 10 for morphine, 15 for dilaudid, and >15 for codeine. Much higher doses were required sublingually because these compounds apparently had low bioavailability by this route. Similarly, plasma ergotamine concentrations were not detectable in 4 subjects taking a 2 mg dose sublingually, but were measurable for at least 2 hours after a 0.5 mg intramuscular dose, indicating low bioavailability of sublingual ergotamine [2]. Sublingual nifedipine had a bioavailability of only 17% relative to oral nifedipine in 11 volunteers [3]. After the buccal administration of a 15 g dose of glucose containing a radiotracer, only 0.1 mg was absorbed, whereas when the dose was swallowed 88% of the glucose was absorbed within 30 minutes [4]. Thus, compounds which may be well absorbed orally are not necessarily well absorbed through the mucosa of the mouth. There are two major reasons for this, (i) the oral mucosal membrane is less permeable than the intestinal membrane; in permeability studies with excised rabbit membranes in vitro, the buccal membrane was at least 5-fold less permeable to carboxyfluorescein and had 5-fold lower electrical conductance than intestinal membranes [5] and (ii) the membrane surface area available for absorption of an applied buccal or sublingual dose is very much smaller than the intestinal membrane surface area available for absorption to the same dose after oral administration.

There is currently a particular interest in delivering peptides via the buccal or sublingual routes. Oral delivery of peptides is often not feasible, in part because of rapid metabolism by gastrointestinal and hepatic proteolytic enzymes. The delivery of peptide drugs by alternative routes offers the possibility of achieving bioavailability and pharmacological activity by a non-injection route. However, many peptides diffuse through epithelial membranes very slowly. Indeed, we can find various illustrations in the literature of relatively low bioavailability of buccally or sublingually administered peptides. Often these studies were done by measuring a pharmacological effect rather than blood levels, and then comparing the relative potencies by buccal or sublingual routes with that after intramuscular, subcutaneous, or intravenous dosing. Thus, thyrotropin releasing hormone [6], oxytocin [7], heparin [8], and insulin [1] were shown to exhibit poor absorption when administered buccally or sublingually. Various peptidases and proteases are present within the oral mucosa and it is possible that metabolism could contribute to the incomplete bioavailability. But poor membrane permeation is a major cause of low bioavailability of peptides administered via the oral mucosa.

The literature briefly summarized above indicates that membrane permeation can be a limiting factor for many drugs administered via the buccal or sublingual routes and that the membranes that line the oral mucosa can be a very effective barrier to the absorption of peptides. For those compounds that penetrate the oral mucosal membranes slowly or incompletely and for which efficient systemic absorption cannot be attained, one strategy that can be used by those interested in their buccal or sublingual delivery is the coadministration of a permeation enhancing excipient.

III. ENHANCEMENT POSSIBILITIES

The literature on oral mucosal permeation enhancement is scant relative to the many published studies on enhancing drug absorption by the nasal, rectal, intestinal, and dermal delivery routes. Therefore, an almost complete listing of the oral mucosal permeation enhancement literature can be provided (Table 1). This survey is useful to illustrate the extent of absorption enhancement that is possible, and to begin to develop an understanding of the types of compounds that act as oral mucosal enhancers and the types of compounds that are enhanced. When possible, Table 1 reports the extent of increase of bioavailability (F) reported. Bioavailability is defined for the purposes of this review to include measures of pharmacological effect relative to some injection route of administration, in addition to the conventional measures of bioavailability based on blood levels of the drug.

Table 1. Summary of Literature on Oral Mucosal Permeation Enhancement.

Drug	Enhancer	Results	Method (ref.)
Lidocaine	0.01%, and 0.1% cetylpyridinium chloride	↑ plasma concentration. 4-5 fold	Dog in vivo (9)
Insulin	Sodium glycocholate	Absorption only in presence of enhancer (F≈0.5%)	Dog in vivo (10)
Butyric acid, butanol, glycerol, urea, glucose, sucrose, inulin	0.025%-1% cetylpyridinium chloride, sodium lauryl sulfate, polysorbate 80	Cetylpyridinium chloride and sodium lauryl sulfate ↑ permeability, polysorbate 80 less effective	Rat in vivo (11)
Propranolol, heptanediol acetamide, urea, glycerol, ethylene glycol, mannitol, sucrose, inulin, dextrans	0.025%-1% cetyltrimethyl-ammonium bromide, cetylpyridinium chloride, sodium lauryl sulfate, benzalkonium chloride	Concentration related increase in permeability for all enhancers. Polysorbate 80 least effective	Dog in vivo (12)
Insulin	5% sodium glycocholate	↑ F sublingual from 0.3% to 12%, ↑ F buccal from 0.7% to 26%	Rat in vivo (13)
Insulin	5% laureth-9, 5% sodium salicylate, 5% sodium EDTA, aprotinin	↑ F from 0.7-3.6% to 27% with laureth-9. Others had no effect	Rat in vivo (14)
Salicylic acid	20 mM sodium lauryl sulfate, cetylpyridinium chloride, 20 mM sodium taurocholate, 5% poly sorbate 80	Sodium lauryl sulfate and cetylpyridinium chloride ↑ absorption. Others had no effect	Hamster in vivo (15)

Table 1. Continued.

Drug	Enhancer	Results	Method (ref.)
Calcitonin	Various saponins, bile salts, fatty acids, sucrose esters, sodium lauryl sulfate	↑ pharmacologic effect	Rat in vivo (16)
Propranolol	5% Azone emulsion	↑ F from 88.5% to 97.1%	Hamster in vivo (17)
Salicylic acid	Azone	↑ flux, ↑ fluidity of membrane lipids	Hamster in vivo (18)
Insulin	40 mM sodium taurocholate, 40 mM dextran sulfate, 40 mM linoleic acid, 5% Labrafil, 5% Transcutol, 1% urea	F ≈ 22% at pH 7.5, not ↑ with enhancers	Dog in vivo (19)
Calcitonin	Various bile salts	↑ pharmacologic effect, ↑ stability in mucosal homogenate	Rat in vivo (20)
Salicylic acid	5% Azone emulsion	↑ F from 51% to 83% at pH 3, ↑ F from 0.4% to 1.4% at pH 7	Hamster in vivo (21)
Insulin	Various bile salts and derivatives, nonionic surfactants, sulfoxides, lauric acid/PG	↑ F from < 1-4% to ≈ 30% maximum. Most effective were deoxycholate, sodium glycholate CHAPS and laureth-9	Rat in vivo (22)
Insulin	Sodium lauryl sulfate, sodium taurocholate, deoxycholate, EDTA, POE 23 lauryl ether, methoxysalicylate, dextran sulfate	Maximum F ≈ 12%	Rabbit in vivo (23)

Table 1. Continued.

Drug	Enhancer	Results	Method (ref.)
Octreotide	3% Azone, 4% sodium glycholate, sodium taurocholate, sodium taurocholate + EDTA	Azone ↑ F from 1.5% to 6%, sodium glycholate ↑ F from ≈ 0.4% to 4.2 %	Dog in vivo (24)
Methyl paraben, theophylline, 5-fluorouracil, sulfanilic acid	Azone, sodium lauryl sulfate	Sodium lauryl SO_4 ↓ electrical resistance and ↑ permeation most for hydrophilic compounds. Azone did not alter electrical resistance and ↑ permeation more for hydrophobic compounds	Hamster in vivo (25)
Propranolol	Methanol, ethanol, lauric acid	↑ permeation at pH where drug was ionized. Lauric acid ↑ partitioning	Hamster in vivo (26)
Salicylic acid	Sodium lauryl sulfate, deoxycholate	↑ flux, ↓ electrical resistance	Rabbit in vitro (27)
Insulin	2% sodium cholate, 3% sodium taurocholate, 2% lysophosphatidyl choline	↓ blood glucose, ↑ glucose back diffusion	Dog in vivo (28)
Interferon	1-4% sodium taurocholate, 5% polysorbate 80, 1% sodium lauryl sulfate, 5% cyclodextrin	↑ F from 0.014% to 0.25 % with sodium taurocholate. Others less effective	Rat in vivo (29)
Insulin	Various alkylglycosides (0.1-0.2 M)	↑ F from 0.8% to ≈ 30% maximum	Rat in vivo (30)

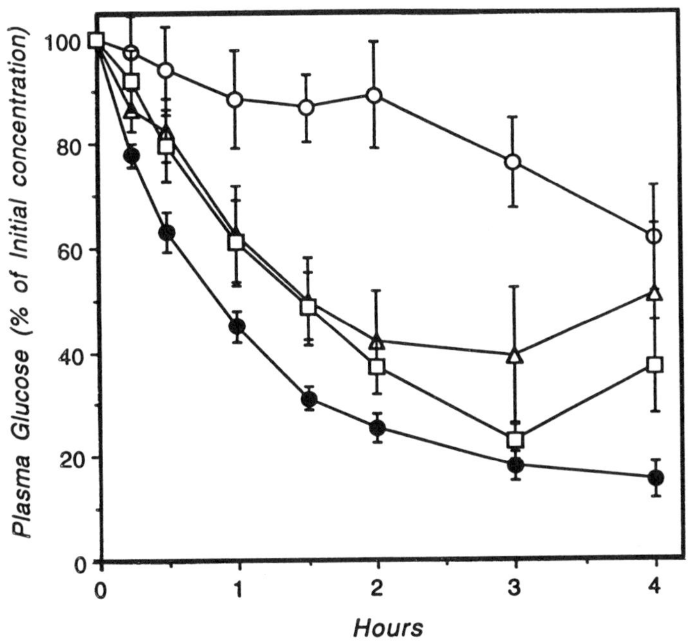

Figure 1. Plasma glucose concentrations in rats (mean ± SEM of 6 or more rats per group) administered insulin 5 U/kg intramuscularly (●), 50 U/kg buccally with no absorption enhancer (O), 10 U/kg buccally with 5% sodium glycocholate (Δ), or 10 U/kg buccally with 5% dodecylmaltoside (□). Results were compiled from references 13 and 30.

A series of studies [13, 14, 30] on buccal and sublingual insulin administration most clearly illustrate the possible utility of oral mucosal absorption enhancers. In these studies insulin was dosed to anesthetized rats that were surgically prevented from swallowing dosing solutions administered to the mouth. Insulin was administered in aqueous solutions in the presence or absence of absorption enhancers. Separate rats were dosed with insulin intramuscularly. Plasma glucose concentrations were measured as an indication of insulin absorption. The cumulative fall of plasma glucose concentrations after buccal dosing were compared to an intramuscular dose versus response curve for insulin, and based on this comparison an estimate of the extent of buccal insulin absorption was obtained. Representative plasma glucose concentration profiles are shown in Figure 1. As shown in Figure 1, a 5 U/kg insulin dose administered intramuscularly produced a substantial pharmacological effect, lowering plasma glucose concentrations in these non-diabetic rats. Buccal dosing with 50 U/kg insulin gave only slight and variable decreases in plasma glucose levels. When effective permeation enhancers were coadministered with insulin, in this case at 5% concentrations, much lower doses of insulin (e.g., 10 U/kg) could be used to produce decreases in plasma glucose concentrations similar to those after intramuscular insulin dosing. When no permeation enhancer was used, the extent of buccal insulin absorption was estimated to be from <1% to 3.6%, depending on the insulin dose. When the most effective absorption enhancers were coadministered, such as sodium glycocholate and dodecylmaltoside (illustrated in Figure 1) the extent of buccal absorption was increased to about 30%. Thus, the feasibility of attaining acceptable bioavailability of a fairly large molecular weight peptide via the oral mucosa has been demonstrated.

Table 1 also gives several examples of studies in which buccal bioavailability of the compound of interest was low, even in the presence of a permeation enhancer. Ishida et al [10] administered insulin to dogs via the buccal mucosa using a patch type formulation containing insulin and 5 mg sodium glycocholate in a lipid core surrounded by a matrix of hydroxypropyl cellulose and Carbopol 934. Only 0.5% of the insulin dose was absorbed. Following buccal administration, octreotide, a cyclic octapeptide, had a bioavailability in dogs of only 6% using a 3% Azone ethanolic solution vehicle, and bioavailability was only 4.2% using a dosing solution containing 4% sodium glycocholate [24]. The buccal bioavailability of α-interferon in rats was 0.25%, using a dosing solution containing 4% sodium taurocholate as an enhancer, although this represented a greater than 10-fold improvement in bioavailability [29]. Certainly α-interferon is a relatively high molecular weight peptide (19.5 kDa), and oral mucosal membrane permeability can be expected to be inversely proportional to molecular weight. But each of these examples points out that even with membrane permeation enhancers, oral mucosal bioavailability may be low. Indeed, the bioavailability of large peptides or proteins may be extremely low. Thus it must be appreciated that oral mucosal delivery may not feasible, even with the coadministration of absorption enhancers.

The compounds listed in Table 1 that have been shown to be responsive to absorption enhancement, are structurally very diverse. They include low molecular weight compounds such as butyric acid and butanol [11], and methyl paraben and theophylline [25]. For the low molecular weight, ionizable drugs salicylic acid [21] and propranolol [26], the extent of enhancement was greatest when the vehicle pH was such that the drug was predominantly ionized. The unionized forms of these compounds were well absorbed through the oral mucosa without permeation enhancement. Also used as model compounds in buccal absorption enhancement studies were the low molecular weight sugars, mannitol and sucrose, and the hydrophilic polymers inulin and dextrans [12]. Perhaps the most useful applications of oral mucosal permeation enhancement may be for relatively low molecular weight peptides and peptidomimetics.

Table 2. Categories and Examples of Membrane Permeation Enhancers.

A. Bile salts and other steroidal detergents
- Sodium glycocholate
- Sodium taurocholate
- Saponins
- Sodium taurodihydrofusidate
- Sodium glycodihydrofusidate

B. Surfactants
1. Nonionics
   - Laureth-9
   - Polysorbate 80
   - Sucrose esters
   - Dodecylmaltoside
2. Cationic
   - Cetyltrimethylammonium bromide
3. Anionic
   - Sodium lauryl sulfate
   - Fatty acids

C. Other enhancers
1. Azone
2. Salicylates
3. Chelating agents
4. Sulfoxides

Examples of peptides having enhanced oral mucosal absorption have been discussed previously.

IV. CHARACTERISTICS OF PERMEATION ENHANCERS

What types of compounds are effective in increasing oral mucosal membrane permeation? This question could be addressed by evaluating studies that have been performed that assess how systematic changes in the structure of absorption enhancers influence permeation enhancement of oral mucosal membranes. However, very few such studies have been performed. There have, however, been many more structure/effect and mechanistic descriptions of the effects of permeation enhancers for other mucosal membranes and for skin.

This information can be applied to some extent to oral mucosal permeation enhancement. However to do this it is necessary to understand the differences between oral mucosal membranes and other epithelial membranes or skin, and the limitations of this approach must be appreciated.

A. Structure/Effect Relationships

Membrane permeation enhancers can be categorized according to their general structural features. These categories are summarized in Table 2. Examples of these structures are given in Figure 2. Many of the oral mucosal enhancers described in the literature (Table 1) fall into the steroidal detergent and surfactant categories. The last group on Table 2 includes additional, structurally diverse compounds which have been frequently used to enhance intestinal, nasal, rectal, or dermal absorption.

Various bile salts and other detergents with the steroidal lipophilic nucleus have been shown to be effective enhancers of oral mucosal absorption. Within this category the most thorough structure/effect study was that of Nakada et al [16], who measured the pharmacological effects of calcitonin after buccal dosing to rats. The bile salt concentrations were 22.5 mg/mL and the dosing solution was at pH 7.4. The enhancement of calcitonin absorption was proportional to the hydrophobicity of the bile salt, as measured by HPLC retention times. Unconjugated bile salts were less hydrophobic by HPLC, and more effective than conjugated bile salts as enhancers. Calcitonin was degraded by proteases in homogenates of the rat oral mucosal membranes, and the bile salts inhibited degradation with the same structure/effect relationship as for in vivo absorption. This may have obscured the relationship between bile salt structure and the membrane permeation enhancing effect in this study.

Nakada et al [16] also compared the effects of other enhancers of calcitonin absorption using rats in vivo. Each additive was again used at a 22.5 mg/mL concentration. The most effective enhancer was sodium lauryl sulfate, followed by sodium deoxycholate and sodium tauroglycocholate, and then sodium myristate, sucrose myristate, and sucrose palmitate. Fatty acids with shorter or longer chain lengths were less effective than myristate, and sucrose esters with shorter or longer chain lengths were not effective.

In our studies on buccal insulin absorption in rats [22, 30], sodium glycocholate, CHAPS, laureth-9, sodium laurate, sodium lauryl sulfate, and dodecylmaltoside were approximately equipotent as absorption enhancers. Various other nonionic surfactants having lauryl (C12) hydrophobic tails were much less effective or were ineffective as enhancers [22]. Thus, the structure of the polar head group of the surfactant strongly influences the effect of the

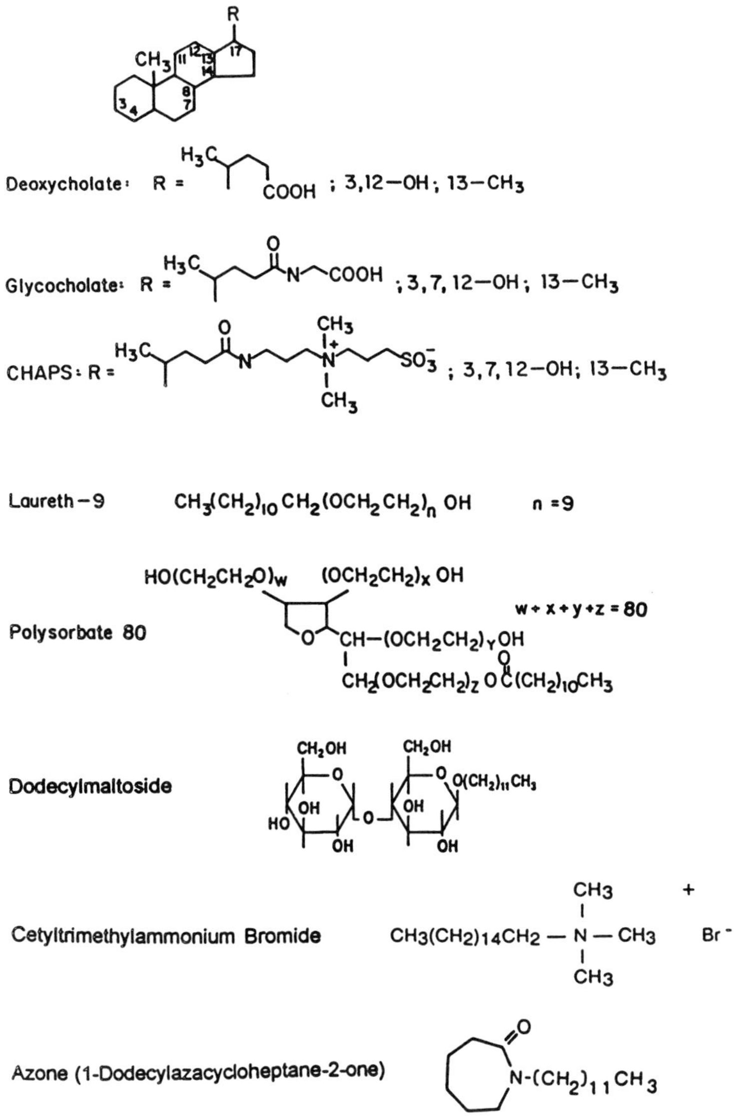

Figure 2. Examples of structures of some known permeation enhancers.

agent on membrane permeability. In addition, absorption enhancement was greater for ether surfactants than for esters with otherwise similar structures. Structure/effect studies of nasal [31], rectal [32], and dermal [33] permeation enhancers have shown maximal effects with enhancers having C10-C12 hydrophobic groups. Such clearly defined structure/effect relationships have not yet been established for oral mucosal absorption.

B. Mechanisms of Enhancement

The oral mucosal membrane is a stratified squamous epithelium, in many ways similar to skin. The spaces separating the multiple layers of flattened cells are packed with lipids and glycolipids that were extruded from the membrane coating granules of the cells. In skin and oral mucosa these lipids may be organized into lamellae with a lipid layer covalently bound to the cell surface, but the intercellular lipids of the oral mucosa are less well structured than in skin [34]. Inside the cells are proteins and, in some areas, keratin, depending on the species. Diffusion of substances through the oral mucosal membrane is principally through the lipid-filled intercellular spaces [34, 35]. The oral mucosal membranes are generally more permeable than skin because its intercellular lipids are less structured [36].

The permeability of stratum corneum has been correlated with the degree of disorder or fluidity of the intercellular lipids, as measured by differential scanning calorimetry (DSC) and infrared spectroscopy [37]. One mechanism of enhancing skin permeability is to administer agents that disrupt the structure of the intercellular lipids. This has been clearly demonstrated with oleic acid and other fatty acids as enhancers. Treatment of stratum corneum with fatty acids increased the fluidity of the intercellular lipids, and the extent of those fluidity changes was proportional to the enhancement of salicylic acid [38] and piroxicam [39] permeabilities. Azone has also been shown to affect stratum corneum lipids, and increased lipid fluidity correlated with changes in skin permeability [40]. Azone also increased the fluidity of lipids extracted from the hamster cheek pouch [18]. Oleic acid, Azone, and dimethylaminoacetate, another known skin permeation enhancer, have been shown to decrease the packing order of lipids of buccal epithelial cells [41]. These studies suggest that the mechanism of increasing the fluidity of intercellular lipids, which is clearly related to skin permeation enhancement, may also apply to the oral mucosal membranes.

Other possible mechanisms of increasing oral mucosal membrane permeation are the alteration of cellular proteins and extraction of intercellular lipids. Sodium lauryl sulfate uncoils the stratum corneum keratin and swells the membrane structure, as shown using DSC [42]. Stratum corneum lipids were also affected by sodium lauryl sulfate. Nonionic surfactants, and presumably ionic surfactants as well, can solubilize and extract stratum corneum lipids [43], a more slowly reversible effect than increased lipid fluidity. The enhancing effects of sodium taurodeoxycholate, sodium lauryl sulfate, cetyltrimethylammonium bromide, and various nonionic surfactants on rat intestinal absorption were related to the release of protein, cholesterol, and phospholipids from the membrane [44]. Similar findings have been reported in the oral mucosal literature; sodium deoxycholate (1%) appeared to denature and extract proteins from rabbit buccal mucosa, and also affected the membrane lipids, using DSC to probe these changes [27].

In addition, for enhancers such as bile salts, other mechanisms of action that have been investigated and confirmed are the formation of micelles, which act to stabilize enzyme-labile drugs, and the inhibition of proteases and aggregation, in the case of proteins.

C. Differences Between Oral Mucosa and Other Membranes

Because there is less information available on oral mucosal absorption enhancement, the previous sections have often described how enhancers affect dermal or non-oral mucosal membranes. This assumed that there is a scientifically rational analogy between the membranes compared. However, there are some clear differences between the oral mucosal membrane and skin or the epithelial membranes of the intestine, nasal cavity, or rectum.

Although epidermis and oral mucosal membranes are both stratified squamous epithelial membranes, the oral mucosal membranes can be considered to be less keratinized and to have more loosely packed intercellular lipids. The intestinal epithelium is, in contrast, a columnar epithelium, so the barrier to drug absorption is a single layer of cells rather than multiple layers. The barrier to paracellular absorption is the network of tight junctions that interconnects the epithelial cells. One mechanism for enhancing permeation through columnar epithelial membranes, like the intestine, is to transiently open the tight junctions. One way this can be accomplished is by exposing the membrane to chelating agents. Since tight junctional permeability is calcium-dependent, calcium chelation with agents like EDTA increases permeability. Since the oral mucosal membranes do not have tight junctions as a major barrier to permeation, enhancers that act primarily on epithelial tight junctions would be expected to not affect its permeability.

The effects of sodium glycocholate, EDTA, salicylate, and laureth-9 on buccal, nasal, and rectal insulin absorption were compared [13, 14]. Results are summarized in Table 3. The nonionic surfactant, laureth-9, and the bile salt, sodium glycocholate, increased insulin absorption from each site from <10% to approximately 25-45%, using pharmacological activity as an index of absorption. In addition, EDTA and salicylate were very effective in enhancing rectal insulin absorption. However, they had essentially no effect on nasal or

Table 3. Comparison of the Effects of Enhancers on Rectal, Nasal, and Buccal Insulin Absorption in Rats. (Compiled from References 13 and 14).

	Pharmacologic activity relative to intramuscular (%)[a]		
Enhancer	Rectal	Nasal	Buccal
None	9.5 ± 2.0	2.0 ± 0.5	1.9 ± 1.3
Na glycocholate (5%)	40.1 ± 8.2	46.8 ± 4.7	25.5 ± 7.5
Laureth-9 (5%)	31.9 ± 11.0	28.7 ± 6.9	27.2 ± 10.3
Na salicylate (5%)	41.7 ± 11.3	4.1 ± 2.4	2.9 ± 2.0
Na_2EDTA (5%)	31.0 ± 6.7	3.5 ± 1.0	2.9 ± 1.4

[a]Mean ± SEM of 6 or more rats per group.

buccal absorption. Thus, although many absorption enhancers for nasal, rectal, and intestinal drug delivery have been described, it should not be assumed that they will have similar effects on oral mucosal drug delivery. This would be particularly true if the mechanism involves opening tight junctions.

V. TOXICITY AND OTHER LIMITATIONS

One of the limitations already mentioned for oral mucosal permeation enhancement is that enhancers may not be very effective in increasing bioavailability, especially for large molecular weight compounds. Although examples have been given where bioavailability was increased from <5% to 30-40%, there are also examples where, even though absorption was increased 2-3 fold, or even 10-fold, bioavailability was still <10%. There have been no examples where the bioavailability of a compound was increased from say 1-5% to 100%, so investigators should not expect this extent of enhancement.

The major limitation of the use of permeation enhancers for oral mucosal drug delivery, indeed all routes of drug delivery, is the potential membrane damage that can be caused by the enhancer. There have been numerous studies using various routes in which increases in permeation enhancement were correlated with damage to the membrane. A few examples will be given in this chapter. A close relationship was demonstrated between insulin absorption enhancement and epithelial damage by histological assessment, for laureth-9, lysophosphatidyl cholide, and a steroidal detergent dosed nasally to rats [45]. A comparison of the toxicity and permeation enhancing effects of Azone and Azone derivatives was made, where, as an indicator of toxicity, several properties of human fibroblasts and keratinocytes were measured in vitro [46]. The study showed a correlation between toxicity and skin permeation enhancement for these compounds. Several bile salts, ionic surfactants, and a fatty acid were evaluated biochemically and histologically for their effects on hamster intestine in vitro, and the effects of those agents on intestinal permeability to various compounds were also determined [47]. Again a relationship was shown between membrane permeation enhancement and membrane damage.

There have only been a few studies of the toxicity of enhancers on oral mucosal membranes. Application of up to 1% sodium lauryl sulfate or cetylpyridinium chloride to the ventral surface of the tongue of dogs caused loss of surface squames and widening and separation of the keratin [11]. Rabbit buccal mucosa treated with 0.5% sodium deoxycholate or 0.1% sodium lauryl sulfate showed loss of surface epithelial layers, which correlated with increased permeability [27]. These studies show that the coadministration of permeation enhancers can potentially cause damage to the mucosa of the oral cavity. This is an important consideration that must be evaluated when using permeation enhancers to optimize the oral mucosal delivery of a drug.

Is it possible to increase membrane permeability without causing a toxic effect on the membrane? This is theoretically possible if (i) the mechanism of permeation enhancement is unrelated to the mechanism of toxicity, or (ii) if the concentration of the enhancer needed to affect permeability is significantly lower than that which causes toxicity. In this respect a transient increase in the fluidity of the intercellular lipids of the oral mucosa could be thought of as a relatively non-toxic effect, whereas extraction of the intercellular lipids or denaturation of cellular proteins may be more damaging.

There is some evidence to suggest that oral mucosal permeation enhancement and membrane damage can be separated. Sodium taurocholate and lysophosphatidyl cholide increased buccal insulin absorption in dogs, and in the same animals the effects on permeability were rapidly reversible and no mucosal irritation was observed [28]. The effects of Azone on the permeability of the hamster cheek pouch were also rapidly reversible [21]. In a study of skin irritation and permeation enhancement using various fatty acids as enhancers, some effective permeation enhancers were irritating, but other very effective enhancers had very low scores on irritation tests [48]. Thus, it appears that it may be possible to develop non-irritating permeation enhancers. However, the toxicity issues should always be raised and addressed.

VI. SUMMARY

Permeation enhancers can be used to increase the rate and extent of absorption of poorly absorbed drugs. Most of the known effective oral mucosal permeation enhancers have structures in either the bile salt, surfactant, or Azone categories. Bioavailabilities of peptide drugs have been increased from <5% to 30-40%. However, some peptides or proteins may still exhibit low bioavailability buccally or sublingually even when coadministered with permeation enhancers. The potential damage to the mucosal membrane caused by the permeation enhancer is a major concern, but there is evidence that permeation enhancement can be achieved without toxicity.

REFERENCES

1. R. P. Walton, and C. F. Lacey, Absorption of drugs through the oral mucosa, *J. Pharmacol. Exp. Ther. 54*:61 (1935).
2. P. Tfelt-Hansen, L. Paalzow, and J. J. Ibraheem, Bioavailability of sublingual ergotamine, *Br. J. Clin. Pharmac. 13*:239 (1982).
3. J. Van Harten, K. Burggraaf, M. Danhof, P. Van Brummelen, and D. D. Breimer, Negligible sublingual absorption of nifedipine, *Lancet:*1363 (1987).
4. R. R. Gunning, and A. J. Garber, Bioactivity of instant glucose - failure of absorption through oral mucosa, *J. Amer. Med. Assoc. 240*:1611 (1978).
5. Y. Rojanasakul, L. -Y. Wang, M. Bhat, D. D. Glover, C. J. Malanga, and J. K. H. Ma, The transport barrier of epithelia: a comparative study on membrane permeability and charge selectivity in the rabbit, *Pharm. Res. 9*:1029 (1992).
6. R. Anders, H. P. Merkle, W. Schurr, and R. Ziegler, Buccal absorption of protirelin: an effective way to stimulate thyrotropin and prolactin, *J. Pharm. Sci. 72*:1481 (1983).
7. R. Warm, and R. Weissbach, Transbuccal administration of oxytocin and induction of labor, *Am. J. Obstet. Gyn. 104*:1174 (1969).
8. E. McDevitt, R. D. Huebner, and I. S. Wright, Ineffectiveness of heparin by sublingual administration, *J. Amer. Med. Assoc. 148*:1123 (1952).
9. S. Bergman, D. Kane, I. A. Siegel, and S. Ciancio, In vitro and in situ transfer of local anesthetics across the oral mucosa, *Arch. Oral Biol. 14*:35 (1969).
10. M. Ishida, Y. Machida, N. Nambu, and T. Nagai, New mucosal dosage form of insulin, *Chem. Pharm. Bull. 29*:810 (1981).
11. I. A. Siegel, and H. P. Gordon, Surfactant-induced increases of permeability of rat oral mucosa to non-electrolytes in vivo, *Arch. Oral Biol. 30*:43 (1985).
12. I. A. Siegel, and H. P. Gordon, Effects of surfactants on the permeability of canine oral mucosa in vitro, *Toxicology Letters 26*:153 (1985).
13. B. J. Aungst, N. J. Rogers, and E. Shefter, Comparison of nasal, rectal, buccal, sublingual and intramuscular insulin efficacy and the effects of a bile salt absorption promoter, *J. Pharmacol. Exp. Ther. 244*:23 (1988).

14. B. J. Aungst, and N. J. Rogers, Site dependence of absorption-promoting actions of laureth-9, Na salicylate, Na_2EDTA, and aprotinin on rectal, nasal, and buccal insulin delivery, *Pharm. Res. 5*:305 (1988).
15. Y. Kurosaki, S. Hisaichi, C. Hamada, T. Nakayama, and T. Kimura, Effects of surfactants on the absorption of salicylic acid from hamster cheek pouch as a model of keratinized oral mucosa, *Int. J. Pharm. 47*:13 (1988).
16. Y. Nakada, N. Awata, C. Nakamichi, and I. Sugimoto, The effect of additives on the oral mucosal absorption of human calcitonin in rats, *J. Pharmacobio-Dyn. 11*:395 (1988).
17. Y. Kurosaki, T. Takatori, M. Kitayama, T. Nakayama, and T. Kimura, Application of propranolol to the keratinized oral mucosa: avoidance of first-pass elimination and the use of 1-dodecylazacycloheptan-2-one (Azone) as an absorption enhancer of bioadhesive film-dosage form, *J. Pharmacobio-Dyn. 11*:824 (1988).
18. Y. Kurosaki, S. Hisaichi, L. -Z. Hong, T. Nakayama, and T. Kimura, Enhanced permeability of keratinized oral mucosa to salicylic acid with 1-dodecylazacycloheptan-2-one (Azone). In vitro studies in hamster cheek pouch, *Int. J. Pharm. 49*:47 (1989).
19. W. A. Ritschel, G. B. Ritschel, H. Forusz, and M. Kraeling, Buccal absorption of insulin in the dog, *Res. Commun. Chem. Pathol. Pharmacol. 63*:53 (1989).
20. Y. Nakada, N. Awata, Y. Ikuta, and S. Goto, The effect of bile salts on the oral mucosal absorption of human calcitonin in rats, *J. Pharmacobio-Dyn. 12*:736 (1989).
21. Y. Kurosaki, S. Hisaichi, T. Nakayama, and T. Kimura, Enhancing effect of 1-dodecylazacycloheptan-2-one (Azone) on the absorption of salicylic acid from keratinized oral mucosa and the duration of enhancement in vivo, *Int. J. Pharm. 51*:47 (1989).
22. B. J. Aungst, and N. J. Rogers, Comparison of the effects of various transmucosal absorption promoters on buccal insulin delivery, *Int. J. Pharm. 53*:227 (1989).
23. C. K. Oh, and W. A. Ritschel, Biopharmaceutic aspects of buccal absorption of insulin, *Meth. Find. Exp. Clin. Pharmacol. 12*:205 (1990).
24. G. J. M. Wolany, J. Munzer, A. Rummelt, and H. P. Merkle, Buccal absorption of Sandostatin® (Octreotide) in conscious beagle dogs, *Proceed. Int. Symp. Control. Rel. Bioact. Mater. 17*:224 (1990).
25. M. Araki, S. Yamashita, T. Nadai, M. Masada, Y. Kurosaki, T. Nakayama, and T. Kimura, Interaction of percutaneous absorption enhancer with stratum corneum of hamster cheek pouch; an electrophysiological study, *Int. J. Pharm. 81*:39 (1992).
26. A. Coutel-Egros, Y. Maitani, M. Veillard, Y. Machida, and T. Nagai,

Combined effects of pH, cosolvent and penetration enhancers on the in vitro buccal absorption of propranolol through excised hamster cheek pouch, *Int. J. Pharm. 84*:117 (1992).

27. R. Gandhi, and J. Robinson, Mechanisms of penetration enhancement for transbuccal delivery of salicylic acid, *Int. J. Pharm. 85*:129 (1992).
28. J. Zhang, S. Niu, C. Ebert, and T. H. Stanley, An in vivo dog model for studying recovery kinetics of the buccal mucosa permeation barrier after exposure to permeation enhancers: apparent evidence of effective enhancement without tissue damage, *Int. J. Pharm. 101*:15 (1994).
29. A. Steward, D. L. Bayley, and C. Howes, The effect of enhancers on the buccal absorption of hybrid (BDBB) α-interferon, *Int. J. Pharm. 104*:145 (1994).
30. B. J. Aungst, Site-dependence and structure-effect relationships for alkylglycosides as transmucosal absorption promoters for insulin, *Int. J. Pharm. 105*:219 (1994).
31. S. Hirai, T. Yashiki, and H. Mima, Effect of surfactants on the nasal absorption of insulin in rats, *Int. J. Pharm. 9*:165 (1981).
32. K. Ichikawa, I. Ohata, M. Mitomi, S. Kawamura, H. Maeno, and H. Kawata, Rectal absorption of insulin suppositories in rabbits, *J. Pharm. Pharmacol. 32*:314 (1980).
33. B. J. Aungst, N. J. Rogers, and E. Shefter, Enhancement of naloxone penetration through human skin in vitro using fatty acids, fatty alcohols, surfactants, sulfoxides and amides, *Int. J. Pharm. 33*:225 (1986).
34. P. W. Wertz, D. C. Swartzendruber, and C. A. Squier, Regional variation in the structure and permeability of oral mucosa and skin, *Adv. Drug Del. Rev. 12*:1 (1993).
35. M. J. Rathbone, and I. G. Tucker, Mechanisms, barriers and pathways of oral mucosal drug permeation, *Adv. Drug Del. Rev. 12*:41 (1993).
36. P. W. Wertz, and C. A. Squier, Cellular and molecular basis of barrier function in oral epithelium, *Crit. Rev. Ther. Drug Carr. Sys. 8*:237 (1991).
37. G. M. Golden, D. B. Guzek, A. H. Kennedy, J. E. McKie, and R. O. Potts, Stratum corneum lipid phase transitions and water barrier properties, *Biochemistry 26*:2382 (1987).
38. G. M. Golden, J. E. McKie, and R. O. Potts, Role of stratum corneum lipid fluidity in transdermal drug flux, *J. Pharm. Sci. 76*:25 (1987).
39. M. L. Francoeur, G. M. Golden, and R. O. Potts, Oleic acid: its effects on stratum corneum in relation to (trans)dermal drug delivery, *Pharm. Res. 7*:621 (1990).
40. J. A. Bouwstra, L. J. C. Peschier, J. Brussee, and H. E. Boddé, Effect of N-alkyl-azocycloheptan-2-ones including Azone on the thermal behavior of human stratum corneum, *Int. J. Pharm. 52*:47 (1989).

41. T. M. Turunen, A. Urtti, P. Paronen, K. L. Audus, and J. H. Rytting, Effect of some penetration enhancers on epithelial membrane lipid domains: evidence from fluorescence spectroscopy studies, *Pharm. Res. 11*:288 (1994).
42. B. W. Barry, Mode of action of penetration enhancers in human skin, *J. Control. Rel. 6*:85 (1987).
43. K. A. Walters, M. Walker, and O. Olejnik, Non-ionic surfactant effects on hairless mouse skin permeability characteristics, *J. Pharm. Pharmacol. 40*:525 (1988).
44. D. A. Whitmore, L. G. Brookes, and K. P. Wheeler, Relative effects of different surfactants on intestinal absorption and the release of proteins and phospholipids from the tissue, *J. Pharm. Pharmacol. 31*:277 (1979).
45. S. G. Chandler, L. Illum, and N. W. Thomas, Nasal absorption in rats. II. Effect of enhancers on insulin absorption and nasal histology, *Int. J. Pharm. 76*:61 (1991).
46. M. Ponec, M. Haverkort, Y. L. Soei, J. Kempenaar, J. Brussee, and H. E. Boddé, Toxicity screening of N-alkylazacycloheptan-2-one derivatives in cultured human skin cells: structure-toxicity relationships, *J. Pharm. Sci. 78*:738 (1989).
47. G. W. Gullikson, W. S. Cline, V. Lorenzsonn, L. Benz, W. A. Olsen, and P. Bass, Effects of anionic surfactants on hamster small intestinal membrane structure and function: relationship to surface activity, *Gastroenterology 73*:501 (1977).
48. B. J. Aungst, Structure/effect studies of fatty acid isomers as skin penetration enhancers and skin irritants, *Pharm. Res. 6*:244 (1989).

5

In Vitro Methods for Measuring Permeability of the Oral Mucosa

Hao Zhang
Anesta Corporation, USA

Joseph R. Robinson
University of Wisconsin-Madison, USA

I. INTRODUCTION

The oral cavity has been used as a site for systemic drug delivery for a long time. Despite the early success of delivering nitroglycerin for angina pectoris [1], the oral mucosa as a route for drug absorption to the systemic circulation has generally been limited to emergency medication. The major problem appears to be that the amount of drug absorbed via this route for most drugs is too low to have clinical efficacy, mainly due to a relatively small surface area and low tissue permeability. Unlike surface area, which is unchangeable, permeability of the oral mucosa can be temporarily altered to allow greater amounts of drug to be delivered to the systemic circulation. Therefore, in recent years considerable effort has been devoted to understanding the mechanism(s) of drug absorption across these tissues both with and without penetration enhancers (see Chapters 3 and 4).

Compared with in vivo assessment, in vitro permeability measurement offers a number of advantages and has been a useful tool to study the mechanism(s) of oral mucosal drug absorption. Experimentally, a piece of freshly dissected oral mucosa from a test animal is used as a membrane to study drug diffusion in a well controlled environment. The experimental set up is simple, because the tissue is isolated from the whole animal, thus restricting the number of variables that need to be controlled. The conditions of the experiment, such as temperature, pH, osmolarity, etc., can be easily controlled, which makes it possible to single out one factor that can influence drug permeation. The permeability of the tissue is measured by the drug concentration on the receiver side, which, by analogy, is equivalent to drug that is available to the circulation. Sample analysis is much easier because the receiver side is a buffer solution rather than blood samples from an in vivo system. Sample purification and preparation before analysis are commonly unnecessary. Of course, there are limitations and problems associated with an in vitro permeability measurement. These will be discussed later in this chapter. In general, in vitro permeability studies are more suitable for studying mechanisms of drug transport across the oral mucosa or perhaps rank order absorption of a series of drugs rather than predicting the actual drug absorption flux in an in vivo system.

II. ANIMAL MODELS

Since human oral mucosa is not widely available, animal oral mucosa is routinely used for in vitro studies. The main concern of choosing a particular animal model is resemblance of the animal mucosa to the oral mucosa of human beings in both ultrastructure and enzyme activity, which represents the physical and metabolic barriers of the oral mucosa. It is important to recognize that no animal model can fully represent human tissue, but what is sought is an animal mucosa that has equivalent physical and biochemical properties to humans. The differences between animal model and human can be corrected for by using a comparative study.

Many laboratory animals have been tested for in vitro oral mucosa permeability studies. The most commonly used animals are dogs [2-6], rabbits [7-10], pigs [2, 8, 11-14], Rhesus monkeys [2, 15], guinea pigs [16-18], rats [19-20] and hamsters [21-22]. Characteristics of oral mucosa from these various species and regions have been discussed in Chapter 1 of this book.

The oral mucosa of dogs, pigs, rabbits and Rhesus monkeys are believed to be similar to the oral mucosa of humans primarily because the epithelia are nonkeratinized. In vivo buccal absorption studies of flurbiprofen in humans and dogs revealed that the permeability of human and dog buccal mucosa are approximately equivalent [23]. In vitro permeability coefficients of tritiated water in human and pig oral mucosa, buccal and floor of mouth, are also similar [24], although this may be an inappropriate probe of comparative permeability since water typically uses a different pathway in mucosal tissue than drugs. Other comparative studies between these animal models have been reported [9, 21]. All these studies demonstrated that dogs, rabbits, pigs and Rhesus monkeys are reasonably good animal models for studying oral mucosal drug absorption. The choice of a particular animal is commonly controlled by cost and availability.

Rats and hamsters, however, have heavily keratinized oral mucosa which differ from the buccal and sublingual mucosa of humans [25]. The permeability coefficients of short chain alcohols and acids are significantly less in hamsters than in dogs, rabbits and humans [21]. The permeability of dextromethorphan in hamsters is not only much lower than in humans, but also has a different pH dependency pattern [21], which implies that the oral mucosa of the hamster is much more lipophilic than that of human and coincides with the fact that hamster oral mucosa is keratinized. Based on this evidence, the use of rats and hamsters as an animal model should be avoided unless the experiment is designed to study the permeability of keratinized oral mucosa [20].

Dogs, rabbits and pigs are the most commonly used animal models to study drug absorption across the oral mucosa in vitro. Rabbits are relatively cheap and easier to handle than dogs and pigs. However, the surface area of the rabbit buccal and sublingual areas is very small and thus the number of experiments that can be performed in one animal is limited. Dogs and pigs have a large mucosal area that permits multiple simultaneous experiments using the same animal, which will minimize individual variation.

III. TISSUE PREPARATION, VIABILITY AND INTEGRITY

A. Tissue Preparation

Tissue preparation for in vitro permeability measurements is not complicated. Animals are sacrificed immediately before the start of an experiment. Oral mucosa with a fair amount of underlying connective tissue is surgically removed from the oral cavity and placed in ice-cold buffer solution. The tissue is then pinned epithelial side down onto a dissecting dish and the connective tissue carefully removed using fine-point forceps and surgical scissors. The connective tissue should be removed as thoroughly as possible, and a dissection scope can be used to facilitate this procedure [7, 9]. The cleaned oral mucosa is then placed in ice-cold buffer before mounting in the diffusion cell.

Although the permeability barrier of the oral mucosa is located on the top one-third of the epithelium [7, 26-27], the connective tissue, like a stagnant layer, may significantly affect permeability if the thickness of the connective tissue is sizable. Therefore, successful removal of connective tissue is essential to minimize variation between tissue specimens.

Since this procedure is time consuming and requires skill and patience, chemical [14, 28-29], thermal [14] and enzymatic [22, 30-31] methods of splitting the oral epithelia and connective tissue have been developed and tested. In chemical splitting, the intact tissue was treated with 0.02M EDTA in PBS (pH 7.4) and incubated at 37°C with agitation for 7 hours. Microscopic examination of these tissues revealed that the separation occurred cleanly at the basement membrane [28] and the basal lamina was removed from the epithelium together with connective tissue [14]. Comparison of the permeability coefficients of horseradish peroxidase for the separated epithelia and intact tissue showed that the separated epithelia was not different from intact tissue. However, using a modified chemical splitting procedures [14], in which the intact tissue was placed in 0.02M EDTA in PBS (pH 7.4) at 60°C for 25-50 minutes, the electrical resistances of separated epithelia was significantly reduced. This result indicates that the permeability of the tissue to ions was significantly increased after chemical splitting of the epithelium and connective tissue. Similar results were found for thermal separation, in which the epithelium was separated from connective tissue by incubating the intact tissue in Krebs buffer solution at 60°C for 25 minutes. It appears that chemical and thermal separation of epithelium and connective tissue may substantially alter the permeability properties of the oral mucosa and should be avoided. Many chemical agents, such as EDTA, have been shown to enhance drug absorption across biological membranes [32-33]. An enzymatic separation method was also developed and tested. In this method, the intact hamster pouch tissue was treated with 0.5% collagenase solution on the endothelial side at 37°C for 20 minutes [30]. The comparison permeability study of intact and separated epithelia with a series of compounds showed that there was no significant difference between these two epithelia [22]. However, for hamster oral epithelium, the rate limiting barrier is the keratin layer. It is possible that the treatment by collagenase affects only the vital portion of the epithelium, but not the keratin layer. In general, these treatments of the tissue are not recommended simply because it is unclear what microscopic changes in the tissue have occurred.

B. Tissue Viability and Integrity Test

In vitro permeability measurement experiments using dissected animal tissue hopefully mimics the oral mucosa of a live animal. How well the dissected tissue is preserved is an important issue, which will directly affect the results and conclusions of studies. However, to date, there are no standard ways to measure the viability or integrity of the dissected tissue. Even "viability" and "integrity" may not be appropriate terms to describe the resemblance of the dissected tissue to its origin. ATP level (nmol/g tissue) has been used to assess the viability and integrity of rabbit oral tissue on several occasions [7, 34]. The problem is that the tissue as a whole may undergo some changes while individual cells may be viable for a much longer period of time. Alternatively, a drop in ATP level may not necessarily mean that the permeability properties of the tissue are changed. The issue of tissue integrity and viability is complicated, and it is therefore difficult to set a universal standard. Fortunately, in the drug delivery field, our interests often lie in the passive drug diffusion process. The tissue is considered "viable" if the barrier function of the tissue is unchanged during the time course of the study. Using diffusion study data in rabbit buccal mucosa, Dowty and Robinson showed that the permeability of thyrotropin releasing hormone remained constant in its initial six hours, then, the permeability started increasing significantly [7]. At six hours, the ATP level in this tissue was reduced by 50%. It appears that the diffusion experiments themselves may be the most useful way of testing whether the tissue is undergoing any change and how long the tissue is viable for the impelled experimental conditions. Note that in the initial phase of the diffusion study, the permeability is not constant due to the fact that the diffusion has not reached steady state.

IV. IN VITRO PERMEABILITY STUDIES

A. Experimental Details

A diagram of a typical plastic side-by-side diffusion cell is shown in Figure 1. There are three components in the system, the donor and receiver chambers

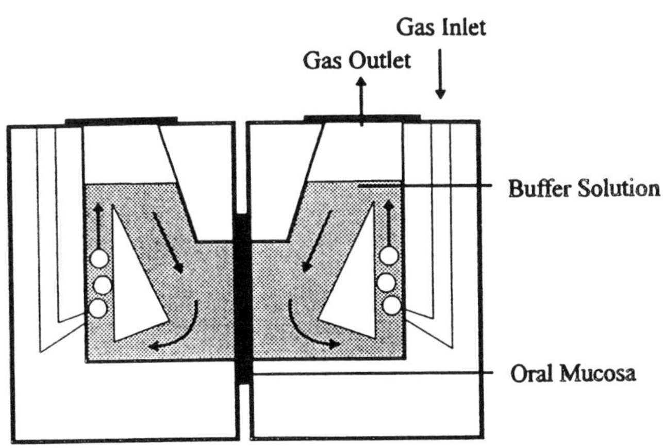

Figure 1. Schematic diagram of the diffusion cell used by Grass and Sweetana. Oxygen gas bubbles provide aeration and agitation.

and the oral mucosa sandwiched in the middle. The donor chamber refers to the side with high drug concentration which mimics the site of drug delivery whereas the receiver chamber mimics the general circulation. The epithelial side of the oral mucosa usually faces the donor chamber except when back diffusion is examined to explore the permeability symmetry of the tissue. In this case, the epithelial side faces the receiver chamber [35]. Solutions in both donor and receiver chambers are agitated by magnetic bars or gas bubbles to reduce the stagnant diffusion layer. Samples are taken periodically from the receiver chamber and replaced by fresh buffer solution.

Although a variety of diffusion cells are commercially available, such as the Franz® cells used by Eggerth [21], small volume diffusion cells used by Grass and Sweetana [36] and Dowty et al [7] (Precision Instrument Design, Los Altos, CA), most people use homemade modified Ussing chambers [37]. We prefer to use the Grass cells because they minimize the stagnant diffusion layer, i.e., gas is bubbled close to the membrane surface, and electrical leads are present to continuously monitor electrical resistance which gives a direct measure of tissue integrity. The key points are that the agitation must be sufficient to minimize the stagnant layer and the seals between tissue and diffusion cells are patent to prevent leakage. Diffusion cells are usually made of glass, Teflon® or plastics. If plastic or Teflon® diffusion cells are used, surface adsorption of lipophilic drug onto the diffusion cell should be tested. Of course, the same concern applies to the Teflon® coated stirring bar. Pre-moisturized oxygen or carbogen gases are often used to supply aeration and agitation for the buffer solution. Experimentalists should be aware that pH shifts do occur for small volume diffusion cells during lengthy experiments if carbogen gas is employed. Because there is 5% carbon dioxide in carbogen gas, the pH may drop caused by dissolving carbon dioxide to form carbonic acid.

B. Permeability Coefficient Measurement

There are many mathematical models to describe the process of drug transport across the oral mucosa. For most drugs, however, absorption via the oral mucosa is a passive diffusion process and can be described by Fick's first law (Figure 2):

$$J = \frac{DK_P}{h} C_D \tag{1}$$

Where J is the flux of the drug absorption defined as the amount of drug moving across the oral mucosa per unit time and area, D is the diffusion coefficient of the drug inside the oral mucosa, K_p is the partition coefficient

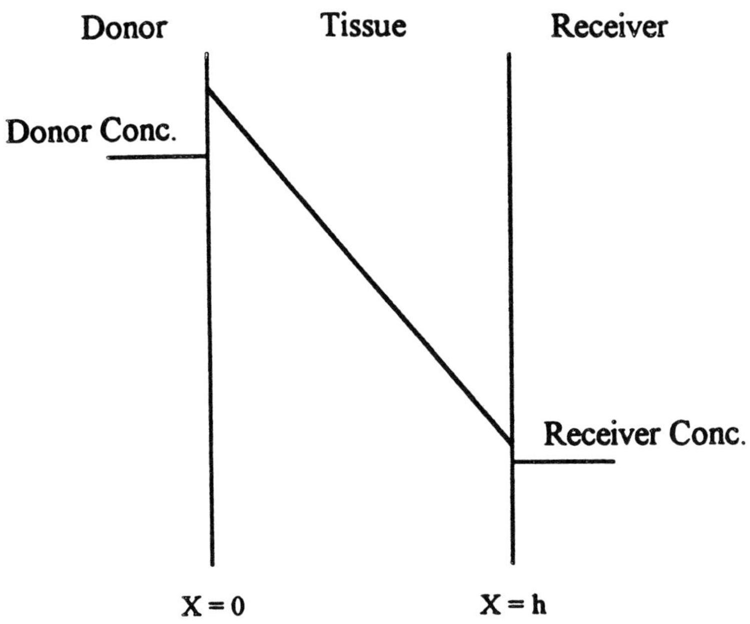

Figure 2. Traditional model of drug passive diffusion across oral mucosa under the assumption that the oral mucosa is a homogeneous hydrophobic membrane which leads to a linear drug concentration gradient and a constant diffusion coefficient inside the oral mucosa. It is also assumed that diffusion has reached steady state, and partitioning between the oral mucosa and donor and receiver solutions are identical.

between the oral mucosa and the buffer solution, h is the effective pathlength of the oral mucosa across which the drug must traverse, and C_D is drug concentration in the donor chamber.

It is impractical to measure diffusion coefficient, partition coefficient and pathlength separately. However, the permeability coefficient, P, which is defined as:

$$P = \frac{DK_P}{h} \tag{2}$$

is easily obtained. In a typical diffusion experiment, the amount of drug (A) moving across the tissue at time, t, is determined by measuring drug concentration on the receiver side. The surface area of the tissue (S) (the opening of the diffusion cell) and the initial drug concentration in the donor chamber are known and remain constant during the course of the experiment. Thus, the flux is:

$$J = PC_D = \frac{A}{St} \tag{3}$$

and the amount of drug transported at time t is:

$$A = PSC_D t \tag{4}$$

Since the total amount of the drug (A_T) on the donor side is:

$$A_T = V_D C_D \tag{5}$$

where V_D is the volume of the donor chamber, the percent of drug transported (T%) at time t is:

$$T\% = \frac{A}{A_T} = \frac{PS}{V_D} t \tag{6}$$

A plot of T% versus t will give a slope of $\frac{PS}{V_D}$, and from this slope the permeability coefficient can be obtained.

Equation (6) shows how to determine the permeability coefficient at steady state. Practically, however, almost all diffusion studies do not begin at steady state, and, as a matter of fact, steady state is theoretically never reached because the donor and receiver drug concentrations are continuously changing. If the concentration changes are small, we can assume that the donor drug concentration is constant and the receiver drug concentration is zero. Under this assumption, the diffusion process can be described in one dimension by Fick's second law [38]:

$$A = (SK_p hC_D)\left[\frac{Dt}{h^2} - \frac{1}{6} - \frac{2}{\pi^2}\sum_{n=1}^{\infty}\frac{(-1)^n}{n^2} e^{\frac{-Dn^2\pi^2 t}{h^2}}\right] \tag{7}$$

As time increases, the series term in equation (7) goes to zero, and equation (7) transforms to equation (8) and (9):

$$A = \frac{SDK_P C_D}{h}\left[t - \frac{h^2}{6D}\right] \tag{8}$$

$$T\% = \frac{A}{A_T} = \frac{PS}{V_D}\left[t - \frac{h^2}{6D}\right] \tag{9}$$

Equation (9) shows that a plot of percent transported versus time has a slope of

$\frac{PS}{V_D}$ and an x-axis intercept of $\frac{h^2}{6D}$. Notice that the difference between equation (6) and (9) is the x-axis intercept, $\frac{h^2}{6D}$, which is also called the lag time. Table 1 shows data for a typical diffusion study, in which six data points were taken during the experiment. It is important to keep in mind that the amount of drug crossing the oral mucosa is cumulative, which means that the amount taken out as a sample must be added back to calculate the amount transported. The T% versus t plot of this data set is shown in Figure 3. The linear portion of the curve is used to calculate the permeability coefficient and lag time.

V. PROBLEMS AND ISSUES ASSOCIATED WITH IN VITRO METHODS

A. Problems of Using Labeled Probes

One of the advantages of using an in vitro permeability measurement is that the drug concentration in the receiver chamber can be measured. However, in many in vitro permeability studies, drug concentration is not measured directly. Instead, radioactivity of a radiolabeled drug is detected [3, 7-9, 12, 15-17, 24, 35]. This is, of course, very convenient because the sample analysis is easy, no sample preparation is necessary and the sensitivity of the assay is high. However, this practice can also introduce problems. The main concern is whether the measured radioactivity is proportional to drug concentration. Under normal condition, this is usually not a problem. A low level of impurity will only introduce a few percent error. The error caused by variation of animal tissues is usually much larger. However, a problem will arise if the permeability of the impurity differs from the drug. The impurities, i.e., contaminations, degradation products and metabolites, are usually smaller than the labeled drugs and have higher permeability. Thus, it is possible that the measured radioactivity in the receiver chamber is not all from the drug, but partially from impurities in the system, which will consequently give false measurement of drug permeability. In addition, tritiated labels will occasionally exchange with solvent and the measurement then becomes tritium labeled solvent diffusion across the tissues. It is suggested that some form of stability indicating assay, over and above that of radioactivity measurement should be used.

If the impurities exist before the experiment, the T% versus time plot will have a negative lag time because impurities commonly have higher

Table 1. Typical Diffusion Study Data. HPLC Peak Heights Were Used to Determine Drug Concentration. The Peak Height to Concentration Conversion Factor is 1.27×10^{-5} mg/mL/mm. Donor Side Concentration is 0.1051 mg/mL. Area is 0.503 cm^2. Volume of Donor and Receiver Chambers are 2.0 mL. Sample Size is 1.0 mL. T% is the Percent of Drug Transported.

Time (minute)	Peak height (mm)	Concentration (mg/ml)	Sample (mg)	Total flux (mg)	T%
15	7.40	9.39×10^{-5}	9.39×10^{-5}	1.88×10^{-4}	0.0894
45	87.90	1.12×10^{-3}	1.21×10^{-3}	2.32×10^{-3}	1.1061
75	165.00	2.09×10^{-3}	3.30×10^{-3}	5.40×10^{-3}	2.5678
105	209.00	2.65×10^{-3}	5.96×10^{-3}	8.61×10^{-3}	4.0953
135	232.00	2.94×10^{-3}	8.90×10^{-3}	1.18×10^{-2}	5.6349
165	237.00	3.01×10^{-3}	1.19×10^{-2}	1.49×10^{-2}	7.0960

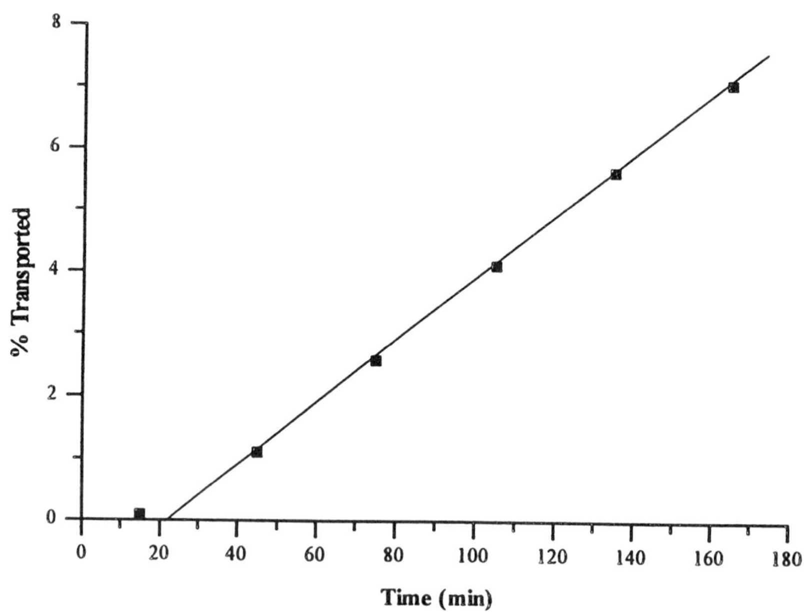

Figure 3. A typical T% versus time plot of a diffusion experiment. The linear portion of the curve is fitted by linear regression to obtain the slope and x-axis intercept, that are used to calculated the permeability coefficient and lag time.

permeability than labeled drugs and the initial radioactivity measurement will be high. The entire curve will move upward resulting in a negative lag time.

The problems outlined above are especially true if the drug is a peptide drug, since it will be readily degraded by enzymes resident in the oral cavity. Indeed, if the drug is metabolized during the diffusion experiment [7, 39], it becomes difficult to detect. Thus before researchers begin permeation studies, they should first investigate the kinetic profiles of degradation and develop means to stabilize the penetrant; this in turn will enable them to obtain meaningful permeation data. As an example, Dowty and Robinson demonstrated that thyrotropin-releasing hormone (TRH) was substantially metabolized during a transbuccal diffusion experiment. In this case, to overcome this problem, a large amount of cold TRH was placed in the system to saturate the metabolic enzyme prior to the experiment. Protease inhibitor may also be used to block the degradation process during the experiment [12].

B. Enzyme Activities

Especially for peptides and protein drugs, there is both a physical and a enzymatic barrier. There are many enzymes in the oral mucosa that have the potential to metabolize peptides and protein drugs [32, 40]. Simultaneous metabolism of thyrotropin releasing hormone [7] and aminopeptidase substrate (L-LPNA) [39] are just two examples of drugs that are substantially metabolized in the oral mucosa. As a first step of characterizing these enzymes, the enzyme activity of the tissue was determined by incubating the drugs in a tissue homogenate [41-43]. These studies provide important initial information about which enzyme is responsible for drug metabolism in the oral mucosa during drug delivery but must be confirmed with whole tissue studies since an homogenate can only tell us the existence of these enzymes, but not their distribution inside the oral mucosa, nor the possibility of their contact with peptides or protein drugs. Some enzymatic barriers extend beyond the oral epithelium itself [32]. Many studies have found enzyme activity in saliva [44, 45] and connective tissues [31].

C. Alteration of the Tissue After Dissection

Although the viability and integrity of the tissue can be tested, the influence of alteration of the tissue by dissection on drug permeability is hard to assess. The alteration may either increase or decrease permeation, depending on the drug delivered. Carefully examining the dissection procedure, it is clear that there are three areas where the oral mucosa can be changed; the mucus and saliva coverage on top of the mucosa, the intercellular interaction or communication, and the capillary blood circulation system underneath the oral mucosa.

The contribution of mucus and saliva to the barrier function of the oral mucosa is not fully understood. Although most in vitro and in vivo studies show that the top quarter to one third of the epithelium is the penetration barrier of the oral mucosa [7, 26-27], some studies have shown that inhibition of salivation increases the penetration of dyes into the oral mucosa in vivo [46-48]. Mucus and saliva also provide a rich media of enzymes to form potential enzymatic barrier. It is possible that the barrier function of mucus and saliva differs from one compound to another depending on the physicochemical properties of the diffusant. In addition, mucus and saliva increases the viscosity on the donor side which will reduce the drug penetration rate, although this resistance may not be the limiting step of penetration.

In a live animal, the intercellular interactions and communications are very active. Upon sacrificing the animal and dissecting the tissue, these interactions will be significantly reduced or stopped in a very short time, although the individual cell may remain viable for a much longer time. This alteration of the tissue may change the properties of the cell membrane, intercellular media, enzyme distributions and activities, etc. It is difficult to know exactly what is changed and to what extent, and how these changes influence permeation. For example, alteration of the distribution of enzymes and their activities will not effect drug permeability if the drug is not metabolized by these enzymes. Conversely, for a drug that is highly metabolized by these enzymes, drug permeation will be sensitive to this alteration.

Capillary blood circulation system extends deep into the conical shaped connective tissue papillae that protrude into the epithelial up to within 0.1 mm from the surface [49]. The purpose of this morphological configuration is to increase material exchange between the epithelial cell and blood circulation. In an in vivo situation, this configuration will also remove the drug once it crosses the oral epithelium. However, in an in vitro system, the tissue is dissected and the capillary circulation no longer exists. If the connective tissue is thoroughly removed, the dissected tissue is able to mimic the tissue in vivo with a rich blood supply or high blood flow. Otherwise, the remaining connective tissue will act as a stagnant layer and reduce permeability. Note that we have assumed that blood circulation is not the rate limiting step of drug absorption. This assumption may not be valid for certain drugs that will cause blood vessel contraction because these drugs will significantly reduce blood flow once the drug reaches blood vessel. This is a rare occurrence since for blood flow to be rate limiting the drug must rapidly cross the buccal tissue and very few drugs will have this ability.

Overall, in vitro methods to study drug permeability can be useful to explore the mechanisms of oral mucosal drug permeation and to obtain a first approximation of the expected in vivo absorption rate. Considerable information regarding the permeability behavior of the oral mucosa to a variety of variables, such as partition coefficient dependency, pH dependency, effect of pH gradient, effect of penetration enhancer, etc., can be determined in vitro and may be useful in subsequent formulation work.

REFERENCES

1. W. Murrell, Nitroglycerin as a remedy for angina pectoris, *Lancet 1*:80-81, 113-115, 151-152, 225-227 (1879).
2. C. A. Squier, and B. K. Hall, The permeability of mammalian nonkeratinized oral epithelia to horseradish peroxidase applied in vivo and in vitro, *Archs. Oral Biol. 29*:45 (1984).
3. W. R. Galey, H. K. Lonsdale, and S. Nacht, The in vitro permeability of skin and buccal mucosa to selected drugs and tritiated water, *J. Invest. Dermatol. 67*:713 (1976).
4. S. Bergman, D. Kane, I. A. Siegel, and S. Ciancio, In vitro and in situ transfer of local anesthetics across the oral mucosa, *Archs. Oral Biol. 14*:35 (1969).
5. N. A. Tobey, V. J. Schreiner, R. D. Readling, and R. C. Orlando, The acute effects of smokeless tobacco on transport and barrier function of buccal mucosa, *J. Dent. Res. 67*:1414 (1988).
6. I. A. Siegel, and H. P. Gordon, Effects of surfactants on the permeability of canine oral mucosa in vitro, *Toxicology Letters 26*:15 (1985).
7. M. E. Dowty, K. E. Knuth, B. K. Irons, and J. R. Robinson, Transport of thyrotropin releasing hormone in rabbit buccal mucosa in vitro, *Pharm. Res. 9*:1113 (1992).
8. I. A. Siegel, and H. P. Gordon, Surfactant-induced alteration of permeability of rabbit oral mucosa in vitro, *Exp. Molecular Pathol. 44*:132 (1986).
9. I. A. Siegel, K. T. Izutsu, and E. Watson, Mechanisms of non-electrolyte penetration across dog and rabbit oral mucosa in vitro, *Archs. Oral Biol. 26*:357 (1981).
10. K. Tolo, and J. Jonsen, In vitro penetration of tritiated dextrans through rabbit oral mucosa, *Archs. Oral Biol. 20*:419 (1975).
11. C. A. Squier, P. Cox, and B. K. Hall, Enhanced penetration of nitrosonornicotine across oral mucosa in the presence of ethanol, *J. Oral Pathol. 15*:276 (1986).
12. C. A. Squier, and B. K. Hall, The permeability of skin and oral mucosa to water and horseradish peroxidase as related to the thickness of the permeability barrier, *J. Invest. Dermatol. 84*:176 (1985).

13. P. P. H. Le Brun, P. L. A. Fox, M. E. de Vries, and H. E. Boddé, In vitro penetration of some β-adrenoreceptor blocking drugs through porcine buccal mucosa, *Int. J. Pharm. 49*:141 (1989).
14. M. E. de Vries, H. E. Boddé, J. C. Verhoef, M. Ponec, W. I. H. M. Craane, and H. E. Junginger, Localization of the permeability barrier inside porcine buccal mucosa: a combination in vitro study of drug permeability, electrical resistance and tissue morphology, *Int. J. Pharm. 76*:25 (1991).
15. M. Mehta, B. W. Kemppainen, and R. G. Stafford, In vitro penetration of tritium-labeled water (THO) and [^{3}H]PbTx-3 (a red tide toxin) through monkey buccal mucosa and skin, *Toxicology Letters 55*:185 (1991).
16. M. C. Alfano, J. F. Drummond, and S. A. Miller, Localization of rate-limiting barrier to penetration of endotoxin through nonkeratinized oral mucosa in vitro, *J. Dent. Res. 54*:1143 (1975).
17. M. C. Alfano, A. I. Chasens, and C. W. Masi, Autoradiographic study of the penetration of radiolabeled dextrans and inulin through non-keratinized oral mucosa in vitro, *J. Periodontal. Res. 12*:368 (1977).
18. K. Tolo, A study of permeability of gingival pocket epithelium to albumin in guinea pigs and Norwegian pigs, *Archs. Oral Biol. 16*:881 (1971).
19. M. A. Hussain, B. J. Aungst, A. Kearney, and E. Shefter, Buccal and oral bioavailability of naloxone and naltrexone in rats, *Int. J. Pharm. 36*:127 (1987).
20. A. Jepsen, An in vitro model of an oral keratinizing squamous epithelium, *Scand. J. Dent. Res. 82*:144 (1974).
21. R. M. Eggerth, Z. A. Rashidbaigi, M. Mahjour, F. W. Goodhart, and M. B. Fawzi, Evaluation of hamster cheek pouch as a model for buccal absorption, *Proceed. Intern. Symp. Control. Rel. Bioact. Mater. 14*:180 (1987).
22. K. W. Garren, and A. J. Repta, Buccal drug absorption II: in vitro diffusion across the hamster cheek pouch, *J. Pharm. Sci. 78*:160 (1989).
23. C. L. Barsuhn, L. S. Olanoff, D. D. Gleason, E. L. Adkins, and N. F. H. Ho, Human buccal absorption of flurbiprofen, *Clin. Pharmacol. Ther. 44*:225 (1988).
24. C. A. Lesch, C. A. Squier, A. Cruchley, D. M. Williams, and P. Speight, The permeability of human oral mucosa and skin to water, *J. Dent. Res. 68*:1345 (1989).
25. C. D. Ebert, V. A. John, P. T. Beall, and K. A. Rosenzweig, Transbuccal absorption of diclofenac sodium in a dog model, *Controlled-Release Technology: Pharmaceutical Applications* (P. I. Lee and W. R. Good, eds.), American Chemical Society, Washington, 1987, p. 310.

26. C. A. Squier, The permeability of keratinized and nonkeratinized oral epithelium to horseradish peroxidase, *J. Ultrastruct Res. 43*:160 (1973).
27. C. A. Squier, and L. Rooney, The permeability of keratinized and nonkeratinized oral epithelium to lanthanum in vivo, *J. Ultrastruct Res. 54*:286 (1976).
28. C. A. Squier, and B. K. Hall, In-vitro permeability of porcine oral mucosa after epithelial separation, stripping and hydration, *Archs. Oral Biol. 30*:485 (1985).
29. S. Scaletta, and D. K. MacCallum, A fine structural study of divalent cation mediated epithelial union with connective tissue in human oral mucosa, *Am. J. Anat. 133*:431 (1972).
30. G. D. McCoy, Respiratory characteristics of mitochondria isolation from squamous epithelium of the hamster cheek pouch, *Proc. Soc. Exp. Biol. Med. 156*:118 (1977).
31. P. Person, J. Felton, and A. Fine, Biochemical and histochemical studies of aerobic oxidative metabolism of oral tissues III. Specific metabolic activities of enzymatically separated gingival epithelium and connective tissue components, *J. Dent. Res. 44*:91 (1965).
32. V. H. L. Lee, and A. Yamamoto, Penetration and enzymatic barriers to peptide and protein absorption, *Adv. Drug Del. Rev. 4*:171 (1991).
33. G. Grass, and J. Robinson, Mechanisms of corneal drug penetration. I: In vivo and in vitro kinetics, *J. Pharm. Sci. 77*:3 (1988).
34. M. A. Longer, Characterization of buccal epithelia relevant to peptide drug delivery, Ph.D. Thesis, University of Wisconsin-Madison, 1988.
35. I. A. Siegel, Effect of chemical structure on nonelectrolyte penetration of oral mucosa, *J. Invest. Dermatol. 76*:137 (1981).
36. G. M. Grass, and S. A. Sweetana, In vitro measurement of gastrointestinal tissue permeability using a new diffusion cell, *Pharm. Res. 5*:372 (1988).
37. H. H. Ussing, Active ion transport through the isolated frog skin in the light of tracer studies, *Acta Physiol. Scand. 17*:1(1949).
38. R. R. Burnette, Theory of mass transfer, *Controlled Drug Delivery-Fundamentals and Applications* (J. R. Robinson, and V. H. Lee, eds.), Marcel Dekker, Inc., New York, 1987, p. 95.
39. K. W. Garren, E. M. Topp and A. J. Repta, Buccal absorption III: simultaneous diffusion and metabolism of an aminopeptidase substrate in the hamster cheek pouch, *Pharm. Res. 6*:966 (1989).
40. G. S. Rao, Drug metabolism in oral soft tissues, *Pharm. Int. 6*:103 (1983).
41. R. E. Stratford, and V. H. L. Lee, Aminopeptidase activity in homogenates of various absorptive mucosa in the albino rabbit: implications in peptide delivery, *Int. J. Pharm. 30*:73 (1986).

42. V. H. L. Lee, S. D. Kashi, R. M. Patel, E. Hayakawa, and K. Inagaki, Mucosal peptide and protein delivery: proteolytic activities in mucosal homogenates, *Proc. Intern. Symp. Control. Rel. Bioact. Mater. 14*:23 (1987).
43. S. D. Kashi, and V. H. L. Lee, Enkephalin hydrolysis in homogenates of various absorptive mucosa of the albino rabbit: similarities in rates and involvement of aminopeptidases, *Life Sci. 38*:2019 (1986).
44. P. Söder, Proteolytic activity in the oral cavity: proteolytic enzymes from human saliva and dental plaque material, *J. Dent. Res. 51*:389 (1972).
45. H. H. Chauncey, F. Lionetti, R. A. Winer, and V. F. Lisanti, Enzymes of human saliva I: The determination, distribution, and origin of whole saliva enzymes, *J. Dent. Res. 33*:321 (1954).
46. D. Adams, The effect of saliva on the penetration of fluorescent dyes into the oral mucosa of the rat and rabbit, *Archs. Oral Biol. 19*:505 (1974).
47. D. Adams, The mucus barrier and absorption through the oral mucosa, *J. Dent. Res. 54*:B19 (1975).
48. L. A. Tabak, M. J. Levine, I. D. Mandel, and S. A. Ellison, Role of salivary mucins in the protection of the oral cavity, *J. Oral Pathol. 11*:1 (1982).
49. S. Y. Chen and C. A. Squier, The ultrastructure of the oral epithelium, *The Structure and Function of Oral Mucosa* (J. Meyer, C. A. Squier, and S. J. Gerson, eds.), Pergamon Press, New York, 1984, p. 7.

6

Buccal Epithelial Cell Cultures as a Model to Study Oral Mucosal Drug Transport and Metabolism

Kenneth L. Audus
The University of Kansas, USA

I. INTRODUCTION

The first 25 years or so in the development of cell and tissue culture systems representative of the oral mucosa was aptly reviewed several years ago by MacCallum et al [1]. Since that review, researchers have directed some attention to a more basic characterization of stratified squamous epithelial cell differentiation markers, alternative growth supports and substrates, and further defining regional classes of epithelium within the oral cavity. Unfortunately, the advancements in understanding the nature of the tissue have not resulted in the establishment of an oral epithelial cell differentiation state in vitro that completely or precisely represents the in vivo ideal. However, the current cell and tissue culture systems successfully mimic many of the features of oral tissues in vivo and have increasing utility. Consequently, some of the applications envisioned by MacCallum et al [1] for these tissue culture systems have been realized and warrant review by researchers in the drug delivery field.

The purpose of this chapter is to review the current state of epithelial cell cultures derived from the buccal region of the oral cavity. In particular, emphasis is placed on potential advantages, disadvantages, an overview of current cell culture types, and applications relevant to drug delivery or closely related problems, expanding on our earlier brief survey of this topic [2]. In this chapter, discussion on establishing buccal epithelial cell cultures will refer strictly to the generation of the complex tissue defined as a nonkeratinized stratified squamous epithelium typical of the buccal regions of the oral cavity (see Chapters 1 and 2).

II. BUCCAL EPITHELIAL CELL AND TISSUE CULTURE SYSTEMS AND APPROACHES

A. Advantages and Limitations

In general, there are several reasons to consider establishing cell and tissue culture systems for a given epithelial cell interface. Some of those reasons include: (i) expanding limited human or animal tissue samples, (ii) the possibility of establishing a cell line which would provide a consistent, continuous supply of tissue, (iii) the ability to readily manipulate experimental conditions (e.g., temperature, pH, irritant conditions, etc.) for characterization of biochemical mechanisms in a living system that is not feasible or possible in an animal or human model, (iv) the opportunity to study cell growth and differentiation processes, (v) the use of small volumes of assay solutions in these systems which allows conservation of costly drugs or agents, (vi) the rapid and convenient assay of permeability and metabolic pathways, (vii) the accessibility to both mucosal and serosal surfaces of tissue in transport or metabolism studies, and (viii) the minimization of extensive and sometimes difficult animal or human studies [2]. These advantages are particularly applicable to the development of tissue culture systems representing the buccal mucosal interface in view of the potential importance of the buccal route for systemic drug delivery.

There remains a formidable challenge to the establishment and development of an appropriate stratified squamous epithelial cell culture systems. The challenge is the defining of conditions for the establishment of a culture system that completely mimics the complex in vivo tissue with respect to cell growth and differentiation, permeability, and metabolism [1-3]. One only needs to look at the broad range of buccal epithelial cell culture systems described in the literature, as well as all of the modifications in culture variables including growth substrates, growth factors tested, serum or serum-free conditions, air-liquid interface growth, and isolation methods for buccal epithelial cells to appreciate the difficulty in this task. On the other hand, the use of different approaches and the manipulation of culture conditions contributes to our understanding of differentiation processes characteristic of stratified squamous epithelium [1, 4]. By analogy, the methodical examination of growth variables and conditions in skin cultures has resulted in the rapid improvement of the in vitro skin model recently described [5] from systems reviewed about five years ago [2].

B. Desirable Characteristics

The use of a particular cell or tissue culture system to mimic a biological barrier in drug delivery studies requires that it fulfill certain criteria with respect to basic anatomy. Although not technically possible for most cell and tissue culture systems in general, ideally, the first requirement would be that the in vitro biological barrier precisely reflects the in vivo biological barrier [2]. Therefore, the desirable morphological and histodifferentiation features of buccal epithelium in vitro would be as described in Chapters 1 and 2 of this book for the tissue in vivo. As stated earlier, many buccal epithelial cell and tissue culture systems have been reported that share similarities with, but do not precisely replicate, the in vivo state with respect to morphology and histodifferentiation. A total and complete replication in vitro is likely to be unrealistic, however, in view of the multitude of interactions that are necessary for normal growth and differentiation of tissues in vivo.

The development of stratified squamous epithelial cell cultures has been aided by the establishment of several specific differentiation parameters and biochemical markers. Cytokeratins 4, 5, 6, 13, 14, 17, and 19 [3, 6-13], involucrin expression [14, 15], lipids [16, 17], phemigus antigen [18], cell surface glycoconjugate [19] or mucin [20] receptors, and blood group markers [21-23], for buccal epithelium have been documented. As a minimum, one can expect to examine the general morphology, stratification/thickness, growth rates, ultrastructural markers, involucrin expression, and keratin profiles as a necessary part of the characterizing a buccal epithelial cell culture system. Additionally, investigators will identify and characterize markers (e.g., enzymes, permeability barrier, antigens, etc.) specific to the intended application of the culture system.

C. Current Cell and Tissue Culture Systems

Explant and conventional dispersed cell culture systems remain the primary methods to establish buccal epithelium in culture. Cell lines also now exist but have fairly specialized applications. Our purpose in this section is to summarize the types of culture systems available and some of the benefits and problems with each type of culture system. A general rule one may apply in the evaluation of these cell culture systems, apparent from development of recent cell culture systems for skin, is that the appearance of appropriate differentiation markers is typically coincident with the development of a permeability barrier and metabolic activity approaching that of the parent tissue [5].

1. Explant Cultures

More than any of the alternative culture systems, the explant type systems have been successfully established and characterized in a number of laboratories. Rabbit [24-26], hamster [27, 28], murine [29], rat [30-34], and human [15, 31, 35-42] systems have been described. To establish an explant culture in primary culture, small samples of excised buccal epithelium are dissected free of underlying submucosa, placed epithelial side up either directly in a culture dish or on a gelatinous sponge support structure [42], and bathed in an appropriate culture medium. This represents an organ-type culture system, generally used in short-term studies. For development of other cultures, after 2-3 weeks, explants that produce outgrowths can be transferred to different dishes to re-establish new primary cultures. Outgrowths can also be collected and dissociated into single cells and grown onto fibronectin/collagen-coated dishes. The latter process can be repeated to produce numerous subcultures or passages. Specific details of these procedures are described for human tissue in recent reports by Sundqvist et al [15] and Liu et al [42]. These studies are noteworthy in that the roles of several growth factors and conditions are examined in the establishment of cultures that approach the in vivo state with regard to morphology, involucrin expression, and cytokeratin profiles.

The advantages of the explants in primary culture are that one maintains the original parent tissue architecture, cell:cell interactions, and cell:matrix contacts of the in vivo state. However, this situation exists only if the explant tissue is maintained under organ culture conditions and as a short term culture. Alternatively, the epithelial cells that are harvested following migration out of explants in long term cultures can be passaged. Therefore, with small tissue samples, one can generate large numbers of pure keratinocytes [42, 43]. A disadvantage of the latter process is the presence of other cell types that, if not controlled, can contaminate the cultures and interfere with the interpretation of the roles of specific cell types. The utility of explant cultures in transepithelial diffusion studies has not been investigated, however, as discussed below, they have found application to the study of metabolism, carcinogenesis, and toxicology of the buccal epithelium.

2. Dissociated Cell Cultures

Buccal epithelial cell cultures may also be generated by dissociation of epithelial cells from freshly excised tissues. Hamster [44, 45] and human [40-

42] systems have been established. To isolate buccal epithelial cells, the surgically excised buccal tissues are treated first with a collagenase to lift the epithelium off underlying connective tissue and then incubated in a trypsin solution to dissociate the epithelial sheets into single cells. The dissociated cells are suspended in an appropriate culture medium and seeded onto a collagen/fibronectin coated surface [40-42, 45]. Alternatively, Percoll gradients can be used to isolate purified subpopulations of cells [44]. Cells may be subcultured or passaged by dissociating subconfluent primary cultures and seeding the cells onto new growth surfaces several times in succession. Sundqvist et al [40] provides a recent detailed protocol for this procedure.

As for the explant cultures, this culture system provides a means to expand a small tissue sample to a larger population of pure keratinocytes. Populations of cells isolated in this manner will form a confluent monolayer, stratify, and differentiate in primary culture to a tissue that retains some of the typical buccal epithelial keratin and enzymatic markers [40, 44, 45]. Comparison studies between explant and dissociated cultures are lacking although there is some indication that the primary cultures derived from dissociated cells have a higher metabolic activity than the primary explant culture type [42]. The short term organ-type explant cultures, however, likely retain more of the parent anatomical structure. Thus, a significant drawback to the dissociated cultures, thus far, is the absence of a precise correlation to the in vivo architecture [2]. Despite the limitations, dissociated type cultures have been used for metabolism, toxicology, and limited permeability studies as discussed in later sections of this chapter.

3. Cell Lines

Several approaches have been taken in the development of appropriate buccal epithelial cell lines. Cell lines have the convenience of being provided as a frozen dissociated cell suspension that can be seeded onto an appropriate growth surface and then passaged multiple times without loss of morphological or biochemical properties. Most of these systems have had specific applications that have required less concern about morphology and histodifferentiation.

In one approach, subpopulations of cells have been isolated by dissociation techniques, cloned out, and studied. Polverini and Solt [44, 46] described the isolation of two subpopulations, subclones I and II, from both normal and carcinogen-treated hamster buccal epithelial cells. In culture, the subclones can be readily distinguished from one another by their morphologies at the light microscope level. The more abundant nonstratifying subclone I has been used further for characterization of normal lipid metabolism of buccal epithelia [17]. The subclone II type was identified as a cell population with preneoplastic properties following exposure to carcinogens. Both subclones retain varying degrees of keratinization [46].

A human buccal carcinoma cell line, SqCC/Y1, has been used to assess the cytotoxicity and genotoxicity of nitrosoamines [40-42]. Sundqvist et al [40] has described the essential characteristics of this cell line. A drawback is that the SqCC/Y1 cell line is apparently defective in its ability to undergo differentiation [41]. Min et al [47] described the establishment of three buccal epithelial cell lines from hamster pouches pretreated in vivo with combinations of the carcinogen 7, 12-dimethylbenz[α]anthracene (DMBA) alone or with type 1 herpes simplex virus (HSV-1) or type 2 HSV (HSV-2). These cells also do not stratify, but exhibit epithelial-like morphology and are keratin positive. The primary application of these cells has been for investigation of the expression of proto-oncogenes following exposure to co-carcinogens DMBA and HSV [47].

Finally, Rupniak et al [48] established a human cell line from a squamous cell carcinoma, TR146, of the buccal mucosa that had infiltrated a lymph node. The cell line retains a squamous cell morphology, are positive for some simple keratins, and undergo stratification in culture. Quite recently, Jacobsen et al [49] described the use of this cell line for permeability studies.

The goal of most cell and tissue culture efforts is to establish an appropriately characterized, homogenous, and stable cell line. The cell line can offer convenient, consistent, and unlimited sources of buccal epithelium. A drawback, unfortunately, is the tendency of cell line properties to undergo differentiation changes with increasing subculture or passage [2]. The buccal epithelial cell lines available currently were developed for specific applications but may represent starting points for the eventual development of appropriate cell lines and therefore, warrant further investigation.

III. APPLICATIONS OF BUCCAL EPITHELIAL CELL AND TISSUE CULTURE SYSTEMS TO DRUG DELIVERY

Drugs applied in the oral cavity are targeted either to local tissue sites or the underlying systemic circulation. Several drug delivery systems have been described for these purposes [50]. Although most of the experimental work with these drug delivery systems has been with in vivo and alternative in vitro models, a few studies summarized here have considered the potential application of buccal epithelial cell culture to evaluate drug delivery systems. Readers are directed to other sources for an extensive consideration of relevant quantitative approaches [51] in applying cell and tissue culture systems to drug transport and metabolism studies.

Table 1. Apparent Permeability Coefficients for the Transfer of Selected Substances Across Hamster Pouch Buccal Epithelial Cells in Primary Culture at 37°C.

Substance	Molecular Weight	Log K_p [a]	P (x 10^5) (cm/second)[b]	Reference
Water	18	-	20.0 ± 1.4	45
Sucrose	342	-	1.1 ± 0.2	45
Fluorescein	376	-	0.6 ± 0.2	45
FITDC[c]	3860	-	0.2 ± 0.1	45
FITDC[c]	40500	-	0.04 ± 0.002	45
Propranolol	259	1.54	21.8 ± 0.2	52
Alprenolol	249	1.23	21.0 ± 0.3	52
Metoprolol	267	0.07	17.1 ± 0.3	52
Pindolol	248	-0.20	13.6 ± 0.1	52
Atenolol	266	-1.40	11.0 ± 0.04	52

[a]Partition coefficient for octanol/buffer, pH 7.4 [45]. [b]Apparent permeability coefficients for buccal epithelial cells (P_{cells}) calculated from the relationship $1/P_{total} = 1/P_{collagen} + 1/P_{cells}$ where P_{total} is the overall permeability coefficient for buccal epithelial cells on collagen-coated polycarbonate filters, $P_{collagen}$ is the permeability coefficient for the collagen-coated polycarbonate filters alone, and P_{cells} is the permeability coefficient for buccal epithelial cells alone [51]. Data represent mean ± SD for $n > 4$. [c]Fluorescein isothiocyanate dextran conjugate (the average molecular weight is listed).

A. Transepithelial Diffusion

Application of buccal epithelial cell cultures to study the transepithelial diffusions of drugs has been limited by the lack of the development of a permeability barrier typical of the in vivo situation. There have been a couple of attempts at characterizing the permeability properties of buccal epithelial cell cultures. Primary cultures of hamster buccal epithelial cells have been successfully grown onto porous, collagen-coated polycarbonate supports [2]. Realistically, excised pieces of hamster pouch buccal epithelium can not be used as explant organ cultures since the tissue is a keratinized interface. On the other hand, primary cultures developed from dissociated hamster pouch buccal epithelium do not fully keratinize, a condition more reflective of the human buccal mucosa [45]. The primary cultures generated by this method expressed the buccal epithelial phenotypic features including stratification, typical desmosomal junctions, interdigitation, tonofilaments, surface microvilli, and keratins, and enzymes typical of the parent tissue after three days in culture [45]. Table 1 summarizes the typical permeability properties for these cultures.

Although the water permeability of the primary cultures was higher than for the parent excised tissue, the primary cultures were essentially impermeable to dextrans with molecular weights greater than about 18 000 [45]. The size cut-off for permeability compares favorably with the observations with excised porcine buccal tissue which was shown to be impermeable to dextrans with molecular weights of 20 000 or greater [52]. The primary culture system also exhibits differential permeability to β-adrenergic antagonists varying in lipophilicity and of different ionization states [53]. Only in a qualitative manner do the latter permeability properties of the in vitro system parallel in vivo observations. Collectively, these results suggested that the intercellular spaces between the stratified cells may be sufficiently developed to restrict diffusion of macromolecules but not developed enough to regulate the diffusion of low molecular weight substances [45, 53].

More recently, Jacobsen et al [49] have established the human cell line, TR146, grown onto transparent permeable teflon supports as an in vitro model for studying transport pathways or mechanisms. Morphological and biochemical properties of the tissue in this orientation were similar to normal human buccal epithelium. These cultures achieved a maximum barrier to permeability after about 30 days in culture as measured by transepithelial electrical resistances and impermeability to mannitol [49]. Based on the numbers reported for mannitol and testosterone, this system appears to form a more restrictive barrier in vitro than the primary cultures of hamster pouch buccal epithelium described above. Although extensive validation of TR146 is required, this cell line should receive immediate consideration by interested researchers for possible applications in drug delivery studies.

The further manipulation of buccal epithelial cell culture conditions should result in a tissue of greater thickness (more layers) and a more representative intercellular barrier. One aspect to consider is that the cellular and lamellar intercellular lipid components of the skin and buccal epithelium have been demonstrated to be critical determinants of the permeability barrier in this tissue [16]. Agents that perturb the lipid components of buccal epithelium generally also have permeability enhancing effects [54], further supporting the importance of lipids in tissue barrier formation. A recent study suggests that understanding sterol metabolism in buccal epithelial cells may be a key in appropriate growth and differentiation, including lipid components [17]. This is consistent with the cholesterol-rich lipid supplements added to growth medium necessary to support proper differentiation of skin in vitro with more restrictive permeability properties [5].

Other considerations in the development of the cultures will be the possible use of a variety of growth surfaces and including establishing cultures at the air-liquid interface. For example, in development of the successful skin model, the establishment of a dermis consisting of neonatal fibroblasts grown on a nylon mesh was required to facilitate deposition of a more natural extracellular matrix. In this configuration, a three-dimensional tissue-like structure is developed and the differentiation of keratinocytes on this extracellular matrix at an air-liquid interface occurs in a manner reflective of the skin. Consequently, the resulting cultures are more representative of the dermal transport and metabolic barrier [5]. Taking the lead from successes with skin cultures, buccal epithelial cell cultures now appear at a point in development where manipulation of lipid metabolism, extracellular matrices, and placement at the air-liquid interface influence development of an appropriate permeability barrier in vitro.

B. Metabolism

The contributions of metabolic pathways in the buccal tissue are of particular and obvious interest in regulating drug delivery [50]. This application is an area where buccal epithelial cell and tissue culture systems have contributed significantly in carcinogenesis studies and presents several possibilities for drug delivery studies. In particular, there remains a very poor understanding of the intracellular or extracellular distribution of the enzymes of the oral mucosa [55].

In primary culture, buccal epithelial cells have been observed to retain the activities of variety of enzyme systems. An example of comparisons between freshly excised hamster pouch epithelium and primary cultures is shown in Figure 1. For the most part, retention of enzyme activities approaching excised

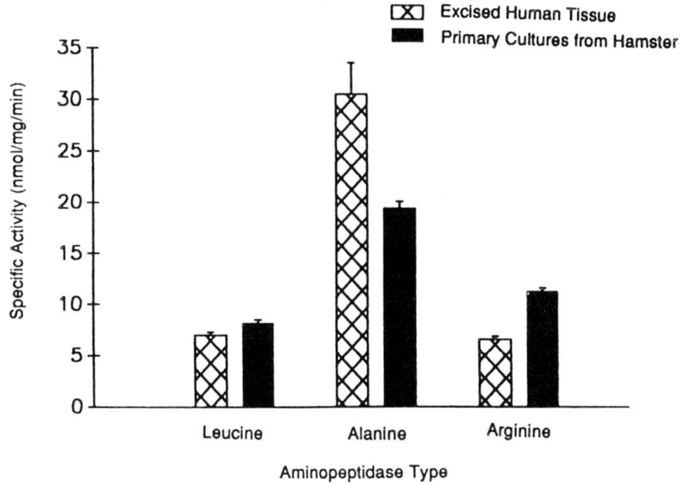

Figure 1. Specific activities of selected enzymes in either primary cultures or freshly excised hamster pouch buccal epithelium. Data points represent mean ± SD. (Compiled from reference 45).

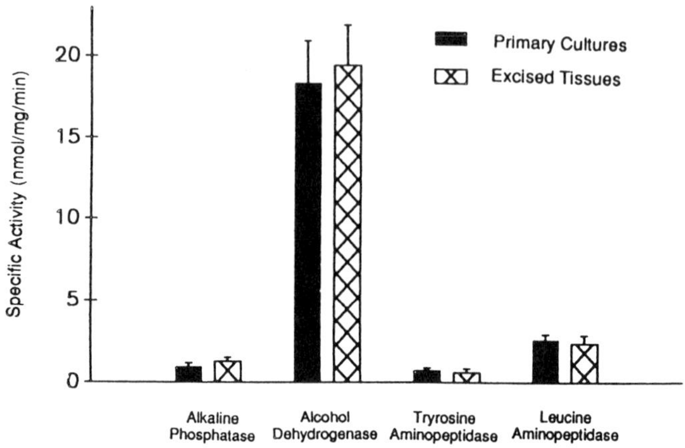

Figure 2. Specific activities of aminopeptidases assayed with indicated 4-methoxy-2-naphthylamide substrates in homogenates of either freshly excised human or primary cultures of hamster buccal epithelium. Data points represent a mean ± SD. (Compiled from reference 56).

tissue levels has been characteristic of primary cultures [42, 44, 45, 56]. Generally, passaging or transformation of buccal epithelialcells in culture, as for other epithelial cell types, results in loss of enzyme activity or expression as reported recently by Liu et al [42]. A few direct comparison studies of species differences in metabolism have been reported. Figure 2 shows that comparable specific activities for aminopeptidases in both primary cultures of hamster and excised human buccal epithelium. In addition, the sensitivity of the aminopeptidases to selected inhibitors in both the rodent buccal epithelial cell cultures and human buccal epithelial cells was comparable [56]. As might be expected, both differences and similarities exist between human and rat in cytochrome P450 pathways. The oxidation of benzy[α]pyrene oxidation [31] and some nitrosoamines [42] in buccal epithelial cell cultures show that both species usually retain similar enzymes but with different levels of activities in some instances.

For many conventional drug molecules, degradation mediated by cytochrome P450 enzymes is a frequent concern of the pharmaceutical scientist. The role of buccal cell culture systems in carcinogenesis studies is worth noting since such studies demonstrated the presence and the retention of cytochrome P450 enzymes. The absence of detoxifying Phase II pathways such as glucuronidation, adds importance to the buccal cytochrome P450 systems

[42]. As alluded to earlier, both human and rodent buccal epithelial cell culture systems have been used to study potent carcinogenic metabolite generation from tobacco products (e.g., chewing or snuff dipping) and betel quid chewing [31-34, 37, 39, 42, 57]. In the more recent of the various reports on these substances, Liu et al [42] were able to demonstrate retention of typical cytochrome P450 pathways for the metabolism of nitrosoamines in human buccal explant, normal dissociated, and transformed epithelial cell cultures. Each of the cell culture systems employed in this study contributed in some way to the characterization of buccal epithelial enzyme pathways [42].

In related work, enzyme expression or secretion by buccal epithelial cells in culture systems has been used as an analytical tool to study neoplastic development in the oral tissues. The expression of gamma-glutamyl transpeptidase by buccal epithelial cells following carcinogen exposure can be used as a marker for the tumorigenic potential of the cells [44, 46]. Similarly, plasminogen activator enzymes secreted by buccal epithelial cells in culture and in vivo have been examined for utility as markers of the neoplastic transformation potential of oral tissue [58, 59].

C. Intraoral Delivery and Pharmacology

Rodent buccal epithelial cell cultures of the explant type have been used to assess and demonstrate the ultrastructural features of colonization and invasion of oral epithelium by *Candida albicans* [24-26]. For the pharmaceutical scientist, this work has established a basis for applying buccal epithelial cell cultures to the in vitro evaluation of the efficacy of antimicrobial agents released from intraoral delivery systems or formulations.

Chlorhexidine and other antifungals have been proposed for inclusion into intraoral controlled release devices for hygiene maintenance in physically and mentally incapacitated or challenged individuals [60]. The activity of both chlorhexidine digluconate solutions and nystatin suspensions against *Candida albicans* in suspensions of isolated human buccal epithelial cells can be readily shown in vitro [61]. However, while human buccal epithelial cells can be readily obtained by gently scraping the buccal regions of volunteers with a wooden spatula, the suspensions of isolated cells are of very low viability and can be contaminated by foods, environmental agents [e.g., smoking, tobacco chewing], and microorganisms that may complicate interpretation and produce considerable variation in experimental results.

Preliminary work in our laboratories suggests that the antimycotic efficacy of chlorhexidine digluconate, released from multilayered bioadhesive drug delivery systems described by Rytting et al [62], can be assessed with cells derived from rodent buccal epithelial cell cultures. On the basis that hamster pouch buccal epithelium in vivo can be infected with *Candida albicans* [63], primary cultures of hamster buccal epithelial cells were established [45]. Chlorhexidine digluconate-induced release of yeasts from the hamster buccal epithelial cells was concentration dependent and similar to previously reported observations with human buccal epithelial cells [61]. Again, the chief advantage of using rodent buccal epithelial cell cultures to generate cells for these studies versus isolated human buccal epithelial cells is that one can work with a viable cell population that has not been exposed to food or other chewed and ingested materials prior to experimentation. In addition, one can assess the effect of any treatment, formulation component, or materials released from the delivery device on the viability of both the buccal epithelial cells and the detached and adherent yeasts.

Potentially, intact cell and tissue cultures could be used to study mechanisms through which drugs might interfere with microorganism colonization and invasion of buccal epithelium.

D. Toxicology

A battery of assays of irritancy, cytotoxicity and genotoxicity have been adapted to buccal epithelial cell culture systems and are summarized in Table 2. As an example of the applications in this area, researchers have shown that nitrosoamines produce DNA damage and effectively suppress buccal epithelial cell growth, differentiation and colony formation [32, 39, 41, 44]. These studies have been important for identifying cytotoxic effects specific to different nitrosoamine metabolites and an aqueous extracted form that proved to be the severely toxic agent and a likely candidate for induction of tumors [39, 41]. In another type of application in this general area, the carcinogenic potential of buccal epithelial cell cultures derived from carcinogen-treated tissues in vivo, has been assessed by determining their ability to stimulate angiogenesis, a requirement for solid tumor growth. Poverini and Solt [46] were able to isolate an angiogenic phenotype of keratinocytes from hamster buccal epithelial cultures with presumptive preneoplastic properties based on stimulation of neovascularization in vivo and endothelial cell migration in vitro.

In our laboratories, the cytotoxic effects of the antifungal drugs, nystatin and chlorhexidine, on buccal epithelial cell cultures has been assayed by colony forming efficiency and hydrolysis of a vital dye, MTT [64]. Typical therapeutic application of chlorhexidine calls for a twice daily rinses of the oral cavity with 0.1 to 0.2% solutions [65, 66], a concentration range considerably higher than the in vitro IC_{50}s of 0.002-0.007% [64]. However, the oral mucosal exposure time to the high concentrations of the drug rinse in vivo, is short (<1 minute), and although chlorhexidine binds to the buccal tissue, the agent does not generally diffuse into the metabolically active, growing basal layers of normal

Table 2. Irritancy, Cytotoxicity, and Genotoxicity Assays Adapted to Buccal Epithelial Cell Culture Systems.

Morphology
Light and electron microscopy [41, 44]
Cell Growth
Colony forming efficiency [15, 39-42, 44, 64]
Thymidine incorporation [39, 45]
DNA binding, damage and repair [31, 32, 41]
Gamma-glutamyl transpeptidase [44]
Vital Dyes
Neutral red uptake [39]
MTT[a] hydrolysis [64]
Trypan blue exclusion [39]

[a]3-(4,5-dimethyl-2-thiazoyl)-2,5-diphenyl-2*H*-tetrazolium bromide

tissue. In vitro we also observed that, the shorter the exposure time, the more resistance buccal epithelial cell cultures show to the cytotoxic effects of chlorhexidine digluconate. Following a five minute exposure to 0.01% chlorhexidine digluconate, for instance, >80% viability of was still observed [64]. Furthermore, drug induced buccal epithelial cell membrane perturbations did not occur except at concentrations >0.15% after the five minute exposure time [61]. In the context of other cytotoxicity studies, buccal epithelial cells were more resistant to the cytotoxic effects of the antifungal drugs than other epithelial and systemic cell types [64].

The cell culture systems offer dynamic, living systems with the added flexibility of permitting manipulation of several experimental variables. Therefore, one might easily envision further exploitation of buccal epithelial cell culture systems to quickly evaluate the irritancy, cytotoxicity, or genotoxicity potential of orally applied drugs or treatments and formulation materials.

IV. FUTURE PERSPECTIVES

Buccal epithelial cell and tissue culture systems have met with some success and have current applications across a number of different disciplines including cell biology, oncology, oral biology, pharmacology, toxicology, and pharmaceutics. Perhaps an additional indication that cell cultures derived from the oral mucosa have made steady progress towards establishing a more in vivo-like state is their application as suitable transplantation tissue for individuals with oral mucosal defects [67]. Clearly, all disciplines will continue to benefit from the future development of systems that more closely mimic the in vivo or ideal state.

Drug delivery research in particular can benefit from buccal epithelial cell and tissue culture systems both now and in the future. Specifically, appropriate tissue culture systems can provide important information on the metabolism, irritancy and biocompatibility potential of orally applied drug formulations and their constituents, absorption enhancers, and bioadhesives, as suggested by MacCallum et al [1]. In the evaluation of some biotechnology products, for instance, preliminary in vitro screening systems using small amounts of product could be important for conservation of an expensive product, reducing animal use and maintenance, and overall, controlling costs. The eventual understanding of the factors necessary for development of the appropriate differentiation, thickness, and permeability barrier in tissue culture will perhaps some day provide a more refined, closer to ideal, tissue culture system for studying transepithelial diffusion.

V. ACKNOWLEDGMENTS

Support for the author's research on topics discussed in this paper was received from INTERx Research Corporation, a Merck & Co. subsidiary, Lawrence, KS, and the National Institute on Dental Research (NIDR NO-DE-92575).

REFERENCES

1. D. K. MacCallum, J. H. Lillie, A. Jepsen, and D. Arenholt-Bindslev, The culture of oral epithelium, *Int. Rev. Cytol. 109*:313 (1987).
2. K. L. Audus, R. L. Bartel, I. J. Hidalgo, and R. T. Borchardt, The use of cultured epithelial and endothelial cells for drug transport and metabolism studies, *Pharm. Res. 7*:435 (1990).
3. A. H. M. Shabana, J. P. Ouhayoun, M. H. Sawaf, and N. Forest, Cytokeratin patterns of human oral mucosae in histiotypic culture, *Arch. Oral Biol. 36*:747 (1991).
4. D. C. Gruenert, Differentiated properties of human epithelial cells transformed in vitro, *BioTechniques 5*:740 (1987).
5. S. R. Slivka, L. K. Landeen, F. Zeigler, M. P. Zimber, and R. L. Bartel, Characterization, barrier function, and drug metabolism of an in vitro skin model, *J. Invest. Dermatol. 100*:40 (1993).
6. R. Moll, W. F. Franke, D. L. Schiller, B. Geiger, and R. Krepler, The catalog of human cytokeratins: Patterns of expression in normal epithelia, tumors, and cultured cells, *Cell 31*:11 (1982).

7. J. P. Ouhayoun, F. Gosselin, N. Forest, S. Winter, and W. W. Franke, Cytokeratin patterns of human oral epithelia. Differences in cytokeratin synthesis in gingival epithelium and the adjacent aveolar mucosa, *Differentiation 30*:123 (1985).
8. H. Clausen, D. Moe, D. Buscard, and E. Dabelsteen, Keratin proteins in human oral mucosa, *J. Oral Path. 15*:36 (1986).
9. H. Clausen, P. Vedtofte, D. Moe, and E. Dabelsteen, Differentiation-dependent expression of keratins in human oral epithelia, *J. Invest. Dermatol. 86*:249 (1986).
10. P. R. Morgan, I. Leigh, P. E. Purkis, I. D. Gardner, G. N. P. van Muijen, and E. B. Lane, Site variation in keratin expression in human oral epithelia - an immunocytochemical study of individual keratins, *Epithelia 1*:31 (1987).
11. M. Juhl, J. Reibel, and K. Stoltze, Immunohistochemical distribution of keratin proteins in clinically healthy human gingival epithelium, *Scand. J. Dent. Res. 97*:159 (1989).
12. A. H. M. Shabana, J. P. Ouhayoun, M. H. Sawaf, and N. Forest, A biochemical and immunological analysis of cytokeratin patterns in the oral epithelium of the minature pig and man, *Arch. Oral Biol. 34*:249 (1989).
13. D. Oda, B. A. Dale, and G. Bourekis, Human oral epithelial cell culture II. Keratin expression in fetal and adult gingival cells, *In Vitro Cell. Dev. Biol. 26*:596 (1990).
14. S. P. Banks-Schlegel, and H. Green, Involucrin synthesis and tissue assembly by keratinocytes in natural and cultured human epithelia, *J. Cell Biol. 90*:732 (1981).
15. K. Sundqvist, Y. Liu, K. Arvidson, K. Ormstad, L. Nilsson, R. Toftgard, and R. C. Grafström, Growth regulation of serum-free cultures of epithelial cells from normal human buccal mucosa, *In Vitro Cell. Dev. Biol. 27A*:562 (1991).
16. C. A. Squier, P. Cox, and P. W. Wertz, Lipid content and water permeability of skin and oral mucosa, *J. Invest. Dermatol. 96*:123 (1991).
17. G. B. Caughman, G. S. Schuster, and T. R. Dirksen, Sterol metabolism and oral epithelial cell growth, *In Vitro Cell. Dev. Biol. 29A*:693 (1993).
18. E. Acosta, and L. Ivanyi, Oral epithelial cells as the origin of phemigus antigen in human saliva, *Arch. Oral Biol. 30*:23 (1985).
19. D. Brassart, A. Woltz, M. Golliard, and J. R. Neeser, In vitro adhesion of *Candida albicans* clinical isolates to human buccal epithelial cells by Fucα1-2Galβ-bearing complex carbohydrates, *Infect. Immun. 59*:1605 (1991).
20. B. L. Slomiany, J. Piotrowski, J. Majka, Y. H. Liau, and A. Slomiany, Identification of buccal mucosal mucin receptor, *Biochem. Mol. Biol. Int. 31*:1091 (1993).

21. E. Dabelsteen, P. Vedtofte, S. -I. Hakomori, and W. W. Young, Carbohydrate chains specific for blood group antigens in differentiation of human oral epithelium, *J. Invest. Dermatol. 79*:3 (1982).
22. U. Mandel, T. F. Orntoft, E. H. Holmes, H. Sorenson, H. Clausen, S. I. Hakomori, and E. Dabelsteen, Lewis blood-group antigens in salivary glands and stratified epithelium - lack of regulation of Lewis antigen expression in ductal and buccal mucosal lining epithelia, *Vox Sanguinis 61*:205 (1991).
23. M. Venegas, A. Schaeffer, E. Navas, and B. Anderson, Detection and quantitation of blood-group antigens in human buccal and vaginal mucous glycoproteins, *FASEB J. 5*:A458 (1991).
24. J. A. Howlett, The infection of rat tongue mucosa in vitro with five species of *Candida*, *J. Med. Microbiol. 9*:309 (1976).
25. J. A. Howlett, Candidal infection of oral mucosa, an in-vitro model, *Proc. R. Soc. Med. 69*:766 (1976).
26. J. A. Howlett, and C. A. Squier, *Candida albicans* ultrastructure: Colonization and invasion of oral epithelium, *Infect. Immun. 29*:252 (1980).
27. D. Mock, and J. H. P. Main, Long term organ culture of hamster pouch mucosa, *J. Oral Pathol. 5*:237 (1976).
28. B. B. Singh, G. S. Schuster, J. F. Erbland, and M. B. Ringler, Effects of calcium ions on hamster cheek pouch epithelium grown in vitro, *J. Oral Pathol. 12*:62 (1983).
29. P. G. Sacks, S. M. Parnes, J. C. Price, H. Risemberg, J. C. Goldstein, M. Marko, and D. F. Parsons, In vitro modulation of differentiation by calcium in organ cultures of human and murine epithelial tissue, *In Vitro Cell. Develop. Biol. 21*:99 (1985).
30. A. Jepsen, An in vitro model of oral keratinizing squamous epithelium, *Scand. J. Dent. Res. 82*:144 (1974).
31. H. Autrup, T. Seremet, D. Arenholt, L. Dragsted, and A. Jepsen, Metabolism of benzo[α]pyrene by cultured rat and human buccal mucosal cells, *Carcinogenesis (Lond.) 6*:1761 (1985).
32. J. L. Autrup, and H. Autrup, Metabolism of tobacco-specific carcinogens in cultured rat buccal mucosal epithelial cells, *Acta Pharmacol. Toxicol. 59*:339 (1986).
33. S. E. Murphy, R. Heiblum, and N. Trushin, Comparative metabolism of N'-nitrosonornicotine and 4-(methylnitrosoamino)-1-(3-pyridyl)-1-butanone by cultured F344 rat oral tissue and esophagus, *Cancer Res. 50*:4658 (1990).
34. J. L. Autrup, C. Hansen, and H. Autrup, Detection of tobacco-smoke carcinogen-DNA adducts in cultured rat buccal mucosal cells following exposure to ethanol and total cigarette-smoke condensate or chewing tobacco, *Chem. Biol. Inter. 85*:141 (1992).

35. B. A. Gusterson, and P. Monaghan, Keratinocyte differentiation of human buccal mucosa in vitro, *Invest. Cell Pathol. 2*:171 (1979).
36. L. Taichman, S. Reilly, and P. R. Grant, In vitro cultivation of human oral keratinocytes, *Arch. Oral Biol. 24*:335 (1979).
37. A. Castonguay, G. D. Stoner, H. A. I. Schut, and S. S. Hecht, Metabolism of tobacco-specific N-nitrosoamines by cultured human tissues, *Proc. Natl. Acad. Sci. USA 80*:6694 (1983).
38. D. Arenholt-Bindslev, A. Jepsen, D. K. MacCallum, and J. H. Lillie, The growth and structure of human oral keratinocytes in culture, *J. Invest. Dermatol. 88*:314 (1987).
39. K. Sundqvist, Y. Liu, J. Nair, H. Bartsch, K. Arvidson, and R. C. Grafström, Cytotoxic and genotoxic effects of areca nut-related compounds in cultured human buccal epithelial cells, *Cancer Res. 49*:5294 (1989).
40. K. Sundqvist, P. Kulkarni, S. S. Hybbinette, F. Bertolero, Y. Liu, and R. C. Grafström, Serum-free growth and karyotype analyses of cultured normal and tumorous (Sqcc/Y1) human buccal epithelial cells, *Cancer Comm. 3*:331 (1991).
41. K. Sundqvist, and R. C. Grafström, Effects of areca nut on growth, differentiation and formation of DNA damage in cultured human buccal epithelial cells, *Int. J. Cancer 52*:305 (1992).
42. Y. Liu, K. Sundqvist, S. A. Belinsky, A. Castonguay, H. Tjalve, and R. C. Grafstrom, Metabolism and macromolecular interaction of the tobacco-specific carcinogen 4-(methylnitrosoamino)-1-(3-pyridyl)-1-butanone in cultured explants and epithelial cells of human buccal mucosa, *Carcinogenesis 14*:2383 (1993).
43. S. M. Fischer, A. Viaje, G. D. Mills, and T. J. Slaga, Explant methods for epidermal cell culture, *Meth. Cell Biol. 21A*:207 (1980).
44. P. J. Polverini, and D. B. Solt, Effect of in vivo carcinogen exposure on colony formation and growth of hamster buccal pouch keratinocytes in culture, *Lab. Invest. 54*:432 (1986).
45. M. R. Tavakoli-Saberi, and K. L. Audus, Cultured buccal epithelium: An in vitro model derived from the hamster pouch for studying drug transport and metabolism, *Pharm. Res. 6*:160 (1989).
46. P. J. Polverini, and D. B. Solt, Expression of the angiogenic phenotype by a subpopulation of keratinocytes derived from 7, 12-dimethylbenz[α]anthracene-initiated hamster pouch buccal epithelium, *Carcinogenesis 9*:117 (1988).
47. B. M. Min, K. Kim, H. M. Cherrick, and N. H. Park, Three cell lines from hamster buccal pouch tumors induced by topical 7, 12-dimethylbenz[α]anthracene, alone, or in combination with herpes simplex virus inoculation, *In Vitro Cell. Dev. Biol. 27A*:128 (1991).

48. H. T. Rupniak, C. Rowlatt, E. B. Lane, J. G. Steele, L. K. Trejdosiewicz, B. Laskiewicz, S. Povey, and B. T. Hill, Characteristics of four new human cell lines derived from squamous cell carcinomas of the head and neck, *J. Natl. Cancer Inst. 75*:621 (1985).
49. J. Jacobsen, B. van Deurs, M. Pedersen, and M. R. Rassing, TR146 cells grown on filters as a model for human buccal epithelium. I: Morphology, growth, barrier properties, and permeability, *Int. J. Pharm. 125*:165 (1995).
50. H. P. Merkle, and G. J. M. Wolany, Intraoral peptide absorption, *Biological Barriers to Protein Delivery* (K. L. Audus and T. J. Raub, eds.), Plenum Press, New York, 1993, p. 131.
51. N. F. H. Ho, T. J. Raub, P. S. Burton, C. L. Barsuhn, A. Adson, K. L. Audus, and R. T. Borchardt, Quantitative approaches to delineate passive transport mechanisms in cell culture monolayers, *Transport Processes in Pharmaceutical Systems* (K. J. Himmelstein, G. L. Amidon, and P. I. Lee, eds.), Marcel Dekker, Inc., New York, 1995, in press.
52. A. J. Hoogstraate, C. Cullander, J. F. Nagelkerke, S. Senel, J. C. Verhoef, H. E. Junginger, and H. E. Boddé, Diffusion rates and transport pathways of fluorescein isothiocyanate (FITC)-labeled model compounds through buccal epithelium, *Pharm. Res. 11*:83 (1994).
53. M. R. Tavakoli-Saberi, and K. L. Audus, Physicochemical factors affecting β-adrenergic antagonist permeation across cultured hamster pouch buccal epithelium, *Int. J. Pharm. 56*:135 (1989).
54. T. M. Turunen, A. Urtti, P. Paronen, K. L. Audus, and J. H. Rytting, Effect of some penetration enhancers on epithelial membrane lipid domains: Evidence from fluorescence spectroscopy studies, *Pharm. Res. 11*:288 (1994).
55. P. K. Gupta, S. -H. S. Leung, and J. R. Robinson, Bioadhesives/mucoadhesives in drug delivery to the gastrointestinal tract, *Bioadhesive Drug Delivery Systems* (V. Lenaerts and R. Gurney, eds.), CRC Press, Boca Raton, Florida, 1990, p. 66.
56. K. L. Audus, A. Williams, and M. R. Tavakoli-Saberi, A comparison of aminopeptidases from excised human buccal epithelium and primary cultures of hamster pouch buccal epithelium, *J. Pharm. Pharmacol. 43*:363 (1991).
57. R. C. Grafström, Carcinogenesis studies in human epithelial tissues and cells in vitro: Emphasis on serum-free culture conditions and transformation studies, *Acta Physiol. Scand. 140(Suppl. 592)*:93 (1990).
58. S. Sindet-Pederson , J. Gram, and J. Jespersen, The possible role of oral epithelial cells in tissue-type plasminogen-activator-related fibrinolysis in human saliva, *J. Dent. Res. 69*:1283 (1990).

59. Y. Barlow and J. C. Southam, Plasminogen activators in normal and malignant oral epithelium in vivo and in vitro, *Arch. Oral Biol. 37*:749 (1992).
60. D. B. Mirth, A. Bartkiewicz, R. J. Shern, and W. A. Little, Development and in vitro evaluation of an intra-oral controlled release delivery system for chlorhexidine, *J. Dent. Res. 68*:1285 (1989).
61. K. L. Audus, M. R. Tavakoli-Saberi, and E. N. Boyce, Chlorhexidine effects on membrane lipid domains of human buccal epithelial cells, *J. Dent. Res. 71*:1298 (1992).
62. J. H. Rytting, J. J. Hefferren, H. Qi, T. Itoh, T. Nishihata, and E. Boyce, Bioadhesive system for intraoral delivery of chlorhexidine, *Proceed. Int. Sym. Control. Rel. Bioact. Mater. 18*:115 (1991).
63. M. D. McMillan, and V. M. Cowell, Experimental candidiasis in the hamster cheek pouch, *Arch. Oral Biol. 30*:249 (1985).
64. H. Zheng and K. L. Audus, Cytotoxic effects of chlorhexidine and nystatin on cultured buccal epithelial cells, *Int. J. Pharm. 101*:121 (1994).
65. H. Loe, Does chlorhexidine have a place in the prophylaxis of dental disease?, *J. Periodont. Res. 8*:93 (1973).
66. G. Grennstein, D. Berman, and R. Jaffin, Chlorhexidine, an adjunct to periodontal therapy, *J. Periodontol. Res. 57*:370 (1985).
67. M. De Luca, E. Albanese, M. Megna, R. Cancedda, P. E. Mangiante, A. Cadoni, and A. T. Franzi, Evidence that human oral epithelium reconstituted in vitro and transplanted onto patients with defects in the oral mucosa retains properties of the original donor site, *Transplantation 50*:454 (1990).

7

In Vivo Techniques for Studying the Oral Mucosal Absorption Characteristics of Drugs in Animals and Humans

Michael J. Rathbone
InterAg, New Zealand

Robert Purves
University of Otago, New Zealand

Firoz A. Ghazali
University of Otago, New Zealand

Ping C. Ho
University of Otago, New Zealand

I. INTRODUCTION

Irrespective of whether a drug is administered to the mouth to treat local conditions of the oral tissues or with the intention to produce a systemic effect, knowledge of the absorption characteristics of the drug are important since, in both cases, it needs to be taken up by the oral mucosa. In the case of local delivery knowledge of how long the drug remains in the mucosa following uptake is an important consideration. In the case of systemic delivery the amount of drug crossing the oral mucosa and entering the blood is an important determinant of drug efficacy. Consequently in the development and assessment of an oral mucosal drug delivery system there is a need for experimental methods which allow the absorption characteristics (rate, extent and mechanisms) of a drug to be determined.

Both in vitro and in vivo methods can be used for this purpose. Both are associated with advantages and limitations. As yet no ideal methodology is currently available but many in vitro and in vivo methods that use animal models or human subjects are described in the literature. In vitro models for measuring the permeability of oral mucosa have been reviewed in Chapter 5 of this book. Such methodologies have played, and will continue to play, an important role in the determination of absorption mechanisms, screening of drug candidates and assessment of permeation enhancers. However, because at this present time we are unsure of the relevance of such in vitro studies in oral mucosal drug delivery due to the lack of in vitro:in vivo correlations, ultimately the absorption characteristics of the drug must be assessed in vivo. It is the purpose of this chapter to review both animal and human in vivo methods currently available for measuring the absorption characteristics of drugs across oral mucosa.

When it comes to the in vivo assessment of the absorption characteristics of a drug the most desirable approach is to perform experiments in human volunteers or patients. However, because of the difficulties of cost, time, limited knowledge of drug properties such as toxicity, ethical considerations etc., it is usually impractical to begin with this approach. We are therefore reliant on the use of animal models and their ability to predict what will happen in their human counterpart.

II. ANIMAL TECHNIQUES

When undertaking an in vivo study in which animals are to be used, considerable attention must be given to the experimental design with a full appreciation of the possible limitations. Probably the most important and difficult aspect of the experimental design is the choice of animal species. Animal models are only appropriate to use for the screening of a series of compounds, investigating the mechanisms and usefulness of permeation enhancers or evaluating a set of formulations, if one is certain that the route of penetration and the structure and composition of the permeation barrier for both the drug and excipients are an exact mimic of its human counterpart. Previous chapters of this book have considered the criteria for selecting the most appropriate animal model as well as the factors that influence this decision and those that should be considered when extrapolating animal data to man. It should be pointed out, however, that many of our current arguments on this topic are based on anatomical viewpoints. Very few, and certainly no extensive, in vivo (animal):in vivo (human) correlations have been reported in the literature which would allow us, using direct evidence, to compare the oral mucosal absorption characteristics of a particular animal with those of its human counterpart.

Animal models such as the dog [1-12], cat [13, 14], rabbit [15-21], hamster [22-30], rat [31-41], and sheep [42, 43] have been used to determine the oral mucosal absorption characteristics of drugs. The methodologies used can broadly be categorized into: application of dosage forms, absorption cells and perfusion cells.

A. Dosage Forms

Several different dosage forms have been applied to oral tissues of various animal species for the purpose of assessing the oral mucosal absorption characteristics of drugs. These include patches [6, 13, 14, 38], bioadhesive tablets [3, 5, 9], non-bioadhesive tablets [19, 42, 43], adhesive film [12, 29], ointments [22, 25, 26], bonded compacts [4], aqueous solutions [11, 20, 21, 23, 24, 27, 28, 30-34, 36] and gels [39]. In almost all of the above cases the buccal membrane was used as the platform upon which the delivery system was placed or attached and the absorption characteristics of the drug across buccal mucosa measured. However, in some cases absorption across the floor of the mouth [11, 32] or tongue [11, 35, 37] was investigated. The absorption characteristics of the drug were assessed either by measurement of the amount of drug reaching the blood or by removal and determination of the amount of drug remaining in the delivery system. In general the animals were immobilized and anesthetized throughout the experiment, however, conscious dogs have been used [6, 38].

B. Absorption Cells

For the purpose of this chapter absorption cells are defined as those techniques which restrict known volumes of an aqueous test solution to a defined area of oral mucosa. The cell can be open or closed to the oral environment, but in either case the test solution within the cell is protected from salivary secretions and therefore does not change in volume. An additional criterion which defines this type of cells is that the test solution is not stirred during an experiment.

Perhaps the simplest example of a method that uses an absorption cell is that described by Siegel and co-workers [35, 37]. To restrict the test solution to a defined surface area of oral mucosa (ventral surface of the rat tongue) Siegel and co-workers used a rubber O-ring with an internal diameter of 2.64 mm which was fixed to the mucosa using a cyanoacrylate adhesive. At the beginning of each experiment, the opening in the O-ring was filled with a small quantity (10 μL) of buffered test solution and the absorption characteristics of the organic solutes under investigation were determined by taking plasma samples and samples of the test solution in the O-ring.

Investigators at the Ciba-Geigy Corporation, New York [12] confined 1 mL of test solution on the buccal mucosa of anesthetized beagle dogs using a glass cell with an internal surface area of 1.5 cm^2 [12]. The dog was positioned on a surgical table, the mouth was braced open and the tongue taped to the upper jaw. The cell was placed on the inner central buccal surface and retained in position using either silicone grease or by mechanical clamping for 4 hours. The extent of drug absorption was assessed by taking plasma samples and in order to quantify the total amount absorbed, at the end of the experiment the drug solution was aspirated from the cell and analyzed for drug content [12].

Quadros briefly described a method involving a "cup" which exposed a surface area of 2.2 cm^2 to investigate the absorption characteristics of a novel angiotensin converting enzyme across the buccal mucosa of anesthetized dogs [7]. The method by which the cup was maintained on the buccal mucosal surface was not described but it was reported that the cup allowed 1 mL of drug solution to remain in contact with the buccal mucosa for 4 hours. The absorption characteristics of the drug were determined by blood samples.

A closed cell made from stainless steel was designed by Ritschel et al [8, 15, 16]. The cell was placed on the buccal mucosa of an anesthetized dog and maintained in position with two alligator clamps (Figure 1). Two holes were included in the top of the donor compartment; one for administration or sampling of the solution (on the outer perimeter) and the other for air ventilation (in the center). The inner surface of the cell exposed the test solution to 1.0 cm^2 of buccal mucosa. To use the cell 0.5 mL of drug solution was added via the peripheral hole using a glass syringe with a blunt needle. After a set exposure period (e.g., 30 minutes) the solution was aspirated and the cell rinsed twice with 0.5 mL normal saline. The solutions were then combined and analyzed to determine the amount of drug that was administered. Blood samples were taken to determine the absorption characteristics of the drug under test.

Oh and Ritschel also designed an apparatus (Figure 2) for retention of solutions on the buccal mucosa of the rabbit [17, 18]. Rabbits were anesthetized and the mouth cavity of the rabbit was cleaned with a cotton ball. The absorption cell (A) was placed in the buccal cavity of the rabbit and firmly attached to the buccal mucosa by tightening the knob (D) of the apparatus. 200 μL of drug solution was administered through the upper opening of the absorption cell (B) using a 250 μL microsyringe. After 1 hour the buccal cell was removed and the mouth cavity cleaned with a cotton wool ball. Drug absorption was measured by blood sampling. The dimensions of the cell were;

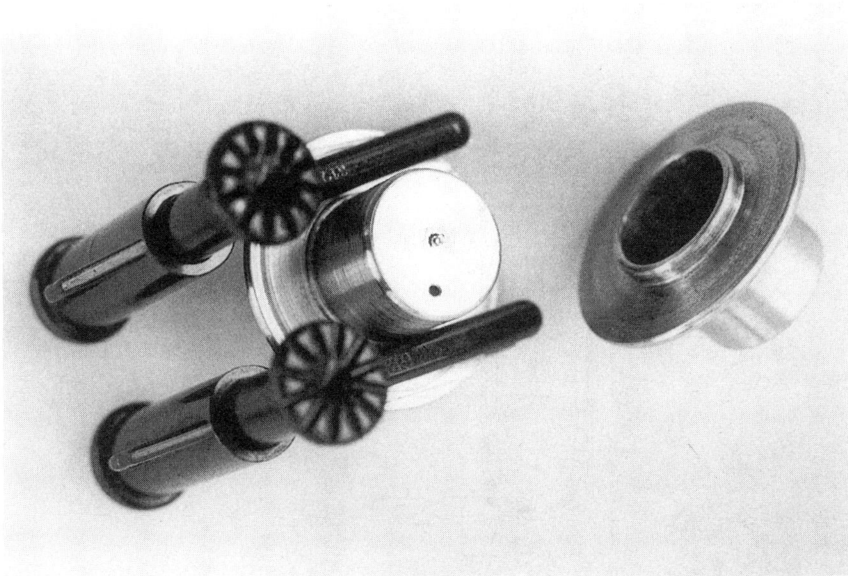

Figure 1. Ritschel's absorption cell [8] manufactured from stainless steel with the following dimensions: diameter of shield: 30 mm, thickness of shield: 1 mm, rim of shield: 1.5 mm, outer and inner diameter of donor compartment 13.4 mm and 11.4 mm respectively, height of sealer ring protruding from the surface of shield 1.5 mm. The figure shows two cells photographed from different angles. The cell on the left shows the position of the inlet and outlet holes on the top of the cell and the two spring clips used to maintain the cell on the oral mucosa of dogs.

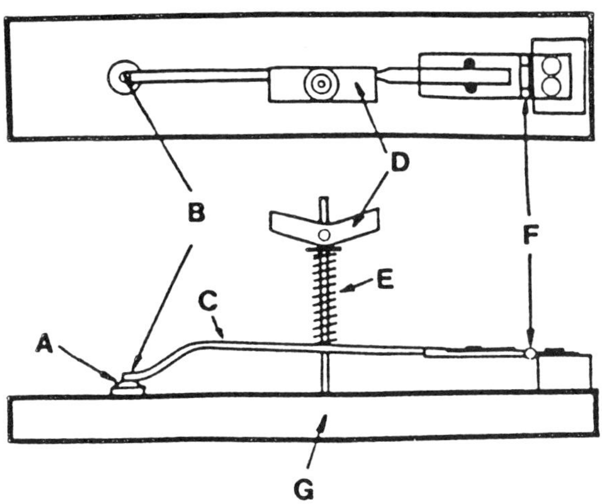

Figure 2. Diagram of the absorption cell applied to the buccal mucosa of rabbit [17, 18]. A: plastic absorption cell, B: upper opening of cell, C: metal arm, D: pressure regulator, E: spring, F: hinge and G: wooden support.

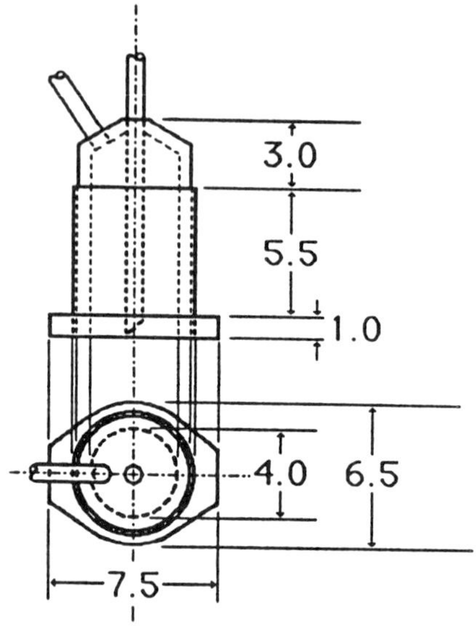

Figure 3. Diagram and dimensions (in mm) of the absorption cell used by Kurosaki et al [29]. Manufactured from the plastic body of a disposable needle for injection, the central tube is used to enter the test solution while the peripheral tube acts as a vent.

12 mm ID, 14 mm OD, height 5 mm, capacity 300 μL and surface area 113 mm^2.

Kurosaki et al [29] prepared a closed absorption cell for use on various mucosa of the anesthetized hamster from the plastic body of a disposable needle for injection (Figure 3). The steel needle was cut off and two polyethylene tubes were fixed in position (Figure 3). The central tube was used as the inlet hole and allowed test solution to be entered into the cell, while the peripheral tube acted as a vent to allow air to escape during addition of the test solution. The cell was fixed to the surface of the oral mucosa with cyanoacrylate tissue cement. Drug absorption was monitored by periodically collecting blood. The dimensions of the cell are given in Figure 3.

Kellaway [13, 14] developed a small cell machined out of a small block of perspex (Figure 4) which comprised two concentric sealed chambers. The inner chamber (0.6 cm diameter, 0.486 cm^3 volume) contained the drug solution, while the outer chamber was used to apply a vacuum which maintained the cell in position on the buccal mucosa of anesthetized cats. The cell exposed an area of 0.33 cm^2 for the duration of an experiment (2 hours). Temporary association of the apparatus with the tissue caused no visible damage during a 2 hour application period. The inner chamber was equipped with two pipes to allow solution to be introduced into the inner compartment. To do this a known concentration of drug solution was injected through the inlet pipe until excess

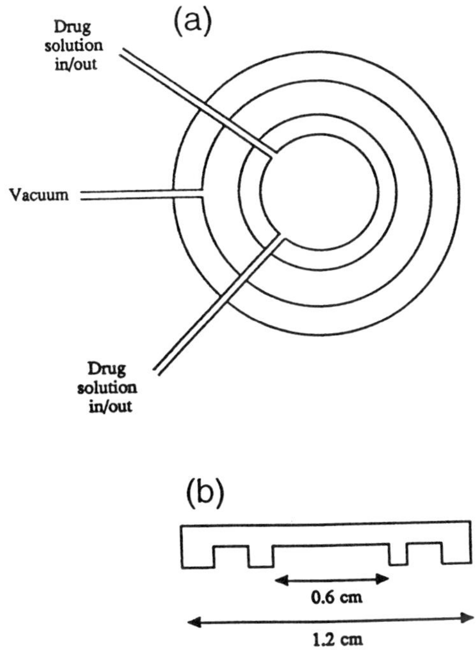

Figure 4. Diagrammatic representation of the perfusion cell used by Kellaway and Warren [13, 14] to deliver a solution of oxytocin to a defined area of cat mucosa; (a) plan view showing relative positions of vacuum chamber and perfusing solution chamber and (b) section through cell showing dimensions.

drained from the outlet tube. The absorption characteristics of the drug under test were determined by blood sampling.

Zhang and co-workers described a cell (Figure 5) which allowed a drug solution to remain in direct contact with a defined area (2.27 cm^2) of the inner side of the cheek of anesthetized dogs [1]. To determine the transbuccal permeation rate of fentanyl the authors introduced a known volume of solution (0.5 mL) containing a known amount of drug into the cell at time t = 0. By taking aliquots of the solution at defined time intervals and analyzing for drug concentration in those samples by HPLC the absorption characteristics of the drug were determined from knowledge of the loss of drug from the cell.

A second absorption cell has recently been described by Zhang et al [10, 44]. The cell was made out of Teflon® (Figure 6) and attached to an adjustable clamp assembly which allowed it to be securely located on the buccal mucosa of anesthetized dogs. Following placement of the cell on the buccal mucosa, 4 mL of drug solution would be introduced into it and retained in direct contact with an 18 cm^2 area of mucosa. Blood samples were collected and analyzed for

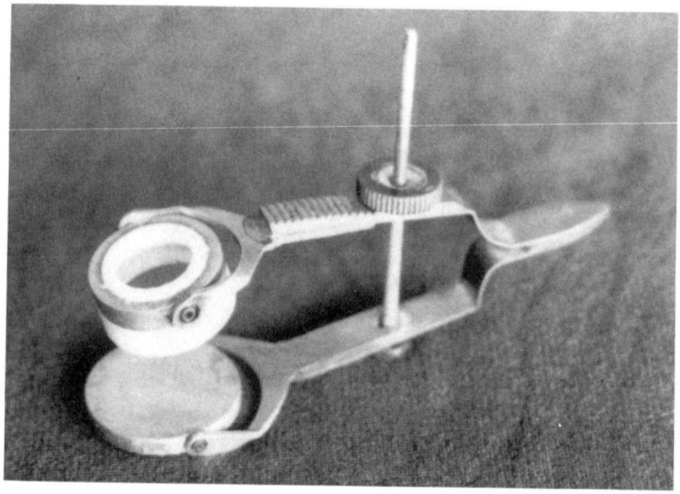

Figure 5. Absorption cell used by Zhang et al to investigate the absorption of fentanyl across dog buccal mucosa [10].

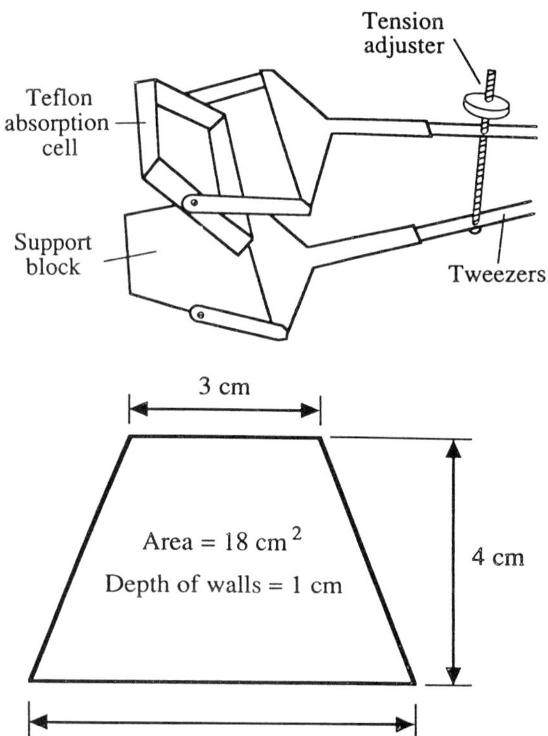

Figure 6. Diagrammatic representation and dimensions of the absorption cell used by Zhang and co-workers [44].

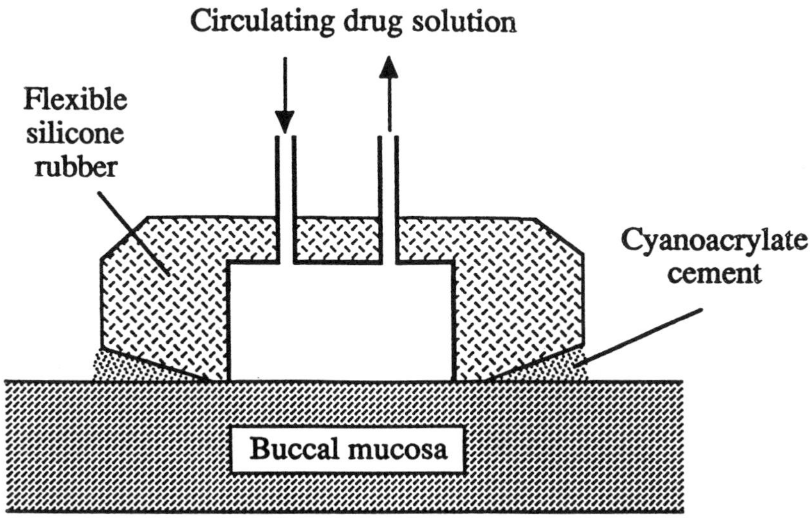

Figure 7. Diagram of perfusion cell used by Veillard et al [45, 46].

drug content to determine the absorption characteristics of the drug under investigation.

C. Perfusion Cells

Perfusion cell techniques are characterized by the restriction of known volumes of an aqueous test solution to a defined area of oral mucosa using cells that are closed to the oral environment. The test solution is therefore protected from salivary secretions and do not change in either volume or pH during an experiment. In contrast to absorption cells the test solution is (i) well stirred and (ii) continually perfused across the mucosal surface throughout the duration of an experiment. In some cases the perfusing solution is continually recirculated over the membrane throughout the experiment, in others the solution passes over the membrane only once and is collected and analyzed for drug content. The absorption characteristics of the drug can be determined either by monitoring drug loss from the perfusing solution or by measurement of blood levels.

Veillard et al [45, 46] developed the perfusion cell shown in Figure 7 which was made from a medical grade silicone polymer. To manufacture a cell the two parts of the polymer were mixed in the correct proportions and added to a specially designed mold. The two halves of the mold were squeezed together and the excess allowed to extrude. After several hours curing time the

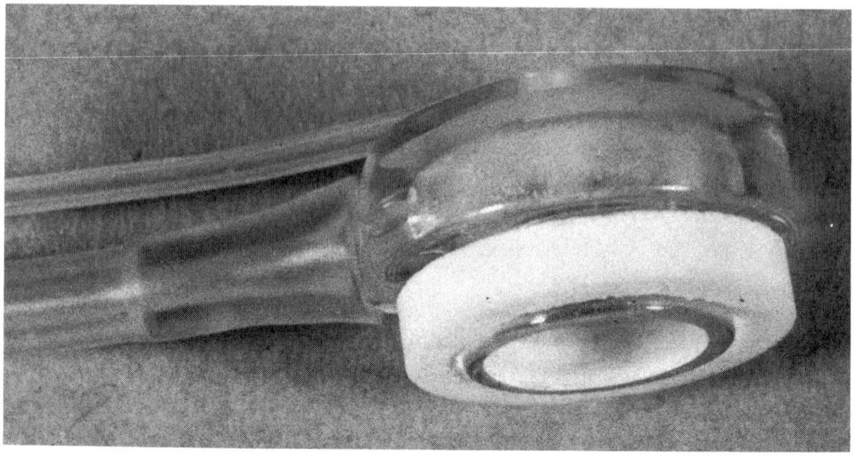

Figure 8. Photograph of the perfusion cell designed by Yamahara et al [47] showing the glass cell and flat-faced bioadhesive polymer ring which was used to attached the glass perfusion cell to the oral mucosa.

mold halves were separated and the cell removed. Holes were added, polyethylene tubes inserted and a dab of glue placed around the holes to prevent leakages. The cell had a volume of 0.075 cm^3 and exposed an area of 0.25 cm^2. It was attached to the buccal mucosa of anesthetized dogs using cyanoacrylate cement. A syringe pump was used to force aqueous drug solution through thermostatted polyethylene inlet tubing (0.75 cm ID), through the perfusion cell and out a polyethylene outlet tube into fraction collector tubes. Aqueous drug solution was perfused through the device for 30 minutes at a rate of 1 mg/mL/5 minutes and collected in 1 mL fractions. Blood samples were taken and used to define the absorption characteristics of the drug investigated.

A glass perfusion cell (Figure 8) was developed by Yamahara et al [47]. A flat faced, non irritating, biocompatible bioadhesive polymer O-ring was attached to the glass cell (Figure 8) which allowed the cell to easily adhere to, and be readily removed from, the oral mucosa. The O-ring comprised a mixture of hydroxypropyl cellulose-M and carboxyvinylpolymer and was manufactured by compressing the polymer powder mixture at 150 kg/cm^2 for 30 seconds using a hand press. The dimensions of the cell are documented in Figure 9. Drug solution was maintained in a reservoir thermostatted to 37°C and recirculated at a rate of 2 mL/minute by a peristaltic pump through Teflon® tubing (2.0 mm OD, 1.0 mm ID). The surface area of membrane exposed to perfusing solution was 0.95 cm^2 and no leakage of the perfusion fluid was reported. Anesthetized male beagle dogs were used in the experiment with up to four cells being attached on a single dog at one time (Figure 10). A

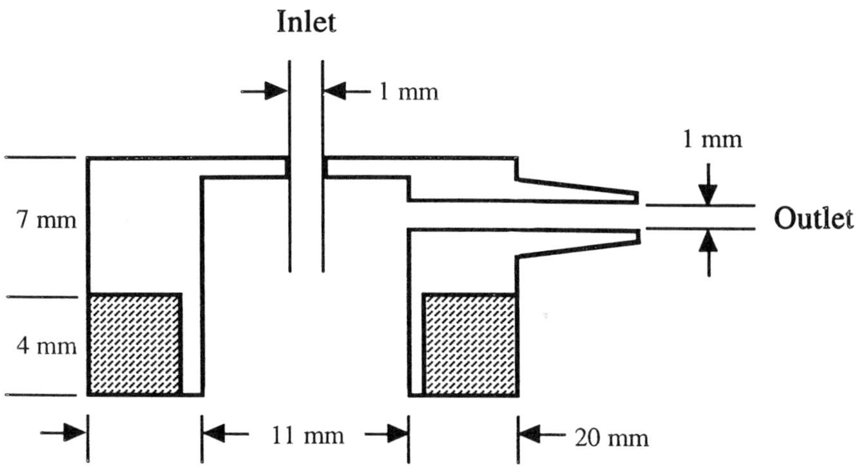

Figure 9. Dimensions of perfusion cell designed by Yamahara et al [47].

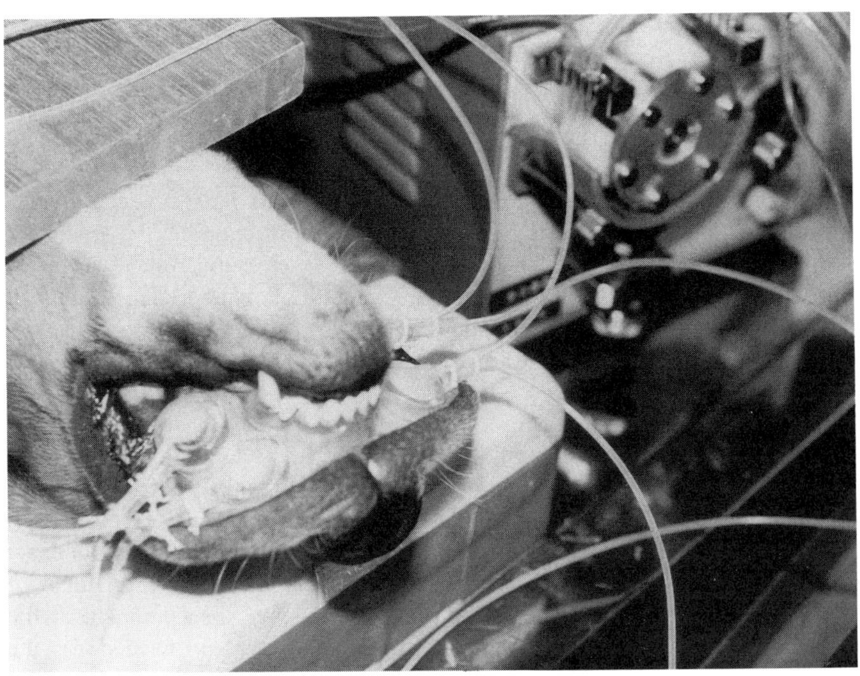

Figure 10. Photograph of four perfusion cells designed by Yamahara et al [47] simultaneously attached to the buccal mucosa of a dog.

2 or 3 hour perfusion time was employed and drug loss was monitored by either taking samples from the reservoir and replacing with fresh solvent or by taking blood samples. In addition to studying the effect of pH on absorption, this method has been used to measure the absorption characteristics of four different oral mucosa including buccal membrane, floor of mouth, dorsum of tongue and ventral surface of the tongue.

Weaver et al [2] reported the use of a Teflon® cell in anesthetized dogs which was held in place against the surface of the buccal mucosa by the use of forceps and a rigid backing held against the cheek. The cell (Figure 11) has a central portion which gives support to the periphery and assures patency of the space for the perfusing drug solution. The cell has an area of 2.8 cm^2 and two 19 gauge needles provide inlet and outlet ports which allow the aqueous drug solution to be flushed across the mucosa. Forceps were used to retain the cell in position on the buccal mucosa with the beaks being held firmly, but not tightly, closed by tape on the forceps (Figure 12). The effluent line from the outlet port flowed to a graduated cylinder which served as a crude check on the pump speed and against leaks. To use the cell it should be orientated with its outlet port at the highest point to minimize air entrapment. A rigid disc (approximately 40 mm in diameter) should be placed on the outside of the cheek in opposition to the cell and the entire assemble held gently in place with the clamp. Gauze can be placed in the throat and behind the cell and used to detect any leakage from the cell (to aid this process a blue dye can be added to the perfusing solution). Initially normal saline should be pumped through the cell at a rate of 0.5 mL/minute and the effluent collected to confirm mass balance. After a minimum of 15 minutes of leak-free operation the saline should be replaced with drug solution and the flow rate reduced to 0.2 mL/minute. The cell effluent should be collected throughout the treatment period and may be analyzed for drug content. Weaver et al [2] have used this procedure for perfusion periods of up to 2.5 hours. Following treatment the cell should be flushed with 5 mL of normal saline.

III. HUMAN TECHNIQUES

Until a suitable animal model is found whose absorption characteristics correlate well with its human counterpart and in which the route of penetration and structure and composition of the permeation barrier are considered an exact mimic of human oral mucosa, the continued development and refinement of human methodologies is of utmost importance. Accurate measurement of the oral mucosal absorption characteristics of drugs in man is needed for the rational design of a delivery system, is invaluable for the clinical evaluation of a new oral mucosal drug delivery system and is required for the validation of an animal model. Several methods have been described in the literature and include the buccal absorption test, disc methods and perfusion cells.

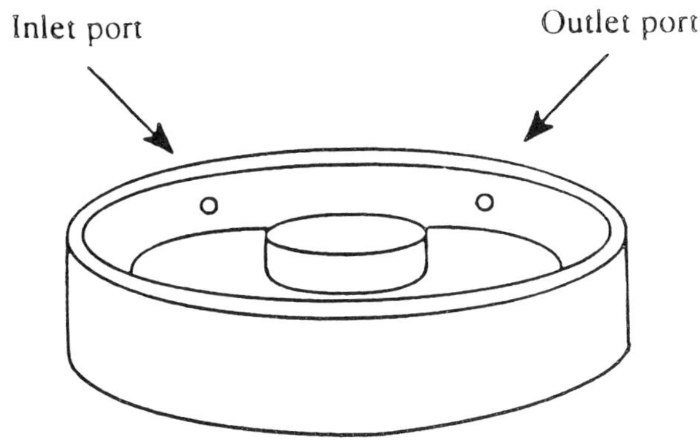

Figure 11. Diagram of perfusion cell used by Weaver et al [2]. The cell was constructed from Teflon® and was 0.94 cm in diameter. The central projection shown in the diagram was included in the design to provide support to the periphery and assure patency of the space for the perfusate.

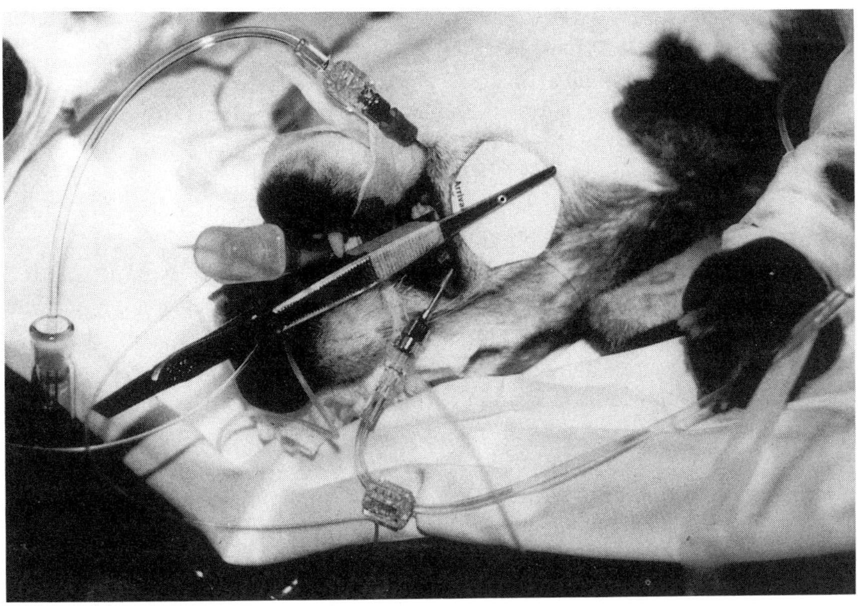

Figure 12. Perfusion cell of Weaver [2] in operation. The cell is held in place by forceps, the beaks of which are held firmly, but not tightly, closed by tape. The rigid backing seen on the outside of the dog cheek serves to support the cell in position. The perfusate is pumped through a line shown passing the snout to the inlet port and the effluent line from the outlet port flows to a graduated cylinder. Other evident (smaller) catheters in the photograph are in the salivary ducts. An endotracheal tube is also evident.

A. Buccal Absorption Test

The buccal absorption test was introduced by Beckett and Triggs in 1967 [48]. The test is a simple, non-invasive method for estimating the rate and extent of drug disappearance from the oral cavity. The method involves controlled swirling of a buffered drug solution of known concentration around the oral cavity by movement of the cheeks and tongue approximately once per second. After a known period of time the solution is expelled and the subject rinses their mouth with an aliquot of either distilled water or an appropriate buffer solution. The drug solution and rinse are then combined, adjusted to volume and analyzed for drug content. The difference between the amount of drug contained in the original solution and the amount recovered is assumed to be the amount of drug lost into the oral cavity mucosa during the test period. Drug loss is usually expressed as a percentage of the original amount entered. If the percentage loss over a fixed time period is measured this provides information on the relative permeability properties of drugs under different conditions [48-57]. If the percentage loss for the same drug is measured over different time periods then kinetic information would be obtained [58-62]. In general a 25 mL volume of test solution was entered [48, 55, 63-69] although some authors have used 20 mL [57, 70-74] or even 10 mL [60]. The original test has been modified by various investigators since its introduction. Dearden and Tomlinson modified the test to correct for the effect of saliva secretion throughout a test [64]. Other authors have modified the test by adding a marker compound e.g., phenol red to monitor for drug dilution by salivary secretion as well as for accidental loss through swallowing [56, 62, 75-78]. The most complex modification was reported by Tucker [62]. He modified the test by adding a marker compound and taking small samples of the swirled solution from the oral cavity every few minutes without removing the test solution. The advantage of this approach is that saliva secretion can be corrected for, accidental swallowing and changes in pH can be made and the absorption kinetics of the drug can be studied in a single 15 to 20 minute test.

Although the buccal absorption test is simple to perform, non-invasive and both the rate and extent of drug loss from the oral cavity from aqueous solutions can be measured, the test does suffer from some disadvantages. The amount of intact drug that reaches the systemic circulation remains unknown as only loss from the oral cavity is monitored and differences in the absorption characteristics of the different membranes that line the oral cavity cannot be determined as absorption simultaneously takes place over all mucosal surfaces. Furthermore the determination of the kinetics of absorption is time consuming because not only has each time point to be determined on separate occasions but also a waiting period must be observed to ensure that at the beginning of each experiment the oral mucosa is void of drug.

B. Disc Methods

These methods have the advantage that absorption across a defined oral cavity mucosa can be studied. Kaaber [79] used a gravimetric method for measuring the uptake or loss of water using a small filter paper disc applied to the mucosal surface. To do this he measured the gain in weight of filter paper discs placed on the surface of carefully dried human palatal or buccal mucosa. The movement of sodium or potassium ions could also be followed by determining the ionic concentrations by flame photometry. Schurr and Ziegler [80] used a Polytef® disc with a diameter of approximately 3.5 cm and height of 1 cm. The disc had a central circular depression depth of 4 mm which left an elevated rim. A water-soaked filter paper disc was placed in the depression and a known amount of drug spread onto the filter paper. Once the drug had dissolved the device was placed on the surface of buccal mucosa. Pimlott and Addy [81] placed a drug soaked filter paper disc of known dimensions onto a defined oral mucosal surface and maintained it in place for 5 minutes. After removal a non-impregnated disc was used to wipe the oral mucosa, the discs combined, analyzed for drug content and the extent of drug disappearance calculated.

C. Perfusion Cells

Two perfusion cells have been used in human volunteers and reported in the literature [82-84] and a third has recently been briefly described [85]. All have utilized the buccal membrane as the platform for perfusion, however, the latest design has also been used on the dorsum of the tongue, ventral surface of the tongue, labial mucosa and floor of the mouth of human volunteers [85].

1. Barsuhn et al

Barsuhn et al [82] constructed a pliable cell made of a hydrophilic vinyl polysiloxane polymer which had an internal volume of 1 mL and allowed a 1.8 cm^2 area of buccal membrane to be perfused (Figure 13). Teflon® recirculation tubing was used in the perfusion circuit which connected the cell to an external reservoir. Stainless steel tubing was included as inlet and outlet tubes to ensure good flow characteristics. Two internal posts were molded into the cell to prevent the buccal membrane from collapsing into the cell void volume and to provide adequate turbulence within the perfusion cell. The design also incorporated a sealing lip to prevent leaks. Before placement of the perfusion cell the membrane of each subject was rinsed with sterile saline solution applied with a cotton gauze. Cells were placed visually and maintained in position by the natural suction created by the perfusion circuit and an extended clamp made from a pair of tweezers (Figure 13). The clamp assembly consisted of a set of 6

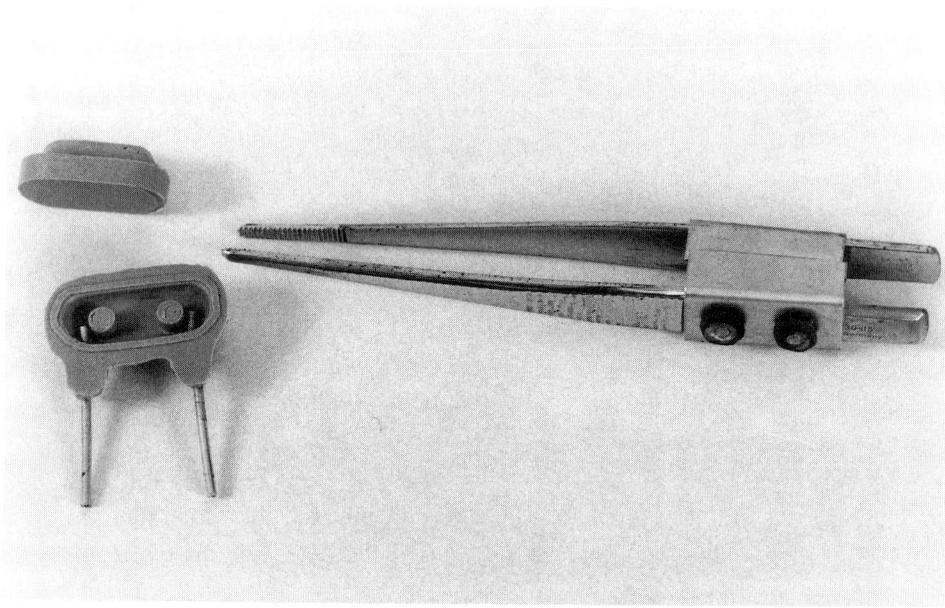

Figure 13. Photograph of the buccal perfusion cell of Barsuhn et al [82] showing the extended clamp and spring bracket assembly, the shape of the cell, the two stainless steel inlet and outlet tubes, the two molded internal posts and the sealing lip.

inch forceps with the hinge end removed and replaced with a spring and bracket assembly. The spring tension was adjusted to ensure that a good seal between the perfusion cell and buccal membrane with minimum discomfort to the volunteers. Perfusing drug solutions were maintained at 37°C and recirculated at 10 mL/minute using a reciprocating piston pump. During a 42 minute perfusion time, 0.05 mL samples were removed from the stirred reservoir every 7 minutes and analyzed for drug content. Absorption of the drug was measured from the rate of disappearance of drug from the reservoir. This method has been successfully been employed to study the effect of pH on the absorption of flurbiprofen in human volunteers.

2. *Rathbone*

Rathbone reported an improved buccal perfusion cell design [83, 84]. In contrast to the one developed by Barshun et al [82] this perfusion cell was constructed from an inflexible material such as nylon or Teflon® (Figure 14)

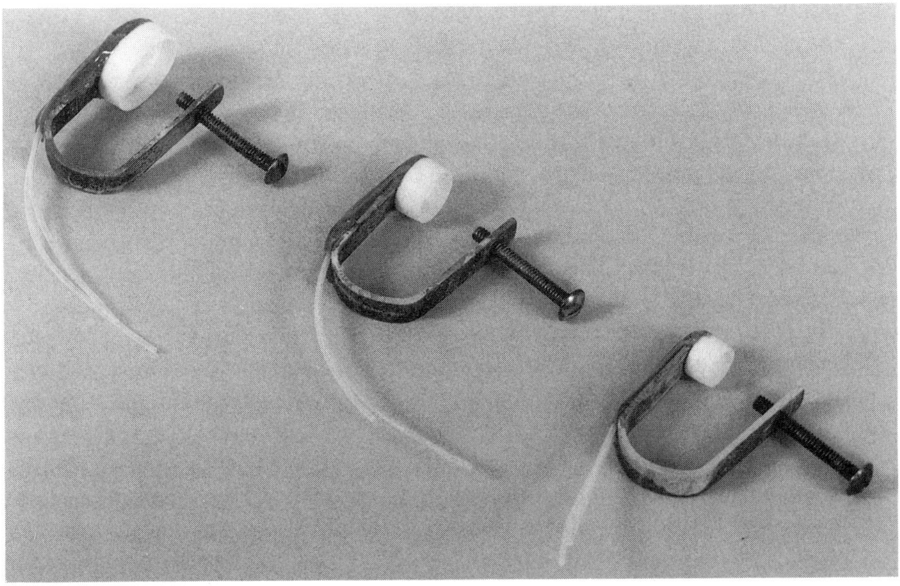

Figure 14. Buccal perfusion cells used by Rathbone [83, 84]. Milled from Teflon® rods, these cells can be made in various diameters. Cells with areas ranging 1 cm^2 to 5 cm^2 have been successfully used. All cells are manufactured with an internal height of 5 mm, 1 mm thickness walls and have 1 mm ID Teflon® circulation tubing entering at opposing sides which act as inlet and outlet holes for the perfusate.

and the perfusion circuit included in-line analysis. The cell is initially held in place by a G-clamp but once an experiment is underway the natural suction pressure of the circuit maintains the cell in position. Several factors should be taken into consideration when manufacturing these cells or designing the perfusion circuit. Our experience has taught us that a wall thickness of about 1 mm is ideal and affords a good seal when in place on the buccal mucosa. A wall thickness of greater than this will tend to result in a poor seal and the possibility of leakage. Our original cell was constructed from nylon but our more recent cells are manufactured from a solid Teflon® rod. This material is softer than nylon and, dependent upon the skills of the miller, a wall thickness of less than ~1.3 mm may not be produced. To overcome this problem we recommend that the walls should be filed down from the outside to a 1 mm thickness using a smooth file. The dimensions of the cell dictate the surface area of exposed buccal mucosa and we have found that cells ranging from 1 to 5 cm^2 in area can be successfully manufactured and used. The position of the inlet and outlet ports are important and the cell should be designed so that the ports are opposite each other and when positioned on the buccal mucosa the outlet port of the cell should be at the highest point of the cell. This avoids air becoming entrapped in the cell and prevents stagnant pools of perfusing solution within the cell. A further design factor that should be taken into consideration is the thickness of the backing on the G-clamp. A very thin backing can result in poor sealing and consequently leakage problems. This problem can be overcome by building up the backing to about 8-10 mm using the epoxy resin compound that is used to adhere the cell to the G-clamp. By building up the back of the cell you also cover the inlet and outlet tubes. They are thus protected from being bitten by the subject during an experiment. We would also recommend that the subject takes on the responsibility of locating the cell in place and should be advised to ensure that the back of the cell is resting on the teeth. If it is resting on the gums the subject may experience discomfort as the cell will rub against the gingiva during the experiment resulting in irritation. The perfusion circuit design should also be given consideration. Of prime importance is the internal suction pressure that the pump creates when it is in operation. This pressure should be great enough to hold the cell in position when the pump is turned on but not too great that it causes the mucosa to be sucked into the cell void which can cause discomfort. The internal suction pressure is a function of the pump itself and the internal dimensions of the circuit tubing. We have found that FMI lab pumps in combination with high flow pump heads are ideal for this purpose [83, 84]. They should be combined with tubing whose internal diameter bore size is between 1 and 2 mm. If all of these factors are taken into account when designing and using the buccal perfusion cell, no leakage from the cell or discomfort to the subject will occur.

We have used the perfusion cell extensively to examine the absorption, and factors affecting the absorption, of a variety of compounds from simple preservatives to more complex drug structures such as β-blockers, triprolidine and opioid analgesics. So far this work has only been published in abstract form but is briefly presented and discussed in this chapter as the results have implications on the use and interpretation of data obtained from perfusion cell studies.

a. Analysis of Loss Data

To date studies using buccal perfusion cells [82-84] have assessed the absorption characteristics of the drug by estimating the disappearance kinetics of the drug from knowledge of the change in drug concentration in the

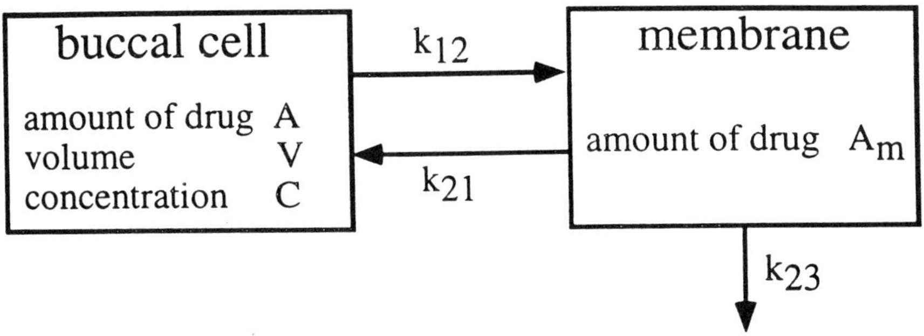

Figure 15. Kinetic scheme ("model III") for modeling the loss of drug from a buccal perfusion cell.

expression with an apparent first-order rate constant for disappearance. We have found that the rate of loss of some drugs cannot be described by this kinetic model. In response to these observations we began to monitor drug loss for two hour periods and analyzed the time course of disappearance of drug from the buccal perfusion cell by least-squares fitting of a compartmental model to the experimental data. This approach has lead us to identify various kinetic models which describe the loss of drug from a buccal perfusion cell. We have considered three models, the most elaborate of which is model III (Figure 15). From inspection of Figure 15 the differential equations that describe the behavior of this model can be written as:

$$\frac{dA}{dt} = -k_{12}A + k_{21}A_m \tag{1}$$

$$\frac{dA_m}{dt} = k_{12}A - (k_{21} + k_{23})A_m \tag{2}$$

With initial conditions set as:

$$A = A_0;\ A_m = 0;\ t = 0 \tag{3}$$

The solution to Equations 1 to 3 giving the concentration of drug in the absorption cell (C) as a function of time is readily found by the Laplace transform method to be:

$$C = C_0 \exp[-(k_{12} + k_{21} + k_{23} + q)\, t/2]\ (\{1 - \exp[qt]\}(k_{12} - k_{21} - k_{23}) + q\{1 + \exp[qt]\})/(2_q) \qquad (4)$$

where

$$q = [k_{12}^2 + k_{21}^2 + k_{23}^2 + 2(k_{21}k_{23} + k_{12}k_{21} - k_{12}k_{23})]^{0.5} \qquad (5)$$

and

$$C = A/V \qquad (6)$$

where A = amount of drug in the perfusing solution and V is the volume of perfusing solution. Model II was a simplified form of that shown in Figure 15 in which the rate constant k_{23} was fixed at zero. This model thus allows for equilibration between the absorption cell and the buccal membrane, but not for subsequent absorption. Model I was even simpler, consisting of a single exponential decay:

$$C = C_0 \exp[-k_{obs}t] \qquad (7)$$

Equation 7 may be derived from model II by setting k_{21} to zero and then either renaming k_{12} as k_{obs}, or allowing k_{12} to tend to infinity and renaming k_{23} as k_{obs}.

The Macintosh non-linear least squares computer program MINIM [86] was used to fit the three models. Errors in the data appeared to have a constant variance, independent of time, and accordingly unweighted fitting was used. The adequacy of fit in each case was primarily judged from randomness (or its lack) of the amplitudes of the residual errors. However, in addition the Akaike Information Criterion (AIC) was also used to compare the outcomes from fitting the three models.

$$AIC = \log[SSE] + 2\, n_{param} \qquad (8)$$

where SSE is the sum of squared residual errors and n_{param} is the number of adjustable parameters in the fitted function [87]. The AIC is a tool to aid the

---

Figure 16. Least-squares fitting of three models to triprolidine data. The upper plot of each pair is the curve-fit and the lower is the residual error plot. Top: model I, showing poor fit. Middle: model II, showing slightly improved fit. Bottom: model III, showing a good fit.

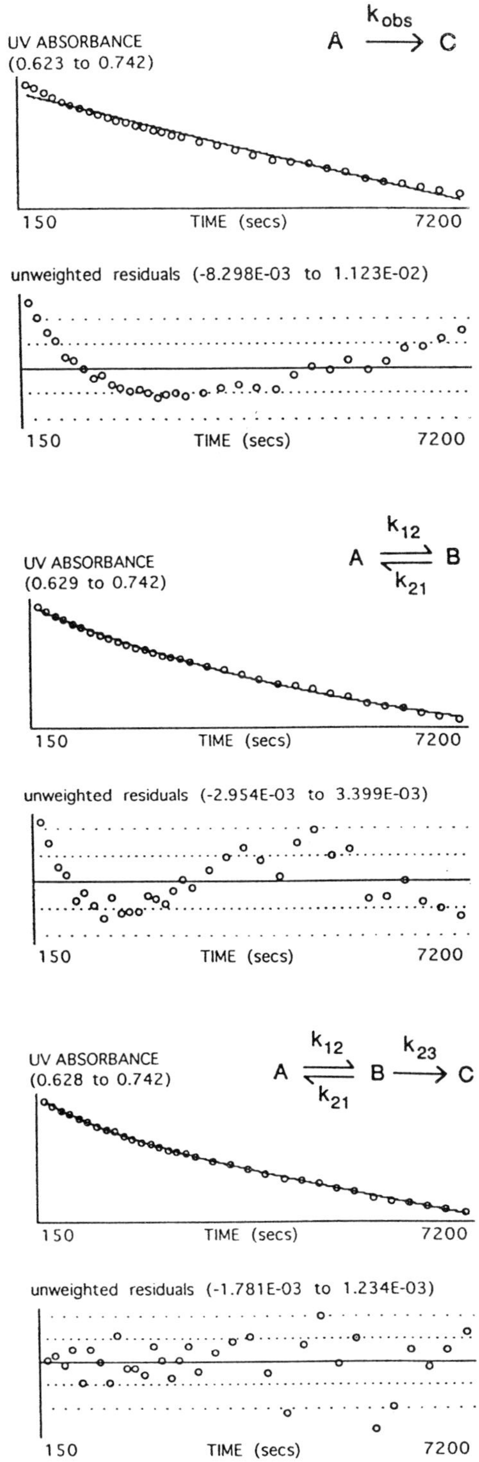

$A \xrightarrow{k_{obs}} C$
UV ABSORBANCE (0.623 to 0.742)
150
TIME (secs)
7200
unweighted residuals (-8.298E-03 to 1.123E-02)
150
TIME (secs)
7200
$A \underset{k_{21}}{\overset{k_{12}}{\rightleftharpoons}} B$
UV ABSORBANCE (0.629 to 0.742)
150
TIME (secs)
7200
unweighted residuals (-2.954E-03 to 3.399E-03)
150
TIME (secs)
7200
$A \underset{k_{21}}{\overset{k_{12}}{\rightleftharpoons}} B \xrightarrow{k_{23}} C$
UV ABSORBANCE (0.628 to 0.742)
150
TIME (secs)
7200
unweighted residuals (-1.781E-03 to 1.234E-03)
150
TIME (secs)
7200

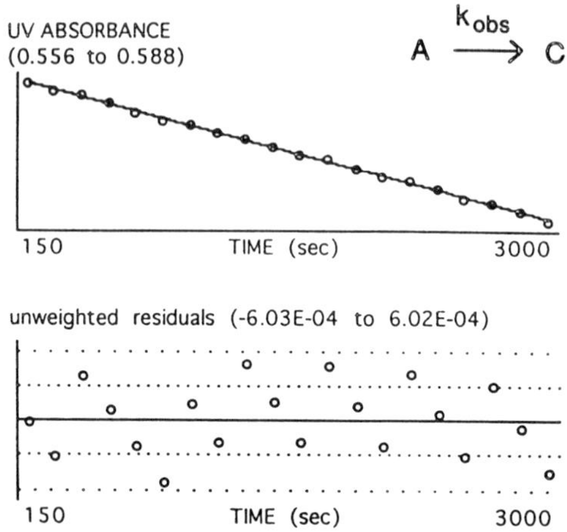

Figure 17. Least-squares curve-fit and residual error plot for butyl para aminobenzoate. Models I, II and III all produced essentially identical plots.

selection of one of a set of rival models, all fitted to the same data set. It attempts to balance two conflicting criteria for a "good" model, namely that the model should be able to fit the data closely (and hence give a small SSE), and that the model should be simple and economical (i.e., have small n_{param}). The model giving the smallest AIC value is considered the 'best'.

Figure 16 shows the results of fitting to a typical set of absorbance data from experiments with triprolidine. Model I gave a poor fit with obvious systematic discrepancies between the data and the fitted curve. Its AIC (-242.6) was the largest of the three models. Model I must therefore be rejected; it cannot adequately describe the experimental findings. Model II gave a better fit (AIC = -308.8) but the residual error plot shows clear patterning. These systematic discrepancies between the model predictions and the measured data mean that model II must also be rejected. Model III gave the smallest AIC (-364.5) and its residual errors show only random-looking deviations from the fitted curve. This model is therefore provisionally accepted.

A different outcome from least-squares curve-fitting was obtained with butyl para aminobenzoic acid. Model I gave an AIC of -260.4; the fitted curve and residual error-plot are shown in Figure 17. No systematic deviation of the fitted curve from the data can be discerned (the remaining semi-regular pattern in the error plot is due to rounding of the raw data to three digits). Model II initially produced a negative estimated value for the rate constant k_{21}. This physically impossible occurrence was then prevented by repeating the fit with a constraint $k_{21} > 0$. The resulting fit had an AIC of -258.4. Attempts to fit Model III initially led to negative values for k_{21} and k_{23}, accompanied by failures of the

Gauss-Marquardt algorithm to converge. Convergence was obtained when both parameters were constrained to be positive, with AIC of -256.4. The fitted curves and residual error-plots for the constrained models II and III were virtually identical with Figure 17. The difficulties encountered with the more complicated models are instructive. They should not be thought of as deficiencies in the software; rather they are 'signs of distress' resulting from fitting a function with too many parameters. The data are very well described by a single exponential decay function (model I) and do not contain the extra information required to fit models II or III. Thus on the basis of the data available there is no reason to prefer any model more complicated than model I, which is therefore provisionally accepted.

The logic of the conclusions reached by model fitting deserves brief discussion. The interest of the experiments lies in the hope of making inferences about the rate of absorption of drug into the blood vascular system. Since the measurements made were not directly of absorption but only of disappearance of drug from the absorption cell, any inference about absorption must necessarily be an indirect one. Modeling with least-squares curve fitting can assist the process of inference, but does not make it more certain. For example, the natural tendency to identify k_{obs} in model I with the rate constant of absorption would be misleading if in fact first-order disappearance of drug from the apparatus were due to chemical destruction or irreversible sequestration in the buccal membrane. Likewise the identification of k_{23} in model III as the rate constant of absorption is natural but unproved. Analysis of the triprolidine data (Figure 16) conclusively shows that models I and II cannot be satisfactory descriptions of buccal absorption of this drug. Model III is not, however, conclusively established as correct. There may be many other models, not considered by us, which would fit as well. The status of model III is that it is (a) physically plausible and (b) consistent with experiment. In contrast, the time course of disappearance of butyl para aminobenzoic acid from the absorption cell is consistent with all three models, but model I provides the most economical description of the present data.

We have shown that it is possible to fit various compartmental models to the experimental data derived from buccal perfusion cell studies. The ability to distinguish between different models is dependent upon assay precision, the availability of early data point and extended (2 hour) perfusion times. The use of curve fitting programs assumes that all data points are valid and may be used directly to calculate a rate constant. Pooling of data from one point sampling procedures may lead to a failure of this premise and to uncertainty in the conclusions which may be drawn from the goodness of fit since replication may increase the scatter around a given measured point resulting in a better fit to the more simpler model. Because of the small percentage drug loss recorded during a buccal perfusion experiment such errors in data precision would lead to the conclusion that disappearance followed a first-order process. A limited number of points measured during the transfer process would also contribute to this problem. We suggest that within the limits of experimental error involved in single point sampling over short time periods it would be difficult to distinguish between the simple and more complex kinetic models using curve fitting techniques. Myhill [88] and Glass and de Garreta [89] performed quantitative theoretical investigations into exponential curve fitting using biexponential functions when controlled random errors were introduced. They concluded that decreasing the error of the raw data and increasing the number of experimental data points decreased the error in the parameter values obtained. This is effectively what is being achieved using the buccal perfusion cell and perfusion circuit design of Rathbone which includes an in-line analysis [83, 84].

We have been pursuing a more precise understanding of oral mucosal drug permeation as this is central to any attempt to build up effective models of the overall absorption process. Our ultimate aim is the prediction of oral mucosal drug absorption in humans, however, the current understanding is limited and provides little or no basis for the quantitative prediction of the absorption characteristics of a new drug molecule. The starting point of our work has been a re-examination of the pH-partition hypothesis of absorption and the validity of Fick's First Law of Diffusion as it applies to the buccal perfusion cell apparatus as we feel that this would be the starting point in the derivation of any theoretical equation which aims to predict absorption across oral mucosa. Assuming that the buccal membrane is the major resistance to drug transfer (i.e., the aqueous diffusion layer offers negligible resistance) for drugs whose disappearance kinetics follow a mono exponential loss, Fick's First Law of Diffusion can be written to show the dependence of k_{obs} on diffusive parameters:

$$k_{obs} = \frac{DAK_p}{Vh} \tag{9}$$

Where D is the diffusion coefficient of the drug in the membrane, A is the area across which transfer can take place, K_p is the membrane/perfusing solution partition coefficient, h is the effective pathlength for diffusion through the membrane and V is the volume of the perfusing aqueous donor phase in the perfusion cell. Our findings are presented below.

b. Effect of Lipid Solubility

The effect of lipid solubility on the rate of absorption of a series of alkyl para hydroxybenzoic acid derivatives was investigated by Rathbone [84]. Figure 18 shows the dependence of the increase in k_{obs} on partition coefficient as the series is ascended.

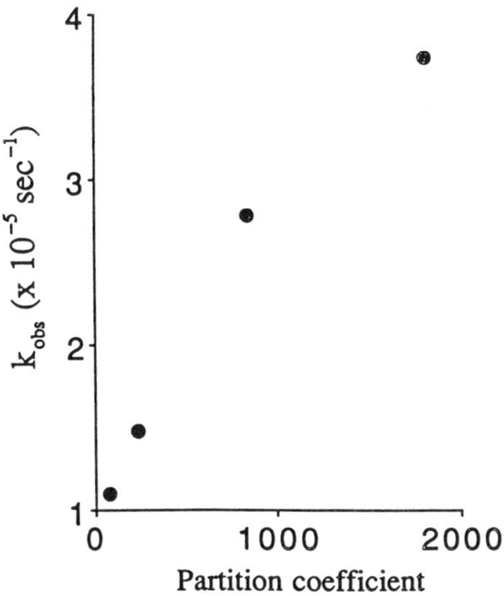

Figure 18. Effect of lipid solubility (as defined by the octanol:water partition coefficient) upon the rate constant for disappearance (k_{obs}) for a series of alkyl hydroxybenzoic acid derivatives.

c. *Effect of pH on Micro Rate Constants*

We have also studied the effect of pH on the micro rate constants for absorption of drugs following different kinetic models. When a simple first-order loss describes the disappearance data the effect of pH on that rate constant is in agreement with the pH-partition hypothesis (Figures 19a and b); absorption is a function of the lipid soluble nonionized drug and the rate of disappearance dependent upon the fraction of nonionized drug (fn) present in the perfusing solution. In contrast when drug loss is described by the more complex model (Figures 20a and b), k_{12} shows a dependence upon pH but in all of the cases studied we have not seen it strictly adhere to the pH partition hypothesis (i.e., the profile is not a function of fn based upon the pKa of the drug). However, in all cases k_{21} and k_{23} remained independent of pH (Figures 20a and b).

d. *Effect of System Dependent Variables*

Several system-dependent parameters were selected from Equation 9 and by modifying either the perfusion cell design or operational conditions we tested to see if, empirically at least, Fick's First Law of Diffusion predicted the

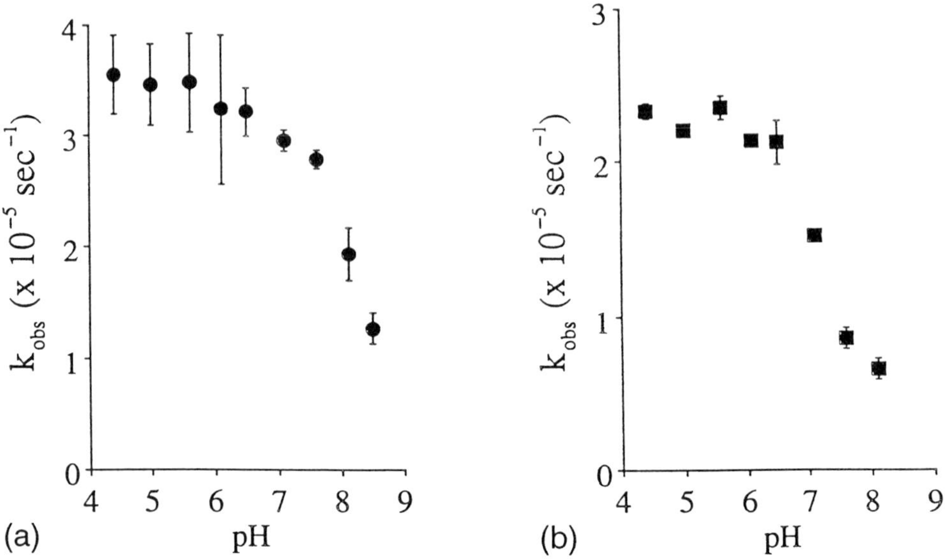

Figure 19. Effect of pH on the experimentally observed first-order disappearance rate constant (k_{obs}) from a human buccal perfusion cell for (a) butyl para hydroxybenzoate [84] and (b) ethyl vanillin.

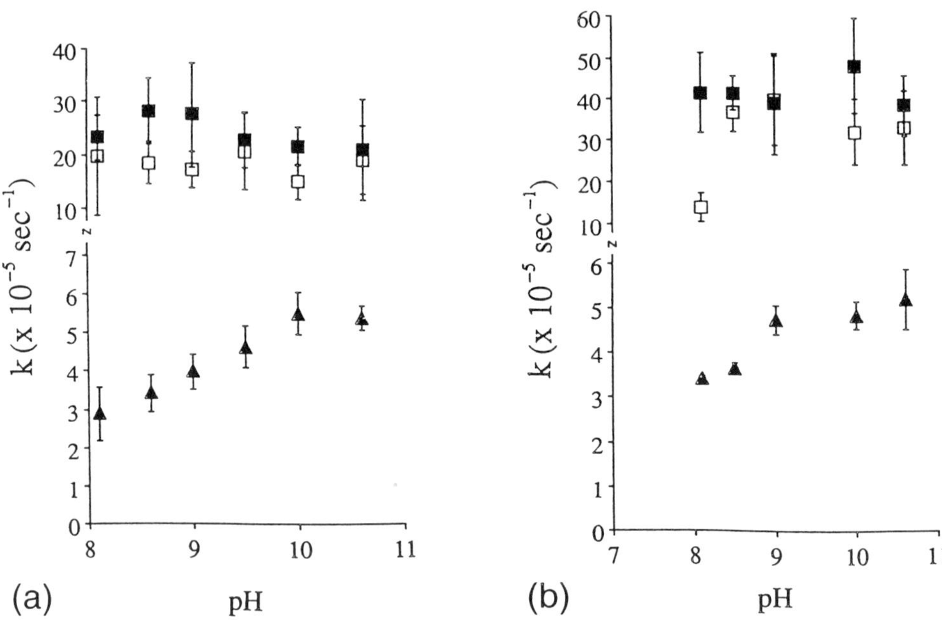

Figure 20. Effect of pH on the micro rate constants k_{12}, k_{21} and k_{23} (Figure 15) for buccal absorption of (a) pethidine and (b) triprolidine.

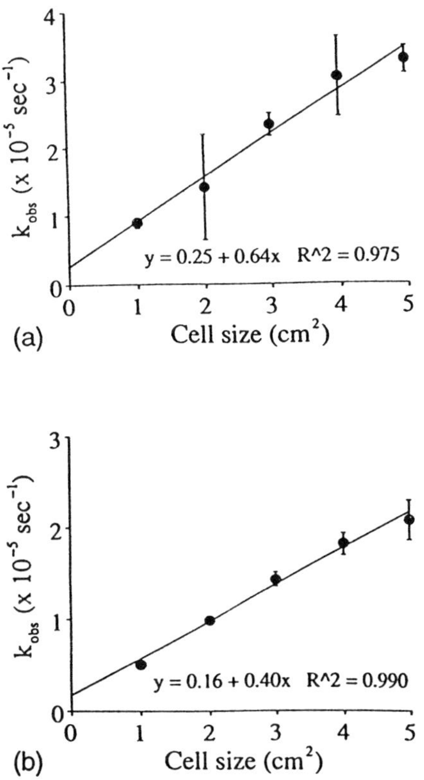

Figure 21. Effect of area of exposed membrane on the experimentally observed first-order disappearance rate constant (k_{obs}) from a human buccal perfusion cell for (a) ethyl vanillin and (b) ethyl para aminobenzoate.

experimentally determined profiles. The parameters tested included area, pump speed and donor phase volume.

Figures 21a and b show the experimentally determined profiles for two compounds as the area of exposed membrane was increased. In both these cases k_{obs} increased linearly with increase in exposed area in agreement with Equation 9.

Figures 22a and b shows the dependence of k_{obs} on pump speed. In both cases k_{obs} remains independent of pump speed and we conclude that the aqueous diffusion layer on the perfusion cell side of the membrane plays an insignificant role in the transfer process. This validates our assumption that, for these drugs at least, the major resistance to drug transfer resides in the membrane.

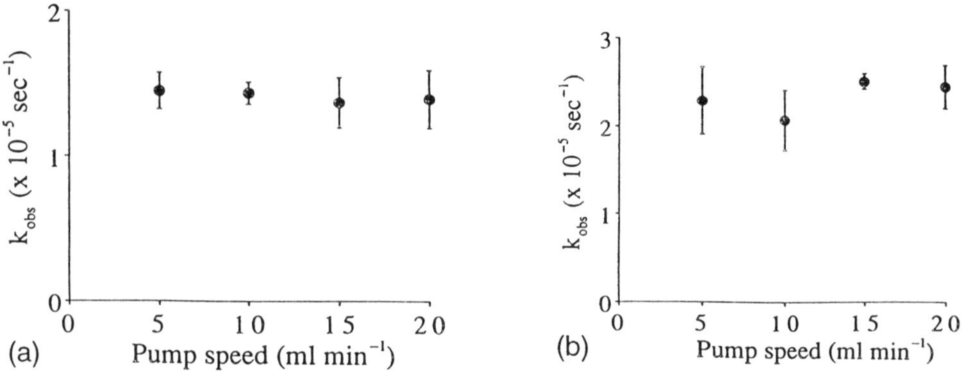

Figure 22. Effect of pump speed on the experimentally observed first-order disappearance rate constant (k_{obs}) from a human buccal perfusion cell for (a) ethyl vanillin and (b) ethyl para aminobenzoate.

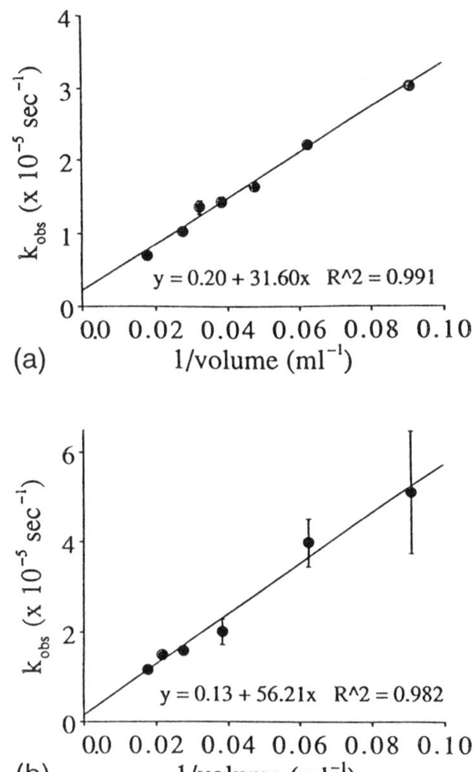

Figure 23. Effect of volume of perfusing donor aqueous phase on the experimentally observed first-order disappearance rate constant (k_{obs}) from a human buccal perfusion cell for (a) ethyl vanillin and (b) ethyl para aminobenzoate.

Figures 23a and 23b show the experimentally determined profiles as the volume of perfusing solution was changed. In all cases k_{obs} increased linearly with 1/V in agreement with Equation 9.

Some interesting profiles have been generated but the work is far from complete. Much remains to be done to develop a satisfactory explanation for the deviations from the basic pH-partition hypothesis for the complex kinetic model (Figure 15). The experimentally determined profiles suggest that when drug disappearance data is described by a simple first-order loss both the pH partition hypothesis and Fick's First Law of Passive Diffusion appear to hold true. These theories may be an appropriate starting point for the derivation of theoretical predictive equations that provide us with a better insight into those factors that govern and control oral mucosal drug absorption.

3. Kurosaki et al

Recently a third perfusion cell, or more correctly a series of perfusion cells, has been reported [85]. Of interest is that in addition to investigating the buccal membrane as the platform for perfusion these authors also studied the absorption characteristics of drugs across the dorsum of the tongue, ventral surface of the tongue, labial mucosa and floor of the mouth of human volunteers [85]. To achieve this three different cell designs were manufactured, each tailored to overcome the problems associated with attachment, available areas, etc., of the different regions that were studied. The cells had inner diameters of 13 or 16 mm, were clamped on the human oral mucosa and 5 mL of test solution was recirculated at a flow rate of 0.8 mL/minute using a peristaltic pump. The absorption characteristics of the drugs were measured by following their disappearance from the perfusing drug solution. The cells were acceptable to volunteers for periods of at least an hour.

IV. CONCLUDING REMARKS

Animal models play an important role in the development of an oral mucosal drug delivery system, in particular when there is relatively limited toxicological data available and when efficacy in man still has to be proven. However, the limitation of animal models still remains their unsuitability for the prediction of human oral mucosal drug absorption. Clearly there are anatomical differences between the animal models and man but with the lack of animal-human correlations debate as to the most appropriate animal model still remains. It would be generally agreed that measurement of oral mucosal absorption of a drug in man is the most satisfactory approach for determining the suitability of a drug for oral mucosal drug delivery, for the clinical evaluation of a new oral mucosal drug delivery system or for the validation of an animal model. Several human methodologies exist. Each has its advantages and disadvantages. Simply constructed perfusion cells offer the possibility of delivering a solution of drug under well defined and controlled conditions across a defined oral cavity membrane and appear to be a useful method for the study of drug absorption across oral mucosa.

V. ACKNOWLEDGMENTS

The authors are grateful for the assistance of James Townshend in the preparation of this manuscript. We are also grateful to Professor Tosikiro Kimura, Professor Wolfgang A. Ritschel, Professor Ian W. Kellaway, Professor Jason M. Tanzer, Dr Hiroshi Yamahara and Dr Jie Zhang for the supply of photographs and descriptions of their absorption and perfusion cells.

REFERENCES

1. J. Zhang, C. E. Ebert, S. McJames, H. J. Gijsman, and T. H. Stanley, Transbuccal permeability of isoproterenol - A dog model, *Pharm. Res. 6*:S-135 (1989).
2. M. L. Weaver, J. M. Tanzer, and P. A. Kramer, Salivary flow induction by buccal permucosal pilocarpine in anesthetized beagle dogs, *J. Dent. Res. 71*:1762 (1992).
3. P. B. Deasy, and C. T. O'Neill, Bioadhesive dosage form for peroral administration of timolol base, *Pharm. Acta Helv. 64*:231 (1989).
4. P. B. Deasy, A. E. M. Collins, F. M. Burke, and D. B. Shanley, In vitro and in vivo evaluation of a bondable compact for the prolonged delivery of triamcinolone acetonide to the oral cavity in patients with lichen planus, *Pharm. Acta Helv. 64*:276 (1989).
5. J. Voorspoels, and J. P. Remon, Buccal absorption of testosterone and testosterone esters using a buccal bioadhesive tablet, *Proceed. Intern. Symp. Control. Rel. Bioact. Mater. 21*:539 (1994).
6. G. J. M. Wolany, J. Munzer, A. Rummelt, and H. P. Merkle, Buccal absorption of Sandostatin (Octreotide) in conscious beagle dogs, *Proceed. Intern. Symp. Control. Rel. Bioact. Mater. 17*:224 (1990).
7. E. Quadros, J. P. Cassidy, K. A. Rosenzweig, and B Berner, Permeation of a novel angiotensin converting enzyme (ACE) inhibitor in vivo and in vitro, *Proceed. Intern. Symp. Control. Rel. Bioact. Mater. 15*:325 (1988).
8. W. A. Ritscel, G. B. Ritschel, H. Forusz, and M. Kraeling, Buccal absorption of insulin in the dog, *Res. Commun. Chem. Path. Pharmacol. 63*:53 (1989).
9. M. Ishida, Y. Machida, N. Nambu, and T. Nagai, New mucosal dosage form of insulin, *Chem. Pharm. Bull. 29*:810 (1981).

10. J. B. Streisand, J. Zhang, S. Niu, S. McJames, R Natte, and N. L. Pace, Buccal absorption of fentanyl is pH-dependent in dogs, *Anesthesiology 82*:759 1995

11. S. Bergman, D. Kane, I. A. Siegel, and S. Ciancio, In vitro and in situ transfer of local anesthetics across the oral mucosa, *Archs Oral Biol. 14*:35 (1969).

12. C. Ebert, A. John, P. T. Beall, and K. A. Rosenzweig, Transbuccal absorption of diclofenac sodium in a dog model, *Controlled-Release Technology Pharmaceutical Applications* (P. I. Lee and W. R. Good, eds.) American Chemical Society, Washington, 1987, Chapter 23.

13. I. W. Kellaway, S. J. Warren, and P. Timmins, Hydrogels for buccal administration, Minutes of the European Symposium on Buccal and Nasal Administration as an Alternative to Parenteral Administration, Editions de Sante, Paris, 1992, p. 101.

14. I. W. Kellaway, and S. J. Warren, Mucoadhesive hydrogels, *Proceed. Intern. Symp. Control. Rel. Bioact. Mater. 18*:73 (1991).

15. C. K. Oh, and W. A. Ritschel, Biopharmaceutic aspects of buccal absorption of insulin, *Meth. Find. Exp. Clin. Pharmacol. 12*:205 (1990).

16. C. K. Oh, and W. A. Ritschel, Absorption characteristics of insulin through the buccal mucosa, *Meth. Find. Exp. Clin Pharmacol, 12*:275 (1990).

17. C. K. Oh, and W. A. Ritschel, Biopharmaceutic aspects of buccal absorption of insulin in rabbits I. Effect of dose size, pH and sorption enhancers: in vivo-in vitro correlation, *Pharm. Res. 5*:S-100 (1988).

18. C. K. Oh, and W. A. Ritschel, Biopharmaceutic aspects of buccal absorption of insulin in rabbits II. Absorption characteristics of insulin through the buccal mucosa. *Pharm. Res. 5*:S-100 (1988).

19. J. Wieriks, Resorption of α-amylase upon buccal application, *Arch. Int. Pharmacodyn. 151*:126 (1964).

20. S. Bergman, I. A. Siegel, and S. Ciancio, Absorption of carbon-14 labeled lidocaine through the oral mucosa, *J. Dent. Res. 47*:1184 (1968).

21. T. S. Miles, and P. G. Dellow, The oral absorption of water, *Can. J. Physiol. Pharmacol. 49*:796 (1971).

22. M. Ishida, N. Nambu, T. and Nagai, Ointment-type oral mucosal dosage form of carbopol containing prednisolone for treatment of aphtha, *Chem. Pharm. Bull. 31*:1010 (1983).

23. Y. Kurosaki, S. Hisaichi, C. Hamada, T. Nakayama, and T. Kimura, Studies on drug absorption from oral cavity II. Influence of the unstirred water layer on absorption from hamster cheek pouch in vitro and in vivo, *J. Pharmacobio-Dyn. 10*:180 (1987).

24. Y. Kurosaki, N. Aya, Y. Okada, T. Nakayama, and T. Kimura, Studies on drug absorption from oral cavity: Physicochemical factors affecting absorption from hamster cheek pouch, *J. Pharmacobio-Dyn. 9*:287 (1986).

25. M. Ishida, N. Nambu, and T. Nagai, Highly viscous gel ointment containing carbopol for application to the oral mucosa, *Chem. Pharm. Bull. 31*:4561 (1983).
26. M. Tanaka, N. Yanagibashi, H. Fukuda, and T. Nagai, Absorption of salicylic acid through the oral mucous membrane of hamster cheek pouch, *Chem. Pharm. Bull. 28*:1056-1061 (1980).
27. Y. Kurosaki, S. Hisaichi, T. Nakayama, and T. Kimura, Enhancing effect of 1-dodecylazacycloheptan-2-one (Azone) on the absorption of salicylic acid from keratinized oral mucosa and the duration of enhancement in vivo, *Int. J. Pharm. 51*:47 (1989).
28. Y. Kurosaki, S. Hisaichi, C. Hamada, T. Nakayama, and T. Kimura, Effects of surfactants on the absorption of salicylic acid from hamster cheek pouch as a model of keratinized oral mucosa, *Int. J. Pharm. 47*:13 (1988).
29. Y. Kurosaki, T. Takatori, H. Nishimura, T. Nakayama, and T. Kimura, Regional variation in oral mucosal drug absorption: Permeability and degree of keratinization in hamster oral cavity, *Pharm. Res. 8*:1297 (1991).
30. Y. Kurosaki, T. Takatori, M. Kitayama, T. Nakayama, and T. Kimura, Application of propranolol to the keratinized oral mucosa: Avoidance of first-pass elimination and the use of 1-dodecylazacycloheptan-2-one (Azone) as an absorption enhancer of bioadhesive film-dosage form, *J. Pharmacobio-Dyn. 11*:824 (1988).
31. Y. Nakada, N. Awata, Y. Ikuta, and S. Goto, The effect of bile salts on the oral mucosal absorption of human calcitonin in rats, *J. Pharmacobio-Dyn. 12*:736 (1989).
32. B. J. Aungst, N. J. Rogers, and E. Shefter, Comparison of nasal, rectal, buccal, sublingual and intramuscular insulin efficacy and the effects of a bile salt absorption promoter, *J. Pharmacol. Exp. Ther. 244*:23 (1988).
33. B. J. Aungst, and N. J. Rogers, Dependence of absorption-promoting actions of laureth-9, Na salicylate, Na_2EDTA, and aprotinin on rectal, nasal, and buccal insulin delivery, *Pharm. Res. 5*:305 (1988).
34. L. B. Hansen, A. Jørgensen, S. N. Rasmussen, L. L. Christrup, and H. Bundgaard, Buccal absorption of ketobemidone and various ester prodrugs in the rat, *Int. J. Pharm. 88*:243 (1992).
35. I. A. Siegel, Permeability of the rat oral mucosa to organic solutes measured in vivo, *Archs Oral Biol. 29*:13 (1984).
36. Y. Nakada, N. Awata, C. Nakamichi, and I. Sugimoto, The effect of additives on the oral mucosal absorption of human calcitonin in rats, *J. Pharmacobio-Dyn. 11*:395 (1988).
37. I. A. Siegel, and H. P. Gordon, Surfactant-induced increases of permeability of rat oral mucosa to non-electrolytes in vivo, *Archs Oral Biol. 30*:43 (1985).

38. H. P. Merkle, R. Anders, J. Sandow, and W. Schurr, Self-adhesive patches for buccal delivery of peptides, *Proceed. Intern. Symp. Control. Rel. Bioact. Mater. 12*:85 (1985).
39. C. R. Bland, S. S. Davis, M. S. Cheema, and D. A. Rawlins, The buccal absortion of two betablocking drugs in the rat, *Proceed. Intern. Symp. Control. Rel Bioact. Mater. 16*:390 (1989).
40. D. H. Dean, and R. N. Hiramoto, Oral mucosal permeability of desalivated rats, *J. Oral Med. 41*:170 (1986).
41. B. J. Aungst, and N. J. Rogers, Comparison of the effects of various transmucosal absorption promotors on buccal insulin delivery, *Int. J. Pharm. 53*:227 (1989).
42. B. A. Burnside, A. D. Keith, and W. Snipes, Microporous hollow fibers as a peptide delivery system via the buccal cavity, *Proceed. Intern. Symp. Control. Rel. Bioact. Mater. 16*:94 (1989).
43. D. H. Maddox, B. A. Burnside, and A. D. Keith, Buccal delivery of progesterone, *Proceed. Intern. Symp. Control. Rel. Bioact. Mater. 17*:291 (1990).
44. J. Zhang, S. Niu, C. Ebert, and T. H. Stanley, An in vivo dog model for studying recovery kinetics of the buccal mucosa permeation barrier after exposure to permeation enhancers: apparent evidence of effective enhancement without tissue damage, *Int. J. Pharm. 101*:15 (1994).
45. M. M. Veillard, M. A. Longer, I. G. Tucker, and J. R. Robinson, Buccal controlled delivery of peptides, *Proceed. Intern. Symp. Control. Rel. Bioact. Mater. 14*:22 (1987).
46. M. M. Veillard, M. A. Longer, T. W. Martens, and J. R. Robinson, Preliminary studies of oral mucosal delivery of peptide drugs, *J. Control. Rel. 6*:123 (1987).
47. H. Yamahara, T. Suzuki, M. Mizobe, K. Noda, and M. Samejima, In situ perfusion system for oral mucosal absorption in dogs, *J. Pharm. Sci. 79*:963 (1990).
48. A. H. Beckett, and E. J. Triggs, Buccal absorption of basic drugs and its application as an in vivo model of passive drug transfer through lipid membranes, *J. Pharm. Pharmacol. 19*:31S (1967).
49. A. H. Beckett, and A. C. Moffat, The influence of alkyl substitution in acids on their performance in the buccal absorption test, *J. Pharm. Pharmacol. 20*:239S (1968).
50. A. H. Beckett, and A. C. Moffat, The influence of substitution in phenylacetic acids on their performance in the buccal absorption test, *J. Pharm. Pharmacol. 21*:139S (1969).
51. A. H. Beckett, and A. C. Moffat, Correlation of partition coefficients in n-heptane-aqueous systems with buccal absorption data for a series of amines and acids, *J. Pharm. Pharmacol. 21*:144S (1969).
52. A. H. Beckett, and A. C. Moffat, The buccal absorption of some barbiturates, *J. Pharm. Pharmacol. 23*:15 (1971).

53. J. C. Dearden, and E. Tomlinson, Buccal absorption as a parameter of analgesic activity of some p-substituted acetanilides, *J. Pharm. Pharmacol. 23*:73S (1971).
54. D. C. Hicks, The buccal absorption of some β-adrenoceptor blocking drugs, *Br. J. Pharmacol. 47*:680P (1973).
55. K. Chan, The effect of physicochemical properties of pethidine and its basic metabolites on their buccal absorption and renal elimination, *J. Pharm. Pharmacol. 31*:672 (1979).
56. W. Schürmann, and P. Turner, The buccal absorption of atenolol and propranolol, and their physicochemical characteristics, *Br. J. Clin. Pharmacol. 4*:655P (1977).
57. D. J. Temple, and K. R. Schesmer, The buccal absorption characteristics of fomocaine, *Arch. Pharm. (Weinheim) 311*:485 (1978).
58. A. H. Beckett, and A. C. Moffat, Kinetics of buccal absorption of some carboxylic acids and the correlation of the rate constants and n-heptane:aqueous phase partition coefficients, *J. Pharm. Pharmacol. 22*:15 (1970).
59. A. H. Beckett, and M. E. Pickup, A model for steroid transport across biological membranes, *J. Pharm. Pharmacol. 27*:226 (1975).
60. R. E. Kates, Absorption kinetics of sublingually administered propranolol, *J. Med. 8*:393 (1977).
61. J. M. Sutherland, W. D. Hooper, M. J. Eadie, and J. H. Tyrer, Buccal absorption of ergotamine, *J. Neurol. Neurosurg. Psych. 37*:1116 (1974).
62. I. G. Tucker, A method to study the kinetics of oral mucosal drug absorption from solutions, *J. Pharm. Pharmacol. 40*:679 (1988).
63. M. H. Bickel, and H. J. Weder, Buccal absorption and other properties of pharmacokinetic importance of imipramine and its metabolites, *J. Pharm. Pharmacol. 21*:160 (1969).
64. J. C. Dearden, and E. Tomlinson, A new buccal absorption model, *J. Pharm. Pharmacol. 23*:68S (1971).
65. A. S. Manning, and D. F. Evered, The absorption of sugars from the human oral cavity, *Clin. Sci. Mol. Med. 51*:127 (1976).
66. I. W. Mathison, P. H. Morgan, N. J. Wojciechowski, J. P. Bandrua, and J. R. Wennemark, Physiocochemical and pharmacological studies of some 8-substituted decahydroisoquinolines, *J. Med. Chem. 19*:385 (1976).
67. M. E. Pickup, A. J. Johnson, C. S. May, J. W. Paterson, and M. P. Harrison, The absorption and elimination of ICI 74,917 in man, *Br. J. Clin. Pharmacol. 4*:357 (1977).
68. G. Edwards, A. M. Breckenridge, K. K. Adjenpon-Yamoah, M. L'E. Orme, and S. A. Ward, The effect of variations in urinary pH on the pharmacokinetics of diethylcarbamazine, *Br. J. Clin. Pharmacol. 12*:807 (1981).

69. A. Odumosu, and C. W. M. Wilson, The buccal absorption of Vitamin C, *Proc. Nutr. Res. 30*:81A (1971).
70. J. A. Henry, K. Ohashi, J. Wadsworth, and P. Turner, Drug recovery following buccal absorption of propranolol, *Br. J. Clin. Pharmacol. 10*:61 (1980).
71. J. C. McElnay, and D. J. Temple, The use of buccal partitioning as a model to examine the effects of aluminium hydroxide gel on the absorption of propranolol, *Br. J. Clin. Pharmacol. 13*:399 (1982).
72. A. Blackett, N. Brion, and P. Turner, Recovery of acetylsalicylic acid and indalpine (LM 5008) after buccal partitioning, *Int. J. Clin. Pharm. Soc. 3*:5 (1983).
73. M. A. Randhawa, and P. Turner, Buccal absorption of drugs: an in vivo measurement of their innate lipophilicity, *Int. J. Clin. Pharm. Res. 8*:1 (1988).
74. M. A. Randhawa, A. N. Blackett, and P. Turner, Spectrofluorimetric analysis and buccal absorption of medifoxamine, *J. Pharm. Pharmacol. 38*:629 (1986).
75. A. G. Arbab, and P. Turner, Influence of pH on absorption of thymoxamine through buccal mucosa in man, *Br. J. Clin. Pharmacol. 43*:479P (1971).
76. W. Meyer, C. M. Kaye, and P. Turner, A study of the influence of pH on the buccal absorption and renal excretion of procainamide, *Eur. J. Clin. Pharmacol. 7*:287 (1974).
77. W. Schürmann, and P. Turner, A membrane model of the human oral mucosa as derived from buccal absorption performance and physicochemical properties of the β-blocking drugs atenolol and propranolol, *J. Pharm. Pharmacol. 30*:137 (1978).
78. T. Past, Zs. Tapsonyi, and I. Hortobagyi, Relationship between the dipole moment and rate of absorption of drugs, *Acta Med. Acad. Sci. Hun. 36*:137 (1979).
79. S. Kaaber, The permeability and barrier functions of the oral mucosa with respect to water and electrolytes, *Acta Odontol. Scand. 32*:7 (1974).
80. W. Schurr, and R. Ziegler, Buccal absorption of protirelin: an effective way to stimulate thyrotropin and prolactin, *J. Pharm. Sci. 72*:1481 (1983).
81. S. J. Pimlott, and M. Addy, Evaluation of a method to study the uptake of prednisolone sodium phosphate from different oral mucosal sites, *Oral Surg. Oral Med. Oral Pathol. 60*:35 (1985).
82. C. L. Barsuhn, L. S. Olanoff, D. D. Gleason, E. L. Adkins, and N. F. H. Ho, Human buccal absorption of flurbiprofen, *Clin. Pharmacol. Ther. 44*:225 (1988).
83. M. J. Rathbone, Human buccal absorption. I. A method for estimating the transfer kinetics of drugs across the human buccal membrane, *Int. J. Pharm. 69*:103 (1991).

84. M. J. Rathbone, Human buccal absorption. II. A comparative study of the buccal absorption of some parahydroxybenzoic acid derivatives using the buccal absorption test and a buccal perfusion cell, *Int. J. Pharm. 74*:189 (1991).
85. Y. Kurosaki, K. Yano, T. Nakayama, and T. Kimura, Regional variation in oral mucosal drug absorption. Presented at the Seventh Japanese-American Conference on Pharmacokinetics and Biopharmaceutics, Japan, 1994.
86. R. D. Purves, Anomalous parameter estimates in the one-compartment model with first order absorption, *J. Pharm. Pharmacol. 45*:934 (1993).
87. J. J. DiStefano, and E. M. Landaw Multiexponential, multicompartmental and noncompartmental modeling, *Amer. J. Physiol. 15*:R651 (1984).
88. J. Myhill, Investigation of the effect of data error in the analysis of biological tracer analysis, *Biophys. J. 7*:903 (1967).
89. H. I. Glass, and A. C. de Garreta, Quantitative analysis of exponential curve fitting for biological applications, *Phys. Med. Biol. 12*:379 (1967).

8

The Flow of Saliva and Its Influence on the Movement, Deposition and Removal of Drugs Administered to the Oral Cavity

John A. Weatherell
Leeds Dental Institute, England

Colin Robinson
Leeds Dental Institute, England

Michael J. Rathbone
University of Otago, New Zealand

I. INTRODUCTION

Dentists and pharmacists have long been interested in the secretion and movement of saliva around the mouth. Dentists are aware that the volumes and quality of the oral secretions are important in dental caries and many other aspects of oral health. On the other hand pharmaceutical scientists involved in optimizing oral mucosal drug delivery have long been frustrated by the presence of saliva in the oral cavity. However, the problems encountered seem not to have been addressed and few fundamental studies have been performed which quantify the role of saliva in oral mucosal drug delivery system design.

Indeed saliva is often only considered in the context of a reason to explain poor release and retention characteristics of delivery systems and/or released drug from developed products. Recently introduced systemic oral mucosal drug delivery systems overcome the problems of saliva by isolating the drug reservoir and releasing surface using water-impermeable backings. Oral mucosal drug delivery systems designed to deliver drugs locally to the oral cavity, however, do not have this option and as such are subject to the influence of saliva.

The view that substances introduced into the mouth are quickly washed away or diluted with saliva and then swallowed is not invariably true. In some instances retention may be prolonged; substances may adhere to oral surfaces, be trapped between teeth or be retained longer at sites where salivary turnover is very small. Alternatively, substances may be removed from the oral cavity by absorption via the oral mucosa into the blood while others may be metabolized by oral bacteria or by enzymes present in the oral fluid. The highly site-specific character of the situation or its implications for delivery system design seems not to have been fully appreciated.

In an attempt to clarify this complicated picture, studies have been carried out investigating the flow of saliva and the distribution and ultimate fate of substances in the mouth, but knowledge about these areas is still incomplete. A flurry of recent investigations on this aspect have come to some interesting conclusions but technical difficulties and a paucity of independent methods still makes the definitive confirmation of some of these findings difficult.

The authors recently made a review of the present state of the art [1]. The present chapter attempts to evaluate further the significance of these and later findings. The principal author (JAW), who has now retired from active research, has taken the liberty of including some preliminary data from work presented at meetings and previously described only in the form of published Abstracts. He has derived some tentative conclusions from this data and attempted to highlight areas which would appear to warrant further work and to offer profitable avenues of exploration.

II. THE SECRETION AND FLOW OF SALIVA

A. Volume of Saliva Present after Swallowing

A consideration about the varying amount of fluid present in the mouth, especially at specific sites of interest, is pertinent to any discussions about drug clearance and retention and consequently drug concentrations and rates of biochemical reaction. Dawes [2] created a useful mathematical model of the mouth in an effort to unravel some the principal factors involved. He and his colleagues then attempted to measure some of the essential variables concerned with the process of salivary dilution and oral clearance. They determined the volume of saliva in the mouths of adults [3] and children [4] after swallowing. To do this, they measured the amounts of endogenous potassium and chloride removed from the mouth by rinsing with water. Using a value for the original concentrations of potassium and chloride in saliva, they were then able to calculate the total volume of saliva in the mouth. Adult males had an average volume of about 0.9 mL and females a slightly smaller average volume of about 0.8 mL. The equivalent value for 5 year-old children was about 0.4 mL.

Replicated values obtained for each volunteer were fairly similar but there were often considerable differences between volunteers, reflecting perhaps individual differences in dental anatomy and the large differences in the rates of salivary secretion reported in the literature [5]. Such differences between volunteers might of course also reflect individual variations in the surface area of the mouth. Collins and Dawes [6] tried to measure this in adults and Watanabe and Dawes [4] in young children by taking dental impressions of their oral surfaces. The total area of the oral cavity normally available to saliva or rinsing solutions was significantly smaller in children than in adults but there seemed to be no sex differences; values were similar for men (217 cm^2) and women (212 cm^2) and for girls (116 cm^2) and boys (119 cm^2).

B. The Salivary Film

Combining the values for the area of the mouth with their data on saliva volumes, Collins and Dawes [6] and Watanabe and Dawes [4] calculated the average thickness of the salivary film covering the oral surfaces after swallowing. When salivary flow was not stimulated to any measurable extent, this would only be about 0.1 mm and it seemed to be similar in both adults and children. The authors did point out that this figure would vary somewhat from time to time and in different regions of the mouth. The salivary film, for instance, would probably be greater near to the ducts of the major salivary glands and it would be tend to be thinner when mucosal layers were separated during speaking or mouth-breathing. These speculations are interesting and certainly the figure of 0.1 mm is of the same order as the value (0.035 mm) obtained by Main et al [7] from direct observation. However, the assumption by Collins and Dawes [6] that all internal surfaces of the mouth are normally in contact with each other when a subject is at rest sits badly with the subjective impression that there is, for instance, considerable space around the tongue. At some sites, such as the floor of the mouth, saliva may also form a pool. There is little direct site-specific information about the distribution of saliva in the mouth after swallowing and hardly any after the stimulation of secretion. Lagerlöf and Dawes' [3] suggestion, that the salivary film would be thicker near to the openings of the major salivary ducts came chiefly from their considerable knowledge of oral anatomy and physiology. Such informed guesses can be made but this is certainly an area where further direct investigation would be valuable.

C. Variations in Saliva Volumes due to Stimulation of Secretion

The introduction of a substance into the mouth or even the anticipation of a meal may stimulate the salivary glands and increase the rate of salivary secretion. This will increase the volume of saliva in the mouth and reduce the concentration of any drug present. It is therefore important in the present context to consider the effects of such salivary stimulation. Much of the data reported in the literature has been obtained by measuring changes in the rates of salivary flow from individual salivary glands. Other data, about the total combined flow from all the major and minor glands, has been obtained by determining how much saliva per minute the patient or volunteer is able to drool into a tared receptacle. Such procedures are time-consuming and often inconvenient. It is also sometimes necessary or desirable to have information about the actual volume of saliva in the mouth at any instant. Lagerlöf and Dawes' [3] values, as mentioned above, were based on measurements of endogenous potassium and chloride present in the mouth. Their method of estimation required a value for the concentrations of endogenous potassium and chloride present in undiluted saliva. Thus their method is limited to measuring volumes of non-stimulated saliva since, during stimulation, the salivary concentrations of potassium and chloride in saliva change.

To overcome this limitation Weatherell et al used an extraneous ion, fluoride, in a simple dilution method [8]. Average values obtained for the volumes of unstimulated saliva in the mouth after swallowing (0.8 mL in adult males and 0.7 mL in adult females) were very similar to those reported by Lagerlöf and Dawes [3]. The average values for 7-14 year old children were 0.7 mL for boys and 0.5 mL for girls.

The accuracy and linearity of test results obtained using this technique (Figure 1) also indicated that when small quantities (1 to 10 g) of water were introduced and gently moved around the mouth for about 15 seconds, they became thoroughly mixed. The linearity of the results in Figure 1 also showed that neither the movement of the mouth, the presence of the small amount of fluoride, nor the presence of different volumes of water in the mouth had detectably stimulated salivary secretion. The fluoride dilution technique procedure was simple, rapid, convenient, fairly accurate (within a standard deviation of $\pm$ 0.1 mL) and very reliable.

In a further check of the fluoride dilution technique, measurements of total fluoride recovery from the mouth were carried out in order to discover whether all the fluoride remained present and available during the rinsing

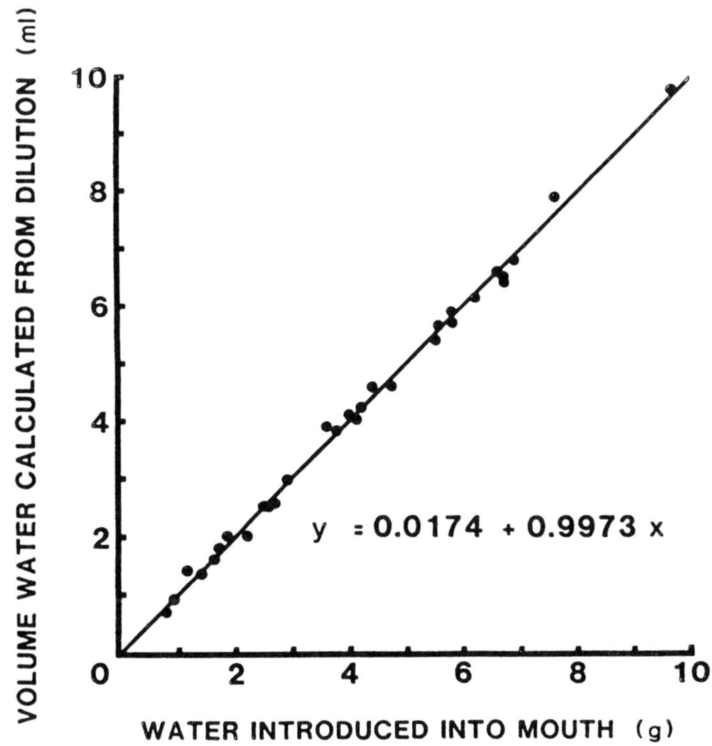

Figure 1. Calibration of the fluoride dilution technique. Weighed amounts of water, introduced into the mouth by pipette, versus volume as determined by fluoride dilution. Combined results from 30 measurements; 5 made on each of 6 volunteers. (From reference 8).

procedure. In neutral pH conditions, this proved to be the case; all the fluoride could be recovered, indicating that it had remained freely available and had thoroughly mixed with the saliva. After stimulation with weak acids, however, only about 80% of the fluoride could be recovered. Whether some of the fluoride had been swallowed prior to complete mixing of the saliva, in a reflex response to the sudden inflow of saliva into the mouth, or taken up by the teeth under the acid conditions, or absorbed through the oral mucosa, this perhaps being facilitated by its conversion to nonionized HF at the low pH of these tests, was not clear; which is why the results have not been formally published. Despite these reservations, the data obtained after acid stimulation was very reproducible; replicate values for the volumes of saliva after stimulation with ascorbic acid were within a standard deviation of ± 10%.

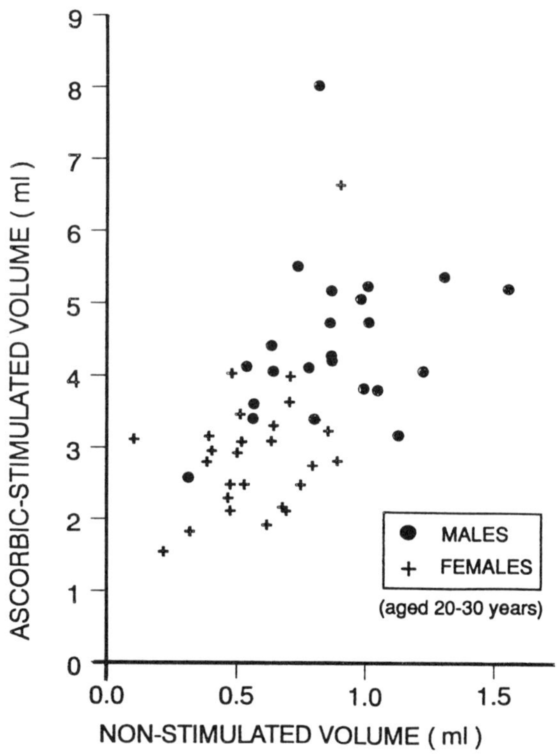

Figure 2. Volumes of saliva in adult volunteers aged 20-30 years, before and after stimulation by ascorbic acid, as determined by the fluoride dilution technique. Both stimulated and non-stimulated volumes were significantly greater in males than in females ($p<0.001$).

D. Variations in Saliva Volumes Between Individuals

The fluoride dilution technique was used in an attempt to compare stimulated and unstimulated secretions between different individuals. The results obtained from a group of about 50 adult volunteers aged 20-30 years are shown in Figure 2. A significant correlation ($p<0.001$) was found between the volume of saliva present before stimulation and the volume after stimulation [9]. This may have been a reflection of body size. A large individual might be expected to have a larger mouth than a small individual and it would seem likely that the amount of saliva in the mouth, stimulated or non-stimulated, would relate to the volume of the oral cavity. In contrast to the experience of Lagerlöf and Dawes [3], the present authors found a significant correlation between the weights of the individuals and the volumes of saliva in the mouth [10].

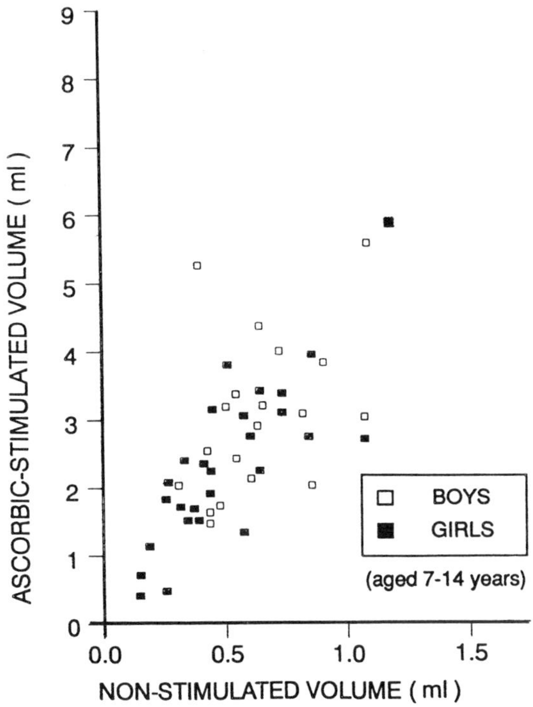

Figure 3. Volumes of saliva in children aged 7-14 years, before and after stimulation by ascorbic acid, as determined by the fluoride dilution technique. Both stimulated and non-stimulated volumes were significantly greater in boys than in girls ($p<0.01$).

There seemed to be no general change with age in the stimulated or non-stimulated volumes of saliva [9]. There was, however, a clear sex difference. The volumes of saliva present both before and after stimulation were significantly greater in males than in females ($p>0.001$) (Figure 2). Collins and Dawes [6] found no difference in the area of the oral cavity (as an indication of volume) of males and females. Ferrario et al [11], using a Euclidian-distance matrix analysis, compared the form of the maxillary- with that of the mandibular-dental arch. They found some sex differences in arch-form but no difference in the size of male versus female arches seem to have emerged from their study. These are, however, difficult measurements and further attempts should perhaps be made to determine mouth size, if possible using other approaches. Another part of the explanation for the above sex difference in the case of the stimulated values, however, might be that the females responded less to salivary stimuli [10].

The investigation of children aged 7-14 years gave analogous results (Figure 3). Volumes of saliva were less in girls than in boys, under both non-stimulated ($p<0.01$) and stimulated ($p<0.01$) conditions. Under stimulated conditions, the volume of saliva was significantly lower in girls than in women ($p<0.01$) and in boys than in men ($p<0.001$) [12].

The responses of patients who complained of a dry mouth were also examined [13]. In a few cases, volumes of saliva under both non-stimulated and stimulated conditions were found to be extremely low and apparently abnormally so. For the great majority of patients, however, non-stimulated volumes were within the normal (control) range and there was also considerable overlap between the "dry mouth" and "normal" groups in the case of the stimulated values. In other words, it would rarely be possible to diagnose or unequivocally to confirm a patient's subjective impression of dry mouth by measuring separately either the non-stimulated or the stimulated saliva volume. This, as suggested earlier, is probably in part because mouth size varies; the volume of saliva present in the mouth of a giant with "dry mouth" would probably flood the mouth of a pygmy. When, however, the above mentioned correlation between stimulated and non-stimulated volumes was taken into account, e.g., by plotting one against the other, as in Figures 2 and 3, a distinction could usually be made between the normal individual and the patient complaining of a dry mouth; the stimulated volume was low relative to the patient's non-stimulated volume.

In view of the accuracy, rapidity and great convenience of this simple fluoride dilution technique (it can be carried out in a matter of seconds even on young children) it would seem worthwhile looking for a marker more suitable than fluoride for use under acidic conditions (see p. 161).

E. The Direction of Salivary Flow in the Oral Cavity

Over 90% of the total volume of saliva in the mouth is made up of secretions from the major salivary glands; usually 7-8% comes from the minor mucous glands; the greatest volume is usually supplied by the submandibular gland although the parotid may respond more to an acidic stimulus [14]. Lecompte and Dawes [15] came to some interesting conclusions about the directional flow of saliva. The overall picture is still sketchy and unclear but seems to be somewhat as follows. On the floor of the oral cavity, on the lingual side of the mandibular dental arch, there would be a major flow from the front towards the back of the mouth; a flow augmented by the saliva from the submandibular and sublingual salivary ducts. A smaller stream would flow in the same anterior to posterior direction on the outer, buccal side of the mandibular dental arch. This might partly explain the high degree of localization of substances placed in the posterior region of the mandibular sulcus [16]. Lecompte and Dawes [15] considered that even the flow of saliva from the opening of the parotid duct in the upper posterior buccal sulcus would still be moving principally in a

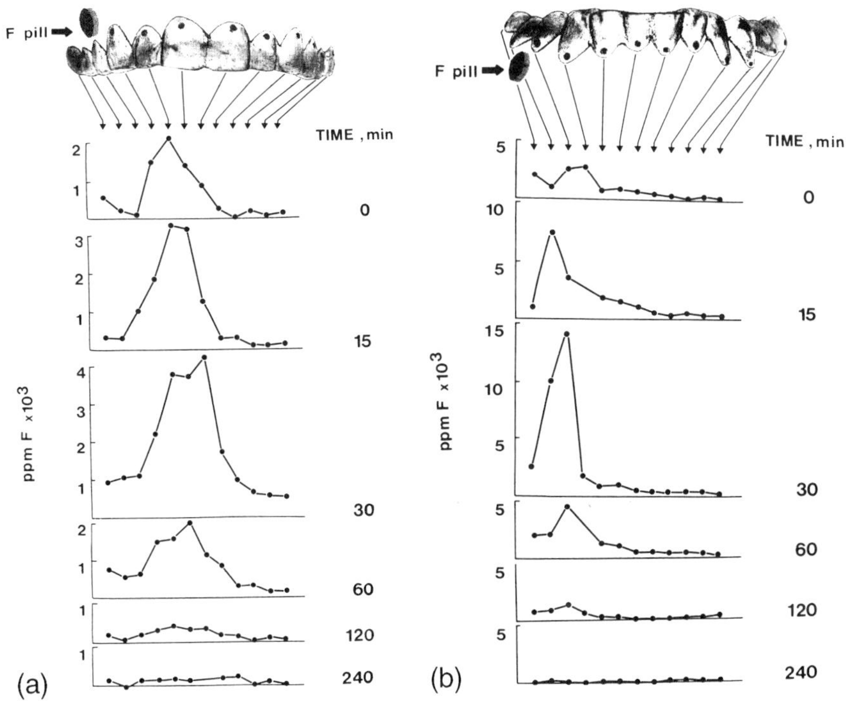

Figure 4. (a) Fluoride released from a tablet placed in the posterior region of the upper (maxillary) buccal sulcus. Fluoride concentrations in saliva became relatively low near the dissolving tablet while in the anterior (labial) part of the sulcus a high concentration developed. (b) Fluoride released from a tablet placed in the posterior region of the lower, (mandibular) buccal sulcus. Fluoride concentrations in saliva increased markedly in the region of the tablet but there was no appreciable overall increase in salivary fluoride levels. (From reference 16).

posterior direction until it arrived at the posterior cul de sac at the end of the maxillary sulcus. From here it would flow over the occlusal surfaces of the molar teeth in a bucco-lingual direction, and then drain down onto the floor of the oral cavity.

On the lingual side of the upper (maxillary) dental arch the saliva would flow downwards from the palate. On the lingual side of the lower (mandibular) arch, some saliva would flow between the teeth into the buccal or labial sulcus while, in the labial region, some would be pushed vertically from the floor of the mouth upwards and over the lingual aspects of the teeth. These vertical streams would meet at the occlusal surfaces of the teeth and tend to flow over these surfaces in a linguo-labial direction. Finally, in order to explain the apparent anterior migration of fluoride from a tablet placed in the upper posterior region of the maxillary sulcus (Figure 4a), it was suggested that a subsidiary stream of parotid saliva may flow along the maxillary sulcus in a posterior-to-anterior direction.

Further work is required to clarify and consolidate this picture of the directional pattern of salivary flow, which is still tentative and unclear.

III. THE ORAL DISTRIBUTION OF SUBSTANCES IN THE MOUTH

A. Movement of Substances Around the Mouth

The view generally held until recently was that substances are distributed easily, rapidly and ubiquitously throughout the oral cavity. This is despite reports as early as 1922 when Bloomfield [17] described how charcoal suspended in saliva exhibited distinct patterns of (restricted) movement around the mouth which were dependent upon the original placement site of the charcoal. Some 47 years later Meyer [18] reported that fluoride from a fluoride tablet dissolving at one site may not move to other regions of the mouth. The full significance of these finding in terms of drug delivery, dental health and salivary flow in general seems not to have been appreciated and it is only following more recent evidence that it is being appreciated that substances dissolved or suspended in saliva seem more reluctant to move around the mouth than might be imagined.

Fluids certainly do mix well in the mouth in some instances. Jenkins [14] thought the fact that the composition of pellicle was the same in different regions of the mouth suggested that submandibular saliva spread over the whole oral cavity. He also demonstrated that powdered charcoal placed under the tongue spread throughout the oral cavity within a few minutes. The linearity of the data presented in Figure 1 showed that when the mouth was rinsed for 15 seconds, fluoride, contained in a milliliter of solution, mixed thoroughly with various other volumes of fluid in the mouth [8].

However, the reports by Bloomfield [17] and Meyer [18] show that mixing does not always take place. These reports were confirmed in later experiments, carried out by Weatherell et al [16], who placed a fluoride tablet in the posterior part of the lower mandibular sulcus (Figure 4b). Fluoride concentrations increased markedly in the region of the tablet but there was no appreciable overall increase in salivary fluoride levels at the other side of the mouth (Figure 4b). Posteriorly, the lower mandibular sulci seemed to be fairly isolated environments. Subsequent investigations by Jenkins and Krebsbach [19] showed that particles of charcoal placed in the posterior mandibular sulcus failed to cross the oral cavity. Other substances tested, e.g., glucose, behaved in a similar way [20] and a recent study by O'Connell et al [21] showed that in rats also there may be little movement of saliva across the midline of the oral cavity. In other sites too, the local release of a substance did not guarantee its

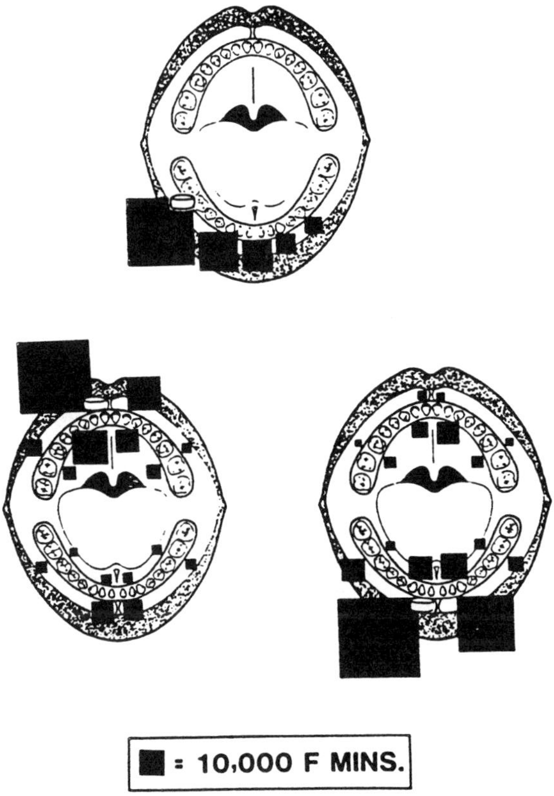

Figure 5. Tablet; passive dissolution. In several sites, the local release of a substance would not guarantee its presence to an appreciable extent elsewhere. The black squares correspond to the areas beneath the fluoride clearance curve at the sites indicated, over a period of 0-120 minutes, as a result of fluoride being released from a tablet at the positions shown in the diagrams. (From a diagram in Weatherell et al [28], constructed from data of Weatherell et al [16] and Primosch et al [35]).

presence to an appreciable extent elsewhere (Figure 5). Hector and Sullivan (1992) [22] showed that even during the unilateral chewing of erythrosin-containing gum, very little erythrosin was present contralaterally. These results are important as they have implications for anyone attempting to deliver drugs from one site to another in the mouth. As Toumba and Curzon [23] pointed out, the position of placement of a delivery system in the mouth was likely to be of considerable importance and although the oral distribution of fluoride from slow-release devices had not been studied, it needed to be.

All sites are not equally restrictive. As mentioned above, Jenkins [14] showed that powdered charcoal placed beneath the tongue spreads rapidly throughout the mouth. Similarly, fluoride released from a tablet placed in the posterior region of the upper, as opposed to the lower, maxillary sulcus seemed to migrate somewhat freely along the maxillary sulcus, away from the tablet towards the anterior region of the mouth. Fluoride concentrations in saliva eventually became relatively low near to the site where the tablet had dissolved while in the anterior i.e., labial part of the maxillary sulcus, a high concentration progressively developed [16] (compare Figures 4a and 4b). Prima facie, it appeared that migration of fluoride from the tablet along the upper, maxillary sulcus had taken place, perhaps together with some trapping of the fluoride ion behind the upper lip. It was suggested that the fluoride was being pushed along the upper labial sulcus in an anterior direction by saliva flowing from the opening of the parotid duct, this being situated near to the dissolving fluoride tablet. Caution is needed in such interpretation, however. It is not possible to make unequivocal deductions about salivary flow from data about regional differences in concentration. A relatively high concentration could mean that salivary turnover was low or that material was being physically or chemically trapped. A low concentration could be due to saliva flowing into the region and reducing local concentrations of a substance by dilution, as probably occurs in the lower labial sulcus. A low concentration could also be due to saliva flowing away from the region and carrying the substance with it, as probably occurs near the opening of the parotid duct in the upper posterior sulcus. Direct evidence of salivary flow is needed before the whole picture can be definitively established.

B. Retention of Substances at Different Sites in the Mouth

Control experiments carried out in parallel with these migration studies, revealed a further curious fact. Analysis of small volumes of saliva sampled from different regions of the mouth after rinsing with a fluoride solution showed that fluoride concentrations varied considerably from place to place in the mouth [24, 25].

While the mouth was being rinsed concentrations were the same at different sites, but after rinsing had stopped a much higher concentration of fluoride was present in the upper than in the lower labial sulcus (Figure 6). Britse and Lagerlöf [26] described a similar distribution of sucrose in the labial sulci after mouthrinsing with sucrose solution. Weatherell et al [20] found a similar pattern with glucose and with the distribution of vegetable dye [24]. In the posterior region the reverse was the case. In general, there was always more fluoride at buccal sites than at lingual sites. The lowest concentration of all was invariably found beneath the tongue. The nature of the substance seemed to be of little significance. The means or manner by which a drug is

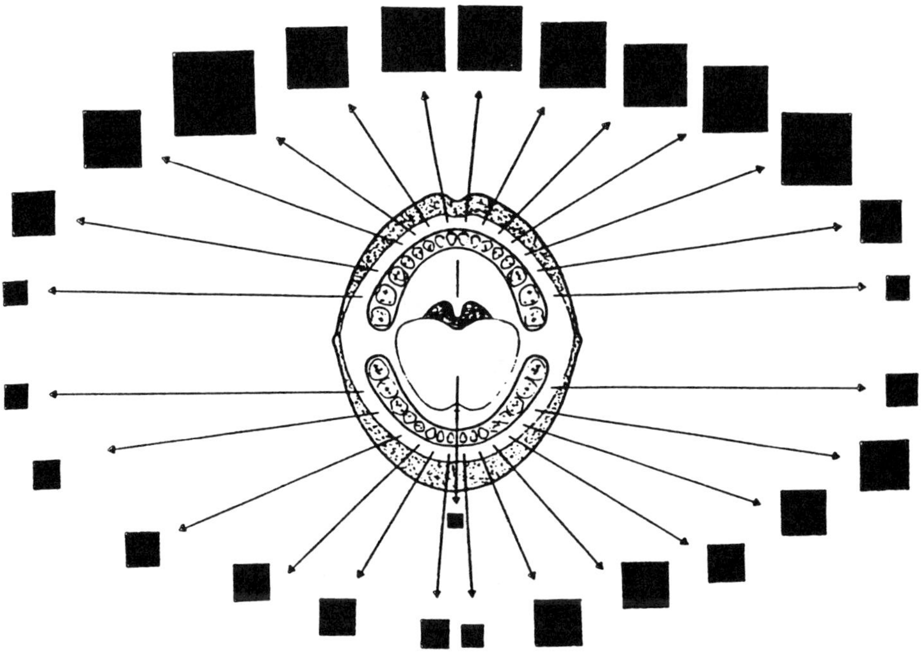

Figure 6. Fluoride retention at different sites in the mouth of one individual after rinsing with a solution containing 1000 ppmF (as NaF). The squares correspond to the areas beneath the fluoride clearance curve at the sites indicated, over a period of 1-15 minutes. (From reference 24).

introduced to a site also appeared to be of no significance to the final pattern. For instance, although fluoride in toothpaste might be applied to specific areas of the dentition by a tooth brush, its ultimate distribution was determined by the physiology of the mouth itself. After brushing had stopped, the fluoride was redistributed according to the typical site-specific pattern for the individual and it was then cleared from each site in the mouth at rates commensurate with this distribution pattern. Studies, unpublished, show that these differential concentration patterns can persist for hours after a substance has been introduced into the mouth.

C. Consistency of Site-Specific Distribution Patterns

The site-specific patterns of substrate distribution and, to some extent, even the rates of clearance were usually fairly consistent from time to time for any one

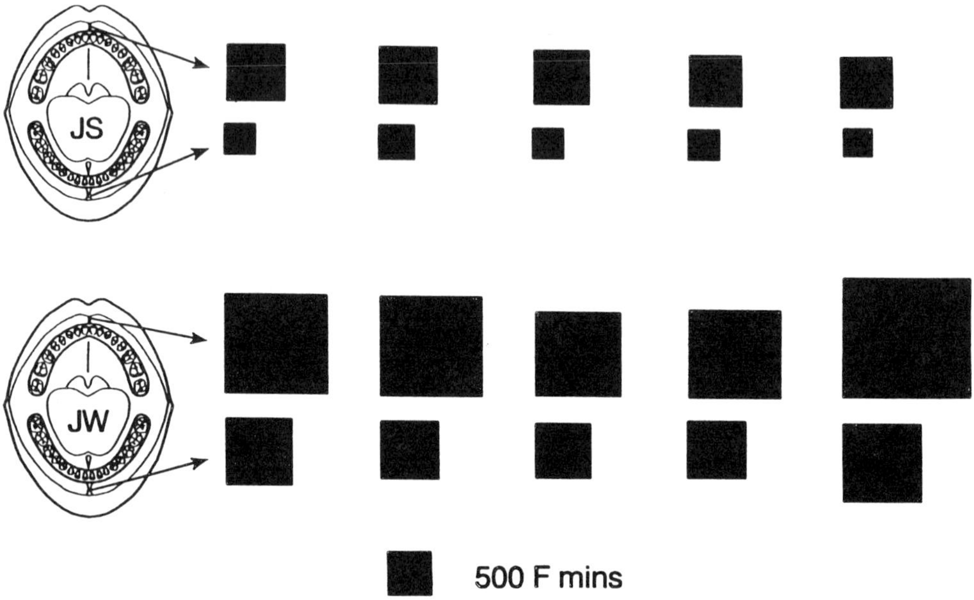

Figure 7. Retention of fluoride by two individuals (JS and JW) measured on five occasions over a period of five months. The squares represent the areas beneath the fluoride clearance curves between 1-15 minutes. The site-specific distribution of fluoride between the upper and the lower labial sulci were consistently similar for both subjects over the test period but much more fluoride was invariably retained by JW than by JS. (From reference 24).

individual. There were, however, often large differences in concentration between individuals. For instance, in the case of the two individuals illustrated in Figure 7, the site-specific pattern of distribution between the upper and the lower labial sulci were similar and consistent over the test period of five months, but much higher concentrations of fluoride were invariably retained by JW than by JS [25]. The retention of fluoride by each volunteer was usually of the same order from one month to the next although concentrations were higher in JW's final test than in his previous four. This was probably an occasion when JW's flow of saliva was low. Even then, however, the distribution pattern between upper and lower labial sulci was very similar. More detailed quantitative studies of glucose clearance [20, 27] again showed that the site-specific patterns of an individual usually remain essentially the same, despite the sometimes large absolute day-to-day variations in oral retention or clearance.

D. Simultaneous Biochemical Reactions and Distribution and Retention

All the above discussions about drug concentration and distribution have made the tacit assumption that changes in concentration are entirely attributable to salivary dilution and swallowing, and are independent of the nature of the substances concerned. There is good evidence that this assumption is largely justified. Britse and Lagerlöf [26] found that, after rinsing the mouth with sucrose solution, sucrose concentrations at a number of sites in the mouth correlated well with induced changes in the salivary flow rate. Weatherell et al [28] found that the site-specific concentration patterns of both glucose and fluoride, when released simultaneously in the mouth, were essentially the same, even though they would behave very differently from a biochemical point of view. Any variations in concentration of these substances due to their biochemical reaction with saliva, with the surfaces of the oral mucosa, with dental or other oral deposits, with oral bacteria or perhaps specifically with diseased sites in the oral cavity, must have been relatively small compared with the changes in concentration brought about by salivary dilution and clearance.

In any study of migration or retention, or in the assessment of a delivery system it is important to know what reactions are occurring, e.g., adsorption, absorption, etc., and to what extent. It is important to confirm that the amounts of drug involved in these processes are minimal compared to those discussed above in relation to the site-specific patterns.

E. The Explanation for the Site-Specific Pattern

Prima facie, the explanation for some of these more general observations seems obvious; they apparently reflect the general anatomy and physiology of the oral cavity.

Concentrations are presumably highest in the upper labial sulcus because this region is distant from any of the openings of the major salivary ducts. Only the viscous secretions from the minor mucous glands are likely to wash and dilute concentrations in this area and the turnover of saliva will consequently be low.

In the lower labial sulcus, on the other hand, concentrations will be relatively low because substances are rapidly diluted by the saliva draining into the lower parts of the mouth and flowing into the region from the submandibular and sublingual glands.

Concentrations are lowest of all beneath the tongue because here too substances will be flushed away and diluted by sublingual and submandibular saliva and by other oral fluids draining into the floor of the mouth. The movement of the tongue will probably further increase salivary turnover.

In the posterior part of the upper (maxillary) buccal sulcus, saliva flows rapidly from the parotid duct. This is situated near to the buccal surfaces of the first or second upper, (maxillary) molar. The parotid saliva will wash away and dilute substances in this area and then drain down into the lower buccal sulcus. As a consequence of this, concentrations are almost always lower at the surfaces of the upper molars than near the lower molars, where substances may tend to be trapped in the cul de sac of the lower posterior sulcus.

As suggested earlier, some of the saliva emerging from the parotid duct might move anteriorly along the upper (maxillary) sulcus and flush substances towards the upper labial region. This could account for the changes in concentration which occur in this region when a fluoride tablet is placed in the posterior maxillary buccal sulcus (Figure 4a).

As suggested above, the action of the tongue will probably increase the turnover of fluid collecting in the floor of the mouth. This could contribute to the lowering of concentrations in this region and help to explain Jenkins' [14] earlier observation that powdered charcoal placed beneath the tongue quickly finds its way to all regions of the mouth. The movement of cheeks and lips could also influence the patterns of salivary flow. Hase and Birkhed [29] mentioned this obvious possibility but little or no work seems to have been carried out on such effects. In the upper anterior sulcus, the lips could, conversely, trap saliva against the surfaces of teeth and gingivae, restricting salivary turnover and contributing to the maintenance of high concentrations in this region.

Once established, such local differences in concentration can persist because migration of substances from one region to another across the oral surfaces can be slow. Lecompte and Dawes [15] investigated the way in which substances were cleared from oral surfaces. They created an artificial intra-oral system in which they measured the diffusion of potassium and chloride ions from layers of agarose placed in acrylic devices at different sites in the mouth. There was a clear correlation between the half-times of diffusion at different regions of the mouth and the site-specific patterns of oral clearance described above. Retention of the potassium and chloride ions was for instance greater in the upper anterior sulcus than in the lower anterior sulcus. They interpreted these findings in the light of their concept of a thin film of saliva covering the oral surfaces, suggesting that the mechanism of clearance of ions from their agarose plaques involved movement of ions into and along these thin films. Differences and variations in the rates of turnover or velocities of the film would account for many features of the site-specific patterns of retention [30].

In summary, the reason these site-specific differences in concentration exist is because (i) mixing of solutions in the mouth is not perfect; substances often migrate with difficulty from one site to another, (ii) there are local differences in rates of salivary flow resulting in differences in concentration due to differences in drug clearance and dilution and (iii) changes in concentrations in one region may or may not affect concentrations in another region. As the work of Collins and Dawes [6] and Watanabe and Dawes [4] has indicated, the saliva covers much of the oral surfaces in the form of a thin film, which is less mobile in some areas than in others [30, 31]. There are also various pockets and cul de sacs in the mouth and even the variation in the width of spaces between the teeth may have a considerable influence on local clearance [32].

F. Divergence from the General Pattern

Very occasionally, major differences from this general site-specific distribution pattern were encountered. This apparently conflicts with the idea of the "general pattern of drug distribution" described above. In a few individuals, the difference between concentrations in the upper versus the lower anterior sulci was not very pronounced. In one of eleven volunteers described in Weatherell et al [25] and in another case encountered (unpublished), fluoride concentrations were lower in the upper compared with the lower labial sulcus! In quite a few individuals, retention was greater in the upper than in the lower posterior buccal sulcus.

These anomalies are difficult to explain with any certainty because as yet an insufficient number of such apparently aberrant individuals have been encountered. Some tentative suggestions can be put forward, however, the tendency to trap substances in the upper labial sulcus may be less in a class II occlusion where the upper incisors protrude outside the lips. Retention could also vary according to the width of the interdental spaces, which will control the flow of saliva between the teeth and the sulcus [32]. Retention in this area may also be less if, perhaps because of idiosyncrasies of speech, the upper lip is more than usually mobile and less persistently or less firmly pressed against the teeth.

In the posterior part of the mouth, minor differences between the rates of clearance from the upper versus lower molar tooth surfaces are easier to explain. They appear to have been due to individual variations in the position of the opening to the parotid duct, relative to the site of sampling, which was generally fixed according to the position of the teeth [27, 33].

Marked differences in concentration between subjects, on the other hand, such as those illustrated in Figure 7 are easily explained; they are most likely due to differences in the overall rates of salivary secretion without concomitant variations in salivary retention.

G. Alterations in the General Pattern by External Intervention

Although the experiment described in Figure 7 and the study of Weatherell, et al [20] suggest that the day-to-day variations in the rate of salivary secretion do not seem to alter the site-specific clearance patterns to any great extent, this is not necessarily the case when the rate of secretion is severely altered by pharmacological intervention. When Hase et al [34] reduced the rate of salivary secretion by submucosal injection of methylscopolamine nitrate, the normal difference in the rates of clearance between a sublingual location and a site in the labial sulcus decreased from about eight fold almost to unity.

The site-specific distribution pattern of a substance may also be temporarily distorted when a substance, e.g., fluoride from a fluoride tablet, is released at a fixed site [16, 35]. How much the normal pattern is distorted will depend upon the rate and amounts of substance released and the site at which it occurs. The disturbance will presumably be greater when the release occurs at a site where retention is relatively high, e.g., in the upper labial sulcus or the posterior part of the lower buccal sulcus and less if the tablet is placed at a site where the turnover of saliva is particularly rapid, e.g., beneath the tongue.

When the local release ceases, the oral distribution will revert to that dictated by the individual's mouth. An illustration of this is presented in Figure 8, which demonstrates the effect a fluoride tablet had on fluoride concentrations in the upper and lower anterior labial sulci. While the tablet was dissolving on the dorsal surface of the tongue, the fluoride would flow downwards. Salivary concentrations were therefore higher in the lower than the upper labial sulcus. After dissolution had finished, the distribution rapidly reverted to the typical pattern; salivary concentrations in the lower sulcus decreased while those in the upper sulcus increased.

H. Alterations in Drug Concentration by External Intervention

Any change in the rate of salivary secretion will affect the intra-oral concentrations of a drug. The drug itself or components of the delivery system could alter the rate of secretion and this may militate against or assist the maintenance of therapeutic drug concentrations.

For instance, most of the commercial fluoride dentifrices are strongly flavored with mint. This stimulates the secretion of saliva which reduces the concentration of fluoride in the mouth. The present authors compared the fluoride concentration in saliva prior to swallowing produced by a well known commercial, mint-flavored fluoride toothpaste, with that produced by a similar volume of water containing the same amount of fluoride. Stimulation of salivation by the toothpaste reduced the concentration of fluoride in the mouth to a level several fold below that of the aqueous solution (Figure 9). Mint

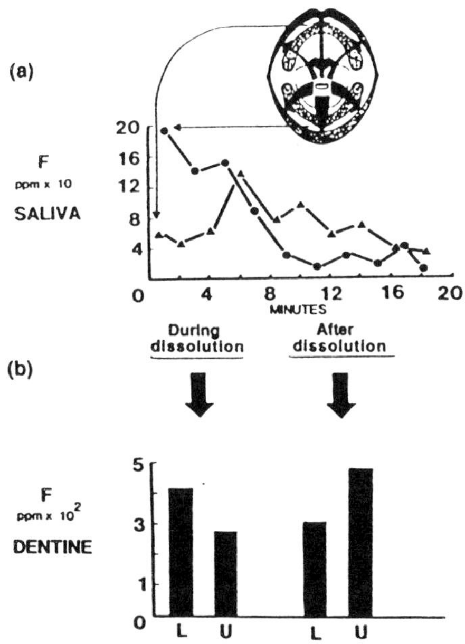

Figure 8. (a) Concentration of fluoride over an 18 minute period in the upper and lower anterior labial sulci during and after dissolution of a fluoride tablet containing 1 mg fluoride (as NaF) placed on the surface of the subject's (JAW) tongue. (b) While the tablet was dissolving, fluoride concentrations were higher in the lower (L) than the upper (U) labial sulcus. After the tablet had dissolved, fluoride concentrations in the lower sulcus decreased while those in the upper sulcus increased, the distribution thereby reverting to the normal site-specific pattern.

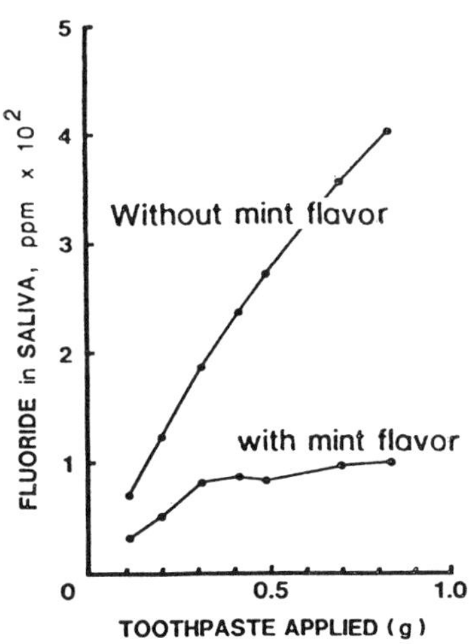

Figure 9. The mint flavor in a commercial dentifrice stimulated the secretion of saliva and greatly reduced the concentration of fluoride in the mouth in the 2 minutes prior to swallowing "with mint flavor", compared with that produced by a similar volume of water containing the same amount of fluoride "without mint flavor".

flavor also encourages the user to swallow, to expectorate and to rinse the mouth with water [36], all of which still further decreases the oral availability of fluoride.

There is a well established positive correlation between the cariostatic action of fluoride and its concentration in dentifrices and in saliva [37-42]. There are, however, strict toxicologically established legal limits to the amount of fluoride which can be put into a commercial dentifrice. Manufacturers use the maximum permitted dose but, having done this, they include the mint flavor. The fluoride concentration achieved in the mouth is then considerably reduced. From a pharmaceutical point of view, it would be rational to remove the mint flavor. Unfortunately, its presence in a dentifrice is closely linked to consumer preference.

Substances which reduce salivary secretion would, conversely, be expected to increase drug concentrations in the mouth. No attempt seems to have been made to exploit this commercially but one of the authors (JW) tested the effect of a travel-sickness tablet containing hyoscine hydrobromide on fluoride concentrations in saliva. After some time, volumes of saliva produced by stimulation had dramatically decreased, as measured by the fluoride dilution technique, and the salivary concentration produced by a standard amount of fluoride increased correspondingly.

IV. TECHNOLOGICAL FACILITIES AND PROBLEMS

Two general methods have been used to determine patterns of movement and retention; qualitative visual and quantitative analytical methods. In the former method substances such as charcoal [14, 17, 19] or dyes [22, 24] are visually observed and their migration recorded. The compounds used in these studies must fulfill certain criteria such as their presence should not stimulate secretion and they should not interact in any way with dental or oral tissues. In the case of glucose, it is possible to demonstrate the site-specific distribution of the molecule visually using the glucose-sensitive strip normally employed for testing blood glucose concentrations in diabetics (Boehringer B M-Test-Glycemie 1-44 test strips). The strips can be used directly as supplied, putting the glucose-sensitive film in contact with the saliva in the mouth or alternatively, thin dental splints can be fitted over the teeth and small squares of glucose-sensitive strip glued to the splints at sites of interest [47, 48]. When removed from the mouth they should be rinsed with water and gently dried with paper tissue. This produces a visual record of glucose distribution at one point in time (Figure 10). The glucose concentrations in saliva can also be estimated either by comparing the color with the visual scale provided with the Boehringer strips or the glucose-sensitive pieces removed from the splint and a

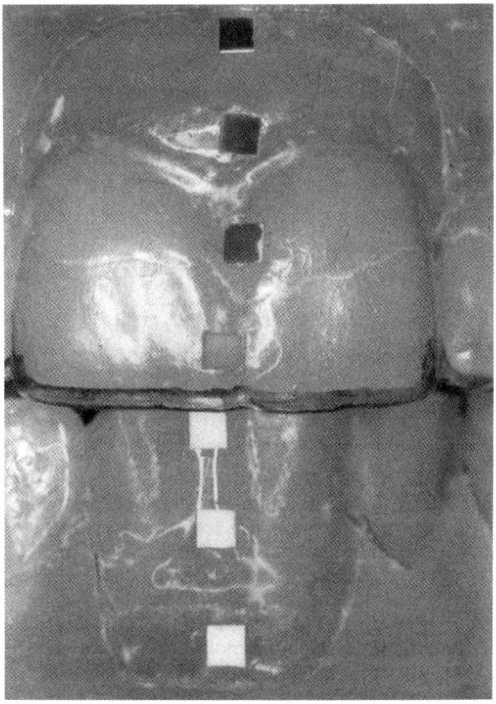

Figure 10. Thin dental splints onto which small squares of Boehringer glucose-sensitive strip had been fixed. The mouth was rinsed for 15 seconds with 10 mL of a 250 mM glucose solution. The splints were placed in the mouth, removed after a minute, rinsed with water and gently dried with paper tissue to produce a visual record of glucose distribution. (From reference 48).

more quantitative determination made using for example a Reflolux IIM analyzer.

In the quantitative analysis of substances at localized sites in the mouth several problems are encountered. These arise due to the small volume of fluid available for sampling. Medlicott et al [43] used Lagerlöf and Dawes' estimate for the volume of saliva in the mouth before and after swallowing and Collins and Dawes' value for the surface area of the adult mouth and thickness of the salivary film to calculate the average amount of saliva for sampling to be about 3.6-5.0 $\mu L/cm^2$. With such small volumes available for sampling it is clear that the analytical procedures used to define site-specific variations need to be very sensitive and, by necessity, depend on sophisticated micro-analytical procedures. The exploitation of fluoride analysis for many of the studies was largely a matter of practical convenience, because of a long experience with the micro-determination of the element.

With the determination of a drug which is slowly released over prolonged periods of time there is the need for sensitive analytical techniques to assess the effectiveness of the system. In this respect, high performance liquid chromatography offers a useful method and has been used for the determination of chlorhexidine concentrations at different sites in the mouth [44].

In quantifying the concentration of a substance at a particular site in the mouth knowledge of the volume of sample taken is required. In this respect two problems must be considered; (i) how to take the sample and (ii) how to determine the volume of the sample. As alluded to above only small (1 μL) samples of saliva from specific sites in the mouth can be taken. The most convenient method is by the use of a small piece of absorbent filter paper. For example, small paper points about 5 mm long were used by Weatherell and co-workers [35], paper discs by Zero et al [45] and Periopaper strips by Medlicott et al [43, 44].

Two methods for determining the volume of sample taken (Periotron and sample mass) were compared by Medlicott et al [43]. These authors demonstrated that sample mass provided a simple and accurate method to determine sample volumes of less than 1 μL. The sample mass technique was similar to that described by Weatherell et al [25] and is described below. The Periopaper strips were retained in small air-tight polypropylene Eppendorf tubes (0.6 mL capacity), the whole being weighed on a 5-place balance to an accuracy of ± 0.02 mg [43]. To sample the oral fluid, the Periopaper was removed from an Eppendorf tube with forceps and placed for a few seconds in contact with the sample site e.g., surface of tooth, tongue, oral mucosa, etc. The Periopaper strip was immediately returned to the Eppendorf tube which was then closed and immediately reweighed to determine the amount of oral fluid absorbed by the Periopaper. The advantages of the sample mass method compared to the Periotron method include that sample loss due to evaporation is minimal since samples are placed immediately after collection into air-tight containers and it is not necessary to construct a standard curve as the density of the sample fluid is known [46].

On occasions when, due to xerostomia, the mouth under investigation is unusually dry, it is not possible to take even the smallest sample of saliva using a paper point. However, Weatherell et al [8] showed that it was still possible to obtain data about the average composition of the saliva, merely by rinsing the mouth gently with 1 mL of standard fluoride solution which was then expectorated. A sample of any saliva present in the mouth would be contained in the expectorated volume of the rinse. From the fluoride concentration of this volume, the amount of saliva present in it could be calculated. The concentration of any other component in the rinse could therefore also be calculated in relation to the original, undiluted saliva present in the "dry" mouth.

In addition to determining the changes in concentration occurring in different regions of the mouth or following release from a drug delivery system due to the influence of saliva, it is often of interest to investigate biochemical events occurring at the oral surfaces, e.g., adsorption, absorption, etc., which may be occurring simultaneously with the effects of saliva. The problem is that it is not possible to use data about the concentrations of reactants or products to obtain definitive information about local biochemical reactions because of the much greater simultaneous changes in concentration taking place due to salivary dilution. In an attempt to overcome this difficulty the authors carried out some preliminary studies [47, 48] on the metabolism of glucose and fluoride in plaque and saliva. The principles of this methodology could be extended to allow investigators to evaluate the contribution of, for example, absorption of a drug to any migration or retention patterns observed following release from a delivery system. The method involved the mouth being rinsed with solutions containing glucose and fluoride at a fixed molar ratio. The idea was that massive changes in substrate concentrations brought about by salivary dilution could not alter a molar ratio, whereas even small changes in the concentration of one of the substrates due to metabolism, absorption, adsorption, etc., would do so. To demonstrate these principles a sample was taken from the cervical surfaces of upper and lower incisors using paper points. This sample would consist of saliva together with any early salivary deposits present on the tooth surface. Samples of saliva were simultaneously taken from the nearby upper and lower labial sulci. The distribution of glucose and fluoride between upper and lower sulci was of course very similar for both types of sample. As, expected, any differential changes in concentration due to biochemical reactions of fluoride or glucose were obscured by the much greater differences imposed by the site-specific differences in salivary dilution. However, an indication of behavioral differences between the two substances was given by the observed changes in the glucose:fluoride molar ratios. In both samples from the upper incisors the ratio was similar to that in the original mouth rinse. This suggested that no detectable metabolic change had occurred. In the samples from the surface of the lower incisor, however, glucose:fluoride ratios were much lower than those in the rinse. Some metabolic change had occurred. Concentrations of glucose in the samples from the surface of the lower incisor were also significantly lower than those in the saliva from the nearby lower labial sulcus. This suggests that the reduction of the molar ratio had been due to a loss of glucose by bacterial metabolism at the surface of the lower incisor.

The above use of molar ratios for the detection of minor changes in concentration due to local biochemical reactions could be extended. The sensitivity of such tests in respect of any particular substrate could be increased merely by reducing the concentration of this substrate in the rinse. Any number of substrates, e.g., a cocktail of different sugars or amino acids at known molar ratios could be used. A metabolically inert molecule such as xylitol could usefully be included in the sugar solution, at a fixed molar ratio, to establish more precisely what changes in concentration are due exclusively to dilution.

These preliminary experiments thus seem to offer a possible approach to the study of metabolic reactions in the oral environment, where salivary dilution changes the concentrations of reactants.

V. IMPLICATIONS FOR DRUG DELIVERY

It is clear from the preceding discussions that the oral cavity is a considerably more complex area for local drug delivery than might first be imagined and the relationship between saliva and oral mucosal drug delivery system design is poorly defined, characterized and controlled. Formulation scientists have, historically, viewed the mouth as an open vessel into which saliva is secreted and then flushed away without giving due consideration to the direction of flow of saliva or its effect on the design of local oral mucosal drug delivery systems. The opinion that saliva exists in the mouth as a free flowing bulk volume is also untrue. In reality it exists as a mobile film of 0.1 mm average thickness. Substances within it seem not to be able to migrate easily from one region of the mouth to another. The view that any substance entering into the mouth is rapidly diluted and removed by swallowing has also had to have been revised in the light of recent investigations. The implications of such site-specific patterns of drug distribution and retention should be considered when designing a local oral mucosal drug delivery system.

Recent studies on the fate of substances dissolved or suspended in saliva have shown that the mouth is a complex area in which the deposition and clearance of drugs is site specific. This picture appears to be substance-independent and largely controlled by the anatomical and physiological conditions of the oral cavity and, although the patterns appear fairly consistent from person to person, the speed of migration [19] and final concentrations (Figure 7) would be expected to vary from individual to individual. This, together with the fact that the area is still in its infancy, means that it is too early to quantitatively use our current knowledge of the area in the design of locally administered oral mucosal drug delivery systems. However, qualitative prediction of sites of migration and retention can be speculated upon.

The aim of local drug delivery is to provide a therapeutic concentration of drug at the required site of action for the desired length of time. Such an aim would be dependent upon the delivery system (its composition and release rate), the site of administration and the anatomical and physiological features of the mouth. It seems to us that an increased knowledge about the relationships between (i) the components of the formulation, release rates and sites of administration and (ii) the various patterns and mechanisms of distribution and retention in the mouth might result in information that provides a scientific rationale for the design, development and use of oral mucosal drug delivery systems for local administration. The former (i) are under the control of the formulation scientist. The latter (ii) appear to be determined by the mouth, and although the formulation scientist has little control over these processes he would need to consider them during preformulation and optimization of any oral mucosal drug delivery system. Whether a local oral mucosal drug delivery system achieves its aim is dependent upon the extent to which released drug in saliva migrates from one site to another in the mouth and how long it is retained there before it is cleared. Recent studies have provided us with some indication of how the type and composition of the delivery system, site of administration and rate of release may affect the fate of drugs administered to sites in the mouth and are discussed below.

The site of placement of a formulation in the mouth appears to be an important consideration in the development of a locally administered oral mucosal drug delivery system since the site of placement of a delivery system will have a marked influence on local concentrations and final deposition of the drug [16-19, 35]. It has become apparent that local release of a substance in some sites in the mouth would not guarantee its presence to an appreciable extent elsewhere (Figures 4 and 5). For example, drug released from a tablet dissolving in the upper buccal sulcus would be expected to migrate in an anterior direction resulting in some transfer from one side of the mouth to the other (Figure 4a). In contrast, if the same tablet were to be placed in the lower buccal sulcus a large local concentration of drug around the delivery system may be observed but little detectable change in drug concentration at any other sites in the mouth (Figure 4b) [16, 18]. Other sites that are restrictive have also been identified, e.g., in the upper labial sulcus or the posterior part of the lower buccal sulcus. Placement at these sites would not result in an increase in concentration of drug elsewhere in the mouth. Also of concern is the possibility that if the release rate from the delivery system was not specifically tailored for these sites, undesirable high local concentrations at these sites may occur [16].

The inability of drugs to transfer across the midline of the oral cavity has been reported by several investigators [17-19, 35]. Such observations have implications when a drug is required to spread throughout the oral cavity. To achieve this requirement the delivery system would probably have to be placed under the tongue [18, 19]. Because of the action of the tongue in the process of swallowing, however, the retention of oral mucosal drug delivery systems in this area is difficult to achieve.

The concentration of drug at a given site will be altered while a substance is being released from the delivery system [16, 35]. An illustration of this is presented in Figure 8. While the tablet was dissolving on the dorsal surface of the tongue, the fluoride would flow downwards. Fluoride concentrations were therefore higher in the lower than the upper labial sulcus. After dissolution had finished, the distribution rapidly reverted to the typical pattern; fluoride concentrations in the lower sulcus decreased while those in the upper sulcus increased. The pharmaceutical implication of these observations is that the concentrations of drug at a given site will depend upon both the site of release and the rate and amounts of substance released. The disturbance will presumably be greater when the release rate is fast or it occurs at a site where retention is relatively high, e.g., in the upper labial sulcus or the posterior part of the lower buccal sulcus and less if the release rate is slow or the tablet is placed at a site where the turnover of saliva is particularly rapid, e.g., beneath the tongue. In this respect the site of placement has also been shown to affect the rate of release of drug from the delivery system. In a study by Hardy et al [49, 50] the release profile of a model substance 99mTc-DTPA was examined from a sustained release dosage form based on a hydroxypropyl methylcellulose polymer matrix. The tablet was placed in the upper buccal cavity, the lower buccal cavity or sublingually. The release rate from the tablet placed sublingually was much faster than for the tablets placed in the upper or lower buccal sulci. This was probably because of dilution by submandibular and sublingual saliva together with the mixed oral fluid which drains into this region of the mouth followed by flushing away by swallowing. Another contributing factor may have been that the turnover of such fluid would be increased by the pressure and movement of the tongue. For two of the four volunteers no difference in release rate between the upper and lower buccal cavities was observed. These results probably reflect differences in anatomical position of the salivary ducts, individual dental anatomy and variations in salivary turnover. For the two subjects whose release rates were very different, release was faster in the upper buccal cavity and presumably arose from the greater salivary turnover in this region associated with the rapid flow of parotid saliva. Movements of the mobile tissues of the buccal mucosa, lips and tongue may also have contributed to the observed differences.

Another factor that could influence the concentration of drug in the mouth is the manner in which a patient administers their delivery system. Upon administration patients may allow the tablet to passively dissolve, or they may actively suck or chew a tablet. Once dissolved, they may swill the solution around the mouth. Individuals will vary in their rate of sucking, chewing, swallowing and salivary flow will influence such results. Primosch et al [35] examined the effect of different methods for dissolving fluoride tablets in the mouth to assess the effect of tablet dissolution on the retention of drugs in the oral cavity. The same tablet was treated in three different ways: active chewing/swishing (where the tablet was dissolved by chewing and swished around the mouth for 1 minute), active sucking (active dissolution)/swishing (active sucking where the tablet dissolved by vigorous sucking and swished around the mouth for 1 minute) and passive dissolution (where the tablet was allowed to dissolve undisturbed in the labial vestibule). Samples taken at various defined sites around the mouth revealed that the passive method resulted in a less homogenous distribution of fluoride around the mouth with a high build up of drug around the region of the dissolving tablet. Tablet chewing and sucking provided a more even distribution of drug around the mouth however, the concentrations at different sites were different and there was a tendency for fluoride to be preferentially retained in the maxillary labial vestibule. Higher maximum fluoride concentrations and longer salivary fluoride retention was consistently observed after tablet chewing compared to tablet sucking. This could be explained by the fact that sucking required more effort and time and thus more greatly stimulated salivary flow. Increased salivary flow would dilute the fluoride concentration faster and create accelerated clearance by subsequent swallowing.

The patterns may also have implications with regard to the best use of pharmaceutical agents [28]. Bloomfield [17] observed that the deposition of charcoal on the tongue was dependent upon the original site of placement. When a suspension of charcoal was placed on the tip of the tongue it migrated in a posterior direction and spread evenly on both sides of the tongue. However, when the charcoal was placed on either the left or right side of the tongue midline its migration in a posterior direction was restricted to the side of the tongue on which it was placed. These observations have implications on the use of pellets administered on the tongue for the treatment of ulcers. Placement of a pellet on the tip of the tongue may result in a reasonable area of both sides of the tongue being covered by drug. However placement of the pellet on one or other side of the tongue midline would not guarantee therapeutic drug concentrations at other areas on the other side of the tongue. Lozenges have been used to administer antibacterial agents over sustained periods to the oral cavity. Patients are directed to suck the lozenge slowly, in order to prolong the release time [1]. Weatherell's work with fluoride [16] and Jenkins and Krebsbach's [19] demonstration with charcoal showed that if the lozenge were to dissolve in the lower left buccal area the active ingredient would remain in the left side of the mouth, the right-hand side of the oral cavity remaining largely void of drug. Pharmaceutically, it may therefore sometimes be more appropriate to move the lozenge frequently from one side of the oral cavity to the other to ensure uniform efficacy. As a result of work performed in this area it has been suggested that the instructions given to patients in the use of fluoride tablets should be revised in order to gain maximum optimal benefit from the released fluoride. Weatherell advised that slow release fluoride tablets should be sucked slowly and that the position of the tablet should be moved frequently, advice which would seem sensible in the light of recent investigations. Whereas Jenkins and Krebsbach [19] suggested that in order to obtain maximum spread of fluoride from a slow release tablet they should if possible be placed under the tongue rather than in the buccal sulcus on one side.

To achieve a uniform distribution of drug around the mouth physical means such as swirling a mouthwash or chewing drug-containing gum would appear to be the most effective way. However, such conditions are short lived with mouthwashes and studies in this area have shown that drug concentrations will only occur uniformly during the act of swirling. When the mouthwash is expelled site specific patterns are quickly reestablished by the mouth. Various studies with mouthrinses [8, 20, 25, 26] have shown that seconds after rinsing with a solution of fluoride or glucose the concentrations of these substances varied markedly from place to place in the mouth, usually according to a general site-specific pattern, as documented in Figure 6. Rates of oral clearance varied enormously and in a site-specific manner (Figure 6) and formulation scientists should be aware of such patterns and their implications.

Likewise, a uniform distribution of drug may not be achieved when chewing gum. A recent report has shown the importance of bilateral chewing to achieve such an aim. In a study of 31 subjects Hector and Sullivan [22] showed that unilateral chewing of gum for 5 minutes resulted in a marker compound being mainly distributed ipsilaterally to the chewing side. In general the marker compound did not cross the midline in either the upper or lower arches; even in the presence of swallowing. Since there is considerable anecdotal evidence that many individuals prefer to chew on one side [22] patients should be instructed to change chewing sides when chewing gum to optimize delivery to the entire oral cavity.

There have been many attempts to administer drugs locally from devices placed in the mouth but the subsequent distribution of the drug within the mouth was rarely accompanied by any serious attempts to establish that such release produced the desired concentration of drug at target sites. As part of the development of any local oral mucosal drug delivery system, the oral distribution of the drug needs to be evaluated. Estimates of the concentration of drugs in the oral fluids have generally been obtained by the analysis of whole saliva either mixed in the mouth or obtained directly from the salivary duct. Such values give little indication of concentrations at any particular site in the mouth [28] and can be very different from, and have very little relevance to drug concentrations at any particular site in the mouth (Figure 11). We would advocate that in the evaluation of any delivery system concentrations at target sites are measured to assess its effectiveness.

VI. GENERAL CONCLUSIONS

The oral cavity is a complex area for local drug delivery. The existence of site-specific patterns of distribution and retention offer challenges to the

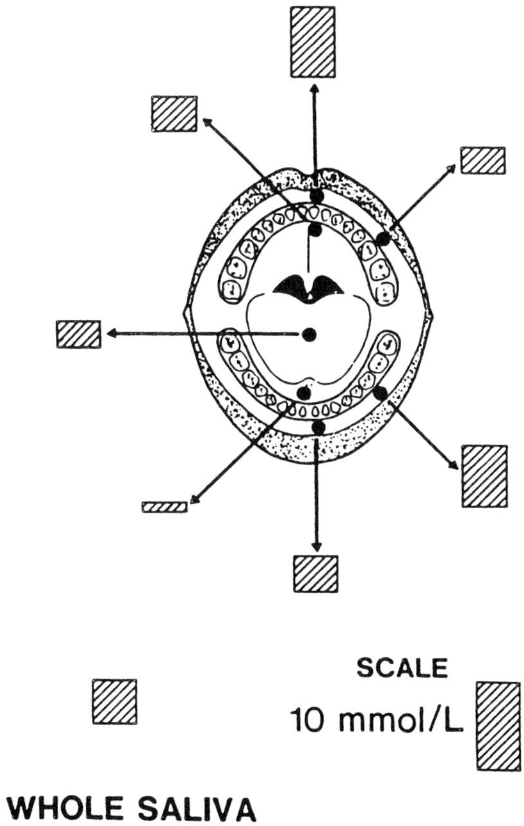

Figure 11. Fluoride concentrations in saliva taken from 7 different sites in the mouth 5 minutes after rinsing the mouth with 20 mL of a 25 mmol/L solution of sodium fluoride. The concentration in whole (mixed) saliva is shown on the lower left on the same scale and is equivalent to about 5 mmol/L. (From reference 28).

formulation scientist. This consideration of recent work has provided an insight into a developing area and its implications for the design and placement of oral mucosal drug delivery systems. We hope that it has also highlighted the possible effect of failing to take note of such fundamental information when attempting to formulate oral mucosal drug delivery systems for local administration.

The anatomical structure of the oral cavity and its physiological mechanisms seem to explain some of these regional variations. Still more experience is required before the situation is fully understood, and more quantitative studies need to be performed before it will possible to predict release rates from delivery systems which provide the desired therapeutic drug levels at selected target sites.

The use of mucoadhesives as platforms for prolonged delivery of drugs in the oral cavity and of controlled-release devices in the treatment of periodontal diseases might especially benefit from more information about the migration and retention of drugs in the oral cavity.

REFERENCES

1. J. A. Weatherell, C. Robinson, and M. J. Rathbone, Site-specific differences in the salivary concentrations of substances in the oral cavity - implications for the aetiology of oral disease and local drug delivery, *Adv. Drug Del. Rev. 13*:23 (1994).
2. C. Dawes, A mathematical model of salivary clearance of sugar from the oral cavity, *Caries Res. 17*:321 (1983).
3. F. Lagerlöf, and C. Dawes, The volume of saliva in the mouth before and after swallowing, *J. Dent. Res. 63*:618 (1984).
4. S. Watanabe, and C. Dawes, Salivary flow rates and salivary film thickness in five-year-old children, *J. Dent. Res. 69*:1150 (1990).
5. H. Becks, A study of rate of flow of resting saliva, *J. Dent. Res. 18*:431 (1939).
6. L .M. C. Collins, and C. Dawes, The surface area of the adult human mouth and thickness of the salivary film covering the teeth and oral mucosa, *J. Dent. Res. 66*:1300 (1987).
7. C. Main, D. A. M. Geddes, S. G. McNee, W. J. N. Collins, D. C. Smith, and D. A. Weetman, Instrumentation for measurement of dental plaque thickness in situ, *J. Biomed. Eng. 6*:151 (1984).
8. J. A. Weatherell, M. Strong, C. Robinson, B. R. Nattress, H. Nakagaki, and D. M. G. Main, Determination of volumes of fluid in the mouth by fluoride dilution, *Caries Res. 26*:94 (1992).
9. J. A. Weatherell, B. R. Nattress, H. Nakagaki, M. Strong, and C. Robinson, Volumes of oral fluid in normal mouths during rest and secretory stimulation, *J. Dent. Res. 69*:965 (1990).
10. J. A. Weatherell, M. Strong, C. Robinson, H. Nakagaki, and B. R. Nattress, Stimulated and non-stimulated volumes of saliva and the greater susceptibility of females to dental caries, *Caries Res. 24*:428 (1990).
11. V. F. Ferrario, C. Sforza, A. Miani. Jr., and G. Tartaglia, Maxillary versus mandibular arch form differences in human permanent dentition assessed by Euclidean-distance matrix analysis, *Arch. Oral Biol. 39*:135 (1994).

12. J. A. Weatherell, B. R. Nattress, E. A. O' Sullivan, M. Strong, and J. T. Wright, Saliva volumes in children measured by fluoride dilution, *J. Dent Res 70*:689 (1991).
13. M. Strong, J. A. Weatherell, and D. M. G. Main, Measurement of total oral fluid under conditions of secretory stimulation and rest, *J. Dent. Res. 68*:566 (1989).
14. G. N. Jenkins, *The Physiology and Biochemistry of the Mouth* 4th Edition, Blackwell, Oxford, 1978, p. 365.
15. P. Lecompte, and C. Dawes, The influence of salivary flow rate on diffusion of potassium chloride from artificial plaque at different sites in the mouth, *J. Dent. Res. 66*:1614 (1987).
16. J. A. Weatherell, C. Robinson, J. P. Ralph, and J. S. Best, Migration of fluoride in the mouth, *Caries Res. 18*:348 (1984).
17. A. L. Bloomfield, The dissemination of bacteria in the upper air passages. I. The circulation of foreign particles in the mouth, *Amer. Rev. Tuberculosis 5*:903 (1922).
18. G. Meyer, *Fluorgehalt der Mundflüssigkeit in Verschiedenen Gebieten der Mundhöle*. Inaugural Dissertation of Medicine, University of Zürich, 1969.
19. G. N. Jenkins, and P. H. Krebsbach, Experimental study of the migration of charcoal particles in the human mouth, *Arch. Oral Biol. 30*:697 (1985).
20. J. A. Weatherell, M. Strong, C. Robinson, H. Nakagaki, and J. P. Ralph, Retention of glucose in oral fluid at different sites in the mouth, *Caries Res. 23*:399 (1989).
21. A. C. O' Connell, S. K. Pearson, and W. H. Bowen, Pilocarpine alters caries development in partially-desalivated rats, *J. Dent. Res. 73*:637 (1994).
22. M. P. Hector, and A. Sullivan, Migration of erythrosin-labeled saliva during unilateral chewing in man, *Arch. Oral Biol. 37*:757 (1992).
23. K. J. Toumba, and M. E. J. Curzon, Slow-release fluoride, *Caries Res. 27*:43 (1993).
24. J. A. Weatherell, M. Strong, C. Robinson, and J. P. Ralph, Migration patterns of substances in the mouth, *Factors Relating to Demineralization and Remineralization of the Teeth* (S. A. Leach, ed.), IRL Press, Oxford, 1986, p. 81.
25. J. A. Weatherell, M. Strong, C. Robinson, and J. P. Ralph, Fluoride distribution in the mouth after fluoride rinsing, *Caries Res. 20*:111 (1986).
26. A. Britse, and F. Lagerlöf, The diluting effect of saliva on the sucrose concentration in different parts of the human mouth after a mouth rinse with sucrose, *Arch. Oral Biol. 32*:755 (1987).

27. M. Hanaki, H. Nakagaki, H. Nakamura, K. Kondo, J. A. Weatherell, and C. Robinson, Glucose clearance from different surfaces of human central incisors and first molars, *Arch. Oral Biol. 38*:479 (1993).
28. J. A. Weatherell, C. Robinson, and B. R. Nattress, Site-specific variations in the concentrations of substances in the mouth, *Br. Dent. J. 167*:289 (1989).
29. J. C. Hase, and D. Birkhed, Salivary glucose clearance, dry mouth and pH changes in dental plaque in man, *Arch. Oral Biol. 33*: 875 (1988).
30. C. Dawes, and L. M. D. Macpherson, The distribution of saliva and sucrose around the mouth during the use of chewing gum and the implications for the site-specificity of caries and calculus deposition, *J. Dent. Res. 72*:852 (1993).
31. L. M. D. Macpherson, and C. Dawes, Distribution of sucrose around the mouth and its clearance after sucrose mouthrinse or consumption of three different foods, *Caries Res. 28*:150 (1994).
32. S. Watanabe, Salivary clearance from different regions of the mouth in children, *Caries Res. 26*: 423 (1992).
33. B. R. Nattress, C. Robinson, and J. A. Weatherell, Site-specific variations in oral retention in relation to patients' individual dentition, *J. Dent. Res. 68*:566 (1989).
34. J. C. Hase, D. Birkhed, F. Lagerlöf, and E. Thornqvist, Oral retention of glucose at pharmacologically reduced salivary flow in man, *Scand. J. Dent. Res. 102*:180 (1994).
35. R. E. Primosch, J. A. Weatherell, and M. Strong, Distribution and retention of salivary fluoride from a sodium fluoride tablet following various intra-oral dissolution methods, *J. Dent. Res. 65*:1001 (1986).
36. C. Bruun, C. Qvist, and A. Thylsrup, Effect of flavor and detergent on fluoride availability in whole saliva after use of NaF and MFP dentifrices, *Caries Res. 21*:427 (1987).
37. H. W. Reed, Clinical evaluation of three concentrations of sodium fluoride in dentifrices, *J. Amer. Dent. Assoc. 87*:1401 (1973).
38. B. Barlage, H. Buhe, and W. Büttner, A 3-year clinical dentifrice trial using different fluoride levels: 0.8 and 1.2% sodium monofluorophosphate, *Caries Res. 15*:185 (1981).
39. C. M. Mitropoulos, P. J. Holloway, T. G. H. Davies, and H. V. Worthington, Relative efficacy of dentifrices containing 250 or 1,000 ppm F in preventing dental caries - report of a 32-month clinical trial, *Commun. Dent. Hlth. 1*:193 (1984).
40. G. K. Stookey, Critical evaluation of the composition and use of topical fluorides, *J. Dent. Res. 69*:805 (1990).

41. C. Bruun, D. Lambrou, M. J. Larsen, O. Fejerskov, and A. Thylstrup, Fluoride in mixed human saliva after different topical fluoride treatments and possible relation to caries inhibition, *Commun. Dent. Oral Epidemiol. 10*:124 (1982).
42. J. M. Ten Cate, and P. P. E. Duijsters, Influence of fluoride in solution on tooth demineralization. I. Chemical data, *Caries Res. 17*:193 (1983).
43. N. J. Medlicott, I. G. Tucker, M. J. Rathbone, and D. W. Holborow, Determination of small sample volumes in the analysis of drugs at specific sites in the oral cavity, *J. Periodont. Res.* In press.
44. N. J. Medlicott, D. G. Ferry, I. G. Tucker, M. J. Rathbone, and D. W. Holborow, High performance liquid chromatographic (HPLC) assay for the determination of chlorhexidine in the saliva film, *J. Liq. Chromatog, 17*:1605 (1994).
45. D. T. Zero, R. F. Raubertas, A. M. Pedersen, J. Fu, A. L. Hayes, and J. D. B. Featherstone, *J. Dent Res. 71*::1546 (1992)
46. Units of measurement, Body Fluids, Composition of the Body Nutrition. *Geigy Scientific Tables 8th Edition*, (C. Lentner ed.), Ciba Geigy Ltd, Basle, Switzerland, 1981, Volume 1, p. 116.
47. J. A. Weatherell, C. Robinson, and B. R. Nattress, The detection of site-specific reactions at the surfaces of oral tissues, *Caries Res. 23*:454 (1989).
48. J. A. Weatherell, C. Robinson, and B. R. Nattress, Site-specific differences in the concentrations of substances which react at tissue surfaces in the mouth, *J. Dent. Res. 68*:561 (1989).
49. J. G. Hardy, J. W. Kennerley, M. J. Taylor, C. G. Wilson, and S. S. Davis, Release rates from sustained-release buccal tablets in man, *J. Pharm. Pharmacol. 34*:91P (1982).
50. S. S. Davis, J. W. Kennerley, M. J. Taylor, J. G. Hardy, and C. G. Wilson, Scintigraphic studies on the in vivo dissolution of a buccal tablet, *Modern Concepts in Nitrate Delivery Systems*, Royal Society of Medicine International Congress and Symposium Series, 1983, p. 29.

9

Salivary Mucins: Their Role in Oral Mucosal Barrier Function and Drug Delivery

Leon C. P. M. Schenkels
State University of New York at Buffalo, USA

Tarikere L. Gururaja
State University of New York at Buffalo, USA

Michael J. Levine
State University of New York at Buffalo, USA

I. INTRODUCTION

Secretory or soluble mucins are the major components of mucous secretions lining the digestive, respiratory, and urogenital tracts. Secretory mucins, which are produced by specialized epithelial cells, can form intermolecular disulfide bridges, resulting in oligomeric or polymeric mucin formation. This property of mucins is primarily responsible for the viscoelastic and lubricating properties of the mucous secretions. Importantly, mucous secretions also serve as a protective cover safe-guarding tissues from noxious environmental agents. In addition to mucin, these secretions contain other macromolecules, water, electrolytes, and cellular remnants. Another class of mucins are those that are membrane-bound or cell-associated. While membrane-bound mucins are, in general, biochemically similar to the secretory mucins, they differ by containing a hydrophobic stretch of amino acids for anchoring into the plasma membrane, and are believed to lack intermolecular disulfide bridges. The functional properties of membrane-bound mucins are still not clearly understood.

Salivary mucins are considered to play a major role in the maintenance of oral health by exhibiting multiple host defense functions [1-4]. Such functions include (i) acting as a permeability barrier against environmental insult at the tissue-environmental interface; (ii) lubricating oral surfaces; (iii) concentrating antimicrobial molecules onto oral surfaces; and (iv) modulating colonization of oral bacteria, fungi, and viruses. These functions are predicated upon the mucin's structure. Recent studies using molecular cloning techniques have greatly increased our insight into the primary structure of mucin's peptide moiety. This information coupled with a knowledge of mucin's oligosaccharide structure now enable us to examine in a detailed and systematic fashion the structure-function relationships of these molecules. This article will first describe the biochemical and biological features of salivary mucins. Subsequent discussion will focus on therapeutic applications of this information to enhance mucin barrier function, augment drug delivery and develop artificial salivas. Finally, what approaches or strategies can be employed to design and develop bioactive mucin analogs for therapeutic application?

II. SALIVA: COMPOSITION, FUNCTION AND CHANGES WITH DISEASE

A. Composition and Function of Saliva

Studies of salivary secretions have established that mucins together with other groups of salivary proteins such as proline-rich proteins, histatins, cystatins, statherins and α-amylases protect the integrity of the hard and soft oral tissues [1-9]. The common functional properties of salivary secretions are summarized in Table 1. It is now apparent that the majority of proteins and glycoproteins in human salivary secretions are produced by salivary acinar cells and occur in secretion as members of "families". In contrast, ductal and stromal products occur primarily as single components. Family members produced by acinar cells share common structural features at the protein and/or DNA level. For example at the protein level, there are at least two groups of salivary mucins; a higher molecular weight oligomeric species (MG1) and a lower molecular weight single subunit species (MG2) [3, 10, 11]. These two groups share common biochemical characteristics such as a high (>50%) content of carbohydrate consisting of O-glycosidic carbohydrate units characterized by a

Table 1. Classification of the Major Salivary Components Based on Cellular Origin and Their Functional Properties.

Salivary proteins occurring as members of families (acinar cell origin)
α-Amylases (digestion, microbial clearance/adherence, pellicle formation)
Carbonic anhydrases (buffering)
Cystatins (anti-microbial, mineralization, pellicle formation)
Histatins (anti-microbial, buffering, mineralization)
Mucins (buffering, digestion, heterotypic complexing, lubrication, microbial clearance/adherence, pellicle formation)
Proline-rich proteins (microbial clearance/adherence, mineralization, pellicle formation)
Salivary peroxidases (anti-microbial)
Statherins (lubrication, mineralization, microbial clearance/adherence, pellicle formation)
Salivary proteins occurring as single species (ductal or stromal cell origin)
Fibronectin (microbial clearance/adherence)
Lactoferrin (anti-microbial)
Lysozyme (anti-microbial)
Kallikrein (proteolytic processing)
Secretory IgA (microbial adherence/clearance)

N-acetylgalactosamine-serine/threonine (GalNAc-Ser/Thr) glycosidic linkage [4]. Further, at least two isoforms of MG2 have been identified that differ in their content of fucose and sialic acid (SA) [12]. At the DNA level, molecular cloning of sequences encoding human submandibular gland statherin and histatin has revealed strong sequence homologies indicating their evolution from a common ancestral gene [13].

The protective properties of salivary proteins and glycoproteins occur when molecules are attached onto oral surfaces (e.g., pellicle) or free in solution. For example, the pellicle provides a selective permeability barrier, moisturizes, lubricates, mineralizes, promotes attachment of a beneficial flora and is antimicrobial to harmful microbes. Molecules in solution may be antimicrobial, initiate digestion, aid in buffering, help in taste and facilitate mechanical flushing of food and debris. Thus, the intra-oral location of a molecule plays a role in biological function.

It has been proposed that salivary proteins and glycoproteins consist of discrete structural domains, each of which may be responsible for a particular biological function. Details on the structure-function relationships of salivary

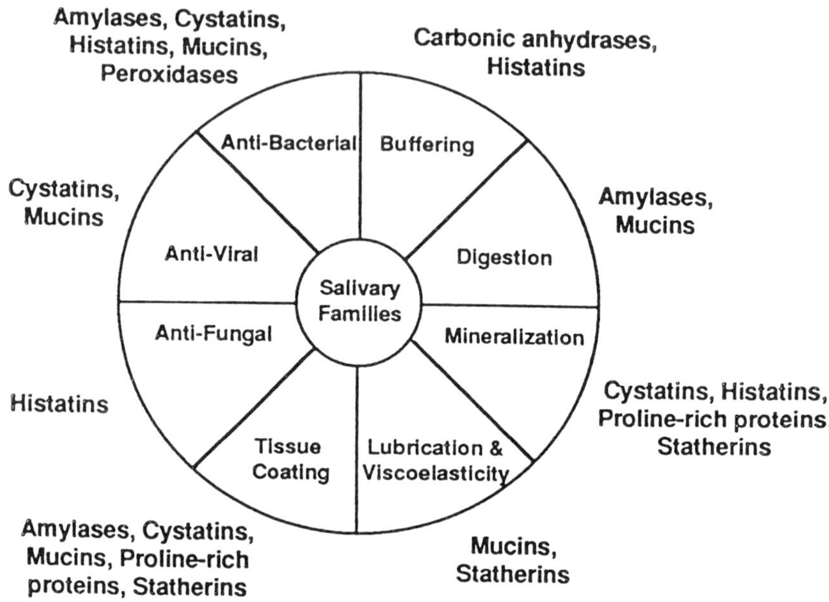

Figure 1. Multifunctional properties of human saliva.

molecules are provided in several recent reviews [4, 14-16]. The highlight of the recent findings from structure-function studies of salivary molecules is that the conformation or shape of a molecule is critical for its biological function. Studies by Gibbons et al [17, 18] demonstrated that salivary proline-rich proteins must be immobilized onto a surface such as hydroxyapatite before they interact with *Actinomyces viscosus* and *Streptococcus gordonii.* It was proposed that a C-terminal glutamine-proline sequence in several acidic proline-rich proteins is exposed upon binding and is important for interaction with these bacteria [17]. Other molecules, such as statherins and histatins also have conformational requirements since they need an α-helical conformation to maximize their biological activity [19-21]. Another molecule with conformational requirements is human salivary α-amylase. Its biological activities include enzymatic digestion of starch, interaction with viridans streptococci and binding to hydroxyapatite [22-24]. Cleavage of this enzyme's disulfide bonds results in the disruption of its suprastructure and in loss of biological activity [23].

Interestingly, most families of salivary molecules have multiple functions (Figure 1). For instance, acidic proline-rich proteins, cystatins, histatins and statherins all adsorb to hydroxyapatite, play a role in mineralization processes and modulate colonization of the oral flora [17, 19-22, 25-30]. While different families participate in these activities to different degrees, this overlap of function provides a redundancy or "protective backup" for the oral cavity. Mucins and statherins also function as lubricants; mucins may serve under light occlusal loads while statherins protect enamel surface under conditions of excess occlusal forces [20]. Another interesting observation regarding saliva is that molecules can interact with one another. Biochemically, non-covalent interactions are known to exist among many salivary molecules. In this manner complexes between different proteins may result in new multifunctional entities.

B. Saliva and Disease

Normal salivation is an essential component of oral health due to its important contributions to oral defense mechanisms [2]. Salivary gland function is frequently compromised as a result of two routinely used therapeutic modalities to treat patients suffering from different types of diseases. The first involves the use of radiation therapy to treat patients having head and neck tumors [31, 32] and the second is the use of pharmaceuticals (e.g., antihypertensives, antidepressants and antihistamines) to treat a variety of systemic and oral diseases [31]. Compromises of oral defenses as a result of these therapeutic methods include interruption of an intact oral mucosa, alterations of salivary flow, inappropriate or inadequate inflammatory responses and diminished soft and hard tissue vascularization. The severity of compromise depends on the type and extent of treatment utilizing radiation and pharmaceutical agents, or the combinations of these modalities. The most common clinical manifestation of this salivary dysfunction is a decreased output of secretion, termed "dry mouth" (also called hyposalivation, xerostomia, or asialorrhea). The consequent xerostomia is usually severe and often permanent, although some recovery of function has been reported. Many clinical problems ensue, including difficulty in chewing, swallowing, talking and inability to wear dentures comfortably. Salivary dysfunction presumably permits colonization of the oral mucosa by opportunistic pathogens such as *Candida sp.*, leading to candidiasis and invasion of tooth structure, often causing rampant caries. Alterations or modifications in salivary gland function have also been correlated to different types of diseases such as cystic fibrosis, autoimmune diseases (e.g., Sjögren's syndrome) and cancer [33]. An extensive article on the etiology and incidence of lost salivary function has been aptly described by Valdez and Fox [34].

III. MUCINS: STRUCTURE-FUNCTION AND THEIR IMPORTANCE IN SALIVARY DYSFUNCTION

The human mucins comprise a family of molecules which share general biochemical and biophysical properties but also possess distinct structural and functional differences. Mucins are the molecules that give all the mucosal secretions their typical viscoelastic character [35, 36]. They are defined as a distinct group of glycoconjugates, differing structurally from serum glycoproteins and proteoglycans. They are highly glycosylated, containing 50-90% carbohydrate by dry weight. The oligosaccharides vary in length from 1 to more than 20 sugar residues, mostly attached by O-glycosidic linkages via GalNAc-Ser/Thr. The character of the mucin is largely determined by the terminal oligosaccharide residues such as sialic acids, sulfate or fucose. An elegant review on mucin structure and biosynthesis has been presented by Strous and Dekker [37]. Characterization of mucin protein backbones (e.g., apo-mucin) has proven to be extremely difficult by classical biochemical techniques because of the high level of glycosylation and large molecular size. These difficulties are probably compounded by the presence of more than one species of mucin in many organs. For these reasons, most of the structural information about mucin protein moiety has been deduced from nucleotide sequences of apo-mucin cDNA. Currently, seven human mucin genes have been identified (Table 2) [38-44].

Table 2. Genes Encoding Human Mucins from Different Tissue(s).

Gene	Tissue type(s)	Number of tandem repeats	Number of amino acids/ repeat	Chromosomal localization	Reference
MUC1[a]	Epithelial	12-125	20	1q21	38
MUC2	Intestinal	~100	23	11p15.5	39
MUC3	Intestinal	?	17	7	40
MUC4	Tracheobronchial	?	16	3	41
MUC5	Tracheobronchial	?	8	11p15	42
MUC6	Gastric	?	169	11p15.4-15.5	43
MUC7[a]	Salivary	6	23	4	44

[a] Gene, completely characterized.

A. Mucin Tandem Repeats

The most characteristic feature of the mucin protein core is the presence of tandem repeat sequences. These repeats, which are located in the central region of the peptide moiety, are rich in the amino acids threonine, serine, proline, alanine, glycine (>50% of the total protein) and poor in aromatic and sulfur containing amino acids. The Ser/Thr residues serve as the anchor for the majority of O-linked carbohydrate units. Sequences rich in proline generally show extended structures, in which these amino acid residues are believed to stabilize the structure. It has been suggested that proline residues must also reside near the serine and threonine, particularly at positions -1 and +3, for the initiation of O-glycosylation [45]. It is noteworthy that the presence of tandem repeats has also been described for several other "proline-rich" proteins, including salivary proline-rich proteins, parasitic circumsporozite protein, cereal storage proteins, a fungal proline-rich protein and elastin [46]. Interestingly, all have the ability to form interlocking networks of high overall strength, a property suitable for coating body surfaces and the irreversible precipitation of harmful toxins. Although the structure and physiology of human mucins are comparable and serve essentially the same functions, their tandem repeats display marked differences in sequence and/or length. This might be due to genetic polymorphisms resulting in additions and deletions in the nucleotide sequence [47]. However, additional studies are required to verify this point.

B. N- and C-terminal Sequences

The N- and C-terminal domains of mucins have a more globular structure, in contrast to the extended structure of the central region containing tandem repeats. The extent of glycosylation is much less in these regions as compared to the tandem repeats. Mucins can contain a small number of N-linked carbohydrate moieties in the N- and C-terminal domains. The role of the N-glycosylation in these molecules is not known. However, it is possible that the N-glycans stabilize the nascent apo-mucin prior to O-glycosylation or they may play a role in the intracellular routing of the mucin. Indeed, recent evidence suggested that presence of significant amount of N-linked oligosaccharide is necessary for maturation of the rat gastric mucin [48]. The cross-linking sites (cysteine residues) are predominantly located in the N- and C-terminal domains, which allow the formation of head-to-tail oligomers and complexing with other non-mucin components. These cysteine residues are also believed to be the basis for the homologies within the mucin family as reported in the case of MUC2 and von Willebrand Factor (vWF) [39]. These two proteins appear to exist as disulfide-linked polymers. Hence, it is likely that the structural similarity of the cysteine-rich regions reflects the common necessity for oligomer formation and/or maintenance. It remains to be determined if additional mucins exhibit sequence similarities to each other or to vWF. While the tandem repeats provide an extended structure with numerous possible sites for O-glycosylation, the N- and C-terminal sequences are important for complexation.

C. Salivary Mucins

Among the various mucins known to be present in different parts of the body, salivary mucins are biologically important because of their immediate exposure to various environmental agents. Also, these molecules can be affected by variations in the oral environment. Current evidence suggests that two mucins exist within submandibular-sublingual saliva; the higher molecular weight mucin glycoprotein 1 (MG1) and the lower molecular weight mucin glycoprotein 2 (MG2) [10, 11, 49]. Immunocytochemical studies using monoclonal antibody probes have localized each of the salivary mucins to mucous acini within human submandibular gland tissues [50]. These studies also demonstrated the existence of distinct cell subpopulations of MG1- and MG2-secreting acini within these glands, thereby suggesting that the two mucins are authentic cell products and not the result of post-translational processing. Important structural features and properties of these salivary mucins are summarized in Table 3.

Structural studies on MG1 have been hindered by the molecule's large size, oligomeric nature and poor solubility in aqueous solutions. The oligomeric nature of mucins is based upon covalent and/or non-covalent associations between monomeric peptide moieties. MG1 consists of multiple disulfide-linked subunits composing a molecule of more than 1000 kDa [11, 51-54]. The protein core of MG1 is responsible for less than 15% of the total weight. Within the protein core, approximately 43% of the total amino acid residues are composed of threonine, serine, proline and alanine. Glycine constitutes 8.6% of the total amino acids. Covalently linked fatty acids are also associated with MG1 [54]. Because of the complexity in molecular structure, the amino acid sequence of MG1 still remains to be determined. Initial characterization of the oligosaccharide units of MG1 has been performed following their release by mild alkaline/borohydride treatment [11]. These studies reveal that the glycopeptide linkage of MG1 involves O-glycosidic bonds between N-acetylgalactosamine and threonine or serine. The major oligosaccharides of MG1 range in size from 4 to 16 sugar residues. These are responsible for 78% of the total weight of this molecule, with sulfate contributing an additional 7%. However, the precise sequences of the MG1 oligosaccharide units have only been partly determined [11]. A representative

Table 3. Important Structural Features and Properties of Human Salivary Mucins.

Properties	MG1	MG2(MUC7)
Biochemical properties		
Protein content	14.9%	30.4%
Carbohydrate content	78.1%	68.0%
Sulfate content	7%	1.6%
Size (kDa)	>1000[a]	Approx. 125
Oligomers	Yes[b]	No
Isoform	?	Yes
O-linked units		
Size of oligosaccharides	4-16 residues	2-7 residues
Number of oligosaccharides	290-300[c]	100[c]
Distribution	Random	Uniform
N-linked units	Yes	Yes
Covalently bound fatty acid[d]	5-10	Negligible
Biophysical properties		
Hydrophobic probe binding[e]	Yes	Yes
Effect of agents on probe binding		
Dithiothreitol		
Increase	None	
Pronase	Decrease	None
Non-glycosylated peptide domains	Yes	No

[a]Estimated by gel-filtration using Sepharose CL-2B. [b]Calculated from the carbohydrate structure and the deduced amino acid sequence. [c]Includes sialic acid-containing, sulfate-containing and neutral chains. [d]Moles fatty acids/mole mucin. [e]1-anilino-8-naphthalenesulfonate and N-phenyl-1-naphthylamine [11].

oligosaccharide unit of MG1 is illustrated in Figure 2 [55]. Biophysical studies using fluorescent probes have demonstrated the existence of hydrophobic pockets associated with MG1 [11]. Treatment of MG1 with dithiothreitol increases binding of these probes, indicating that cleavage of disulfide bridges exposes additional hydrophobic domains. On the other hand, treatment of MG1 with pronase results in diminished probe binding, implying destruction of hydrophobic domains associated with naked peptide regions [11]. Circular dichroism studies have revealed that the carbohydrate units of MG1 may be arranged in a biased (as opposed to random) configuration about the core peptide [11].

MG2, the other human salivary mucin member, is a molecule of approximately 125 kDa. It is composed of a single peptide chain of ~37 kDa

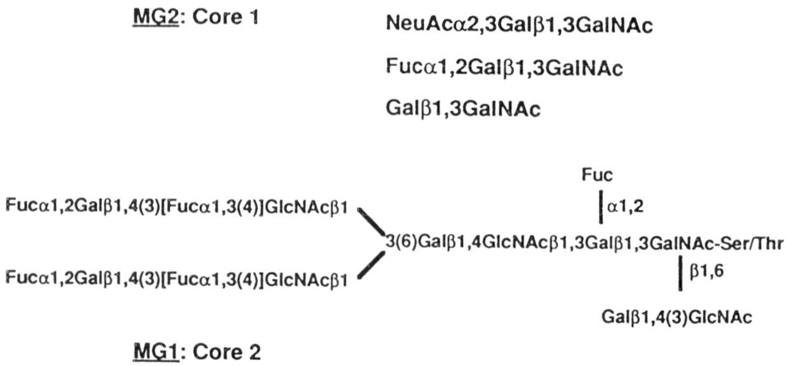

Figure 2. Representative oligosaccharide structures of human salivary mucins.

which accounts for 30% of the total composition [11, 49]. Approximately 75% of the total amino acid residues are accounted for by threonine, serine, proline and alanine, while glycine contributes only 1.4%. The carbohydrate content of MG2 is about 68% and consists of a high density of carbohydrate units attached via O-glycosidic linkages to the peptide core. The major O-linked carbohydrate units of MG2 have been structurally defined and range from 2-7 residues [56]. The structures of the major neutral and acidic oligosaccharides from MG2 have been determined and are presented in Figure 2. We have reported recently the isolation of two isoforms of MG2, designated as MG2a and MG2b which differ in their content of terminal sialic acid and fucose residues (Table 4) [12, 57]. Also, the sequence of the MG2 peptide backbone (e.g., apo-MG2) has been determined using recombinant techniques [44]. The sequence data confirmed and extended a number of features characteristic for mucins. A salient feature is the presence of tandem repeats located in the central region of the peptide chain; a feature common to all mucins [37]. Based upon current information, a hypothetical model for MG2 is shown in Figure 3.

Table 4. Composition of MG2a and MG2b.

Component	MG2a	MG2b
Protein	25.2	20.3
N-acetylgalactosamine	15.6	17.2
N-acetylglucosamine	12.0	15.4
N-acetylneuraminic acid	14.4	26.2
Fucose	16.2	6.9
Galactose	15.1	12.8
Mannose	1.4	1.2

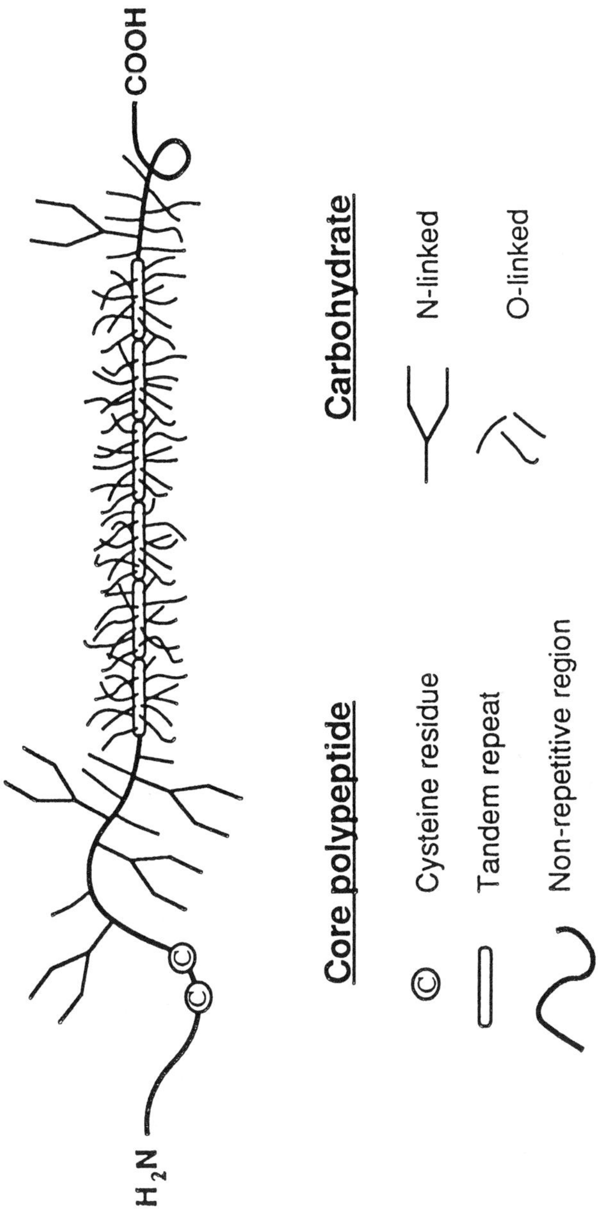

Figure 3. Hypothetical model for the salivary low molecular weight mucin, MG2.

In MG2, there are 6 tandem repeats, each containing 23 amino acid residues. There are a total of 102 potential sites available for O-glycosylation. Out of 102 sites, 51 sites are located on the tandem repeat sequence itself. In addition, MG2 has five potential N-glycosylation sites; four sites are at the N-terminal end and the fifth site at the C-terminal end [44]. Although much is known about the O-linked units on the peptide chain, the patterns of O-glycosylation still remain unknown. MG2 does not bind fluorescent hydrophobic probes, implying the absence of hydrophobic regions [11]. Preliminary circular dichroism studies of MG2 have suggested that this mucin exists primarily as a random coil, displaying little organized secondary structure. Clearly, our knowledge of the complex structure of human salivary mucins is far from complete. Although various structural domains have been identified, their spatial relationships to each other on the parent molecule has yet to be determined. In addition, the conformational structure of these molecules remains to be examined. A general description of salivary mucins including structure, biosynthesis and their functions has recently been reviewed [58].

D. Properties and Functions of Salivary Mucins

The salivary mucins possess unique multifunctional properties such as their role in lubrication, tissue coating, digestion and microbial interactions with bacteria, fungi and viruses [4]. This functional diversity of salivary mucins is predicted, in part, upon the carbohydrate content of these molecules [59]. In concert, both the apo-mucin and numerous oligosaccharide side chains provide a permeability barrier against environmental insult at tooth and soft tissue interfaces and function as a lubricant between enamel surfaces. The ability of a (glyco)protein to function as a lubricant in the oral cavity depends on forming a boundary interface at opposing surfaces moving relative to each other. Mucins and their complexes provide thin film lubrication under dental conditions of low occlusal load and high sliding speed. A physicochemical factor that contributes to this lubrication is water retention due to solvation of carbohydrate residues [60].

Several studies have demonstrated that salivary mucins can form non-covalent interactions or complexes with other salivary molecules. This complexation provides a mechanism whereby mucins concentrate protective molecules at different tissue-environmental interface. For example, salivary mucins undergo non-covalent interactions with sIgA [61], lysozyme and cystatins, all of which have anti-microbial properties [4, 30]. In this type of complexing, mucins may act as "molecular chaperones" by protecting other molecules from enzymatic degradation or concentrating antimicrobial molecules to oral surfaces.

Table 5. Summary of Human Salivary Mucin-Microbial Interactions.

Microorganism	MG1	MG2	Reference
Staphylococci	?	+	61
Candida albicans	?	+	62,63
Pseudomonas	+	+	61, 64, 65
Actinomyces	?	+	65-67
Porphyromonas	?	+	68
Haemophilus	+	-	69
Eikenella	?	+	70
Streptococci	+	+	71-74
HSV	?	+	75
HIV	?	+	76

In the interaction of mucins with bacteria, mucins are "amphifunctional" meaning, a molecule may be harmful or protective depending upon its intraoral localization. If mucin coats bacteria while in solution, potential attachment sites are masked and the microbes swallowed or cleared from the oral cavity; a protective event. In contrast, when mucins are part of the acquired enamel pellicle, they may promote attachment of microorganisms involved in dental plaque formation. Studies by numerous investigators have shown that salivary mucins can interact with many different microorganisms, including *Candida albicans* [62, 63], *Pseudomonas aeruginosa* [61, 64, 65], *Staphylococcus aureus* [61], *Actinomyces viscosus* [65-67], *Porphyromonas gingivalis* [68], *Haemophilus parainfluenzae* [69] and *Eikenella corrodens* [70]. In general, these are protein-protein or protein-carbohydrate interactions. However, the mucin-bacterial interaction that has been most extensively studied involves binding of sialic acid containing oligosaccharides with adhesins on oral streptococci. Numerous in vitro assays have been used to define this interaction [71-74] and it should be noted that results reported from different laboratories are “assay sensitive”. For example, MG2 interacts with *Streptococcus gordonii* when this mucin is immobilized onto a solid surface but not in solution. The specificity of salivary mucin (both MG1 and MG2) interactions with different microorganisms are summarized in Table 5. It is interesting to note that MG2 interacts with many microorganisms including *Herpes simplex* virus (HSV) [75] and human immunodeficiency virus (HIV) [76]. MG1 was found to interact with *Streptococci*, *Pseudomonas aeruginosa* and *Haemophilus parainfluenzae*, while MG2 did not bind *Haemophilus parainfluenzae*. The binding of MG2 to *Pseudomonas aeruginosa* and *Staphylococcus aureus* has been shown to occur due to its association with secretory IgA [61].

E. Mucins and Salivary Dysfunction

As described above, therapy to combat head and neck tumors can result in the cessation of salivary function and as a consequence the protective mucin coating of the oral epithelium and enamel is lost. Such alterations lead to reduced mucosal barrier function. The affected tissues lose their ability to resist the entry of pathogens, thus increasing the risk of systemic infections [77]. In certain diseases, secondary effects result in changes in the quality and amount of mucins secreted. For example, mucins can be over-produced in airway disorders such as cystic fibrosis and chronic bronchitis [78]. A reduction in saliva production, and hence mucin, is a common side effect of many medications [33, 34]. A reduction in salivary mucin secretion with aging has also been described [79]. This may result in a painful mucosa and an enhanced vulnerability to infections by bacteria, viruses and fungi. Some agents are known to specifically alter mucin biosynthesis. Aspirin for instance, is well known to reduce mucin secretion, and thus has been associated with diminished gastric mucosal protection and ulcer formation [80]. Mucins have also been associated with malignancy [81]. Apart from increased synthesis/secretion of mucins, altered glycosylation may be responsible for many antigenic differences between carcinomas and adjacent epithelial tissue. These differences have led to new diagnostics and tumor typing.

IV. THERAPEUTIC USE OF MUCINS: ROLE IN BARRIER FUNCTION, DRUG DELIVERY AND ARTIFICIAL SALIVAS

Mucins are the actual components that cause mucous secretions to form a viscous gel. This is demonstrated by the fact that purified mucins free from detectable protein, lipids and nucleic acid, form a gel with the same rheological properties as the native mucous secretion [82]. These properties are predominantly caused by the functional configuration of the secretory mucins as disulfide-linked oligomers [83], since the gel-forming ability is completely lost upon treatment with reducing agents. Thus, mucins in mucus can form intertangled networks in which the rigid chains hinge at the disulfide-connected peptide extensions. In these networks, oligosaccharide chains contribute to the viscosity not only by size, but also by intermolecular interactions. In the oral cavity, other salivary components (e.g., amylase, secretory IgA, cystatins, lysozyme) may be selectively adsorbed to the mucin gel through non-covalent associations. In addition, salivary components such as proline-rich proteins, may be covalently linked to the epithelial cell surface by the action of an epithelial transglutaminase [84, 85]. Together this surface layer on epithelial cells is referred to as the mucosal pellicle.

A. Barrier Function

In the oral cavity, the buccal mucosa is an excellent surface for the targeted delivery and subsequent absorption of drugs. This is particularly true for metabolically unstable drugs such as peptides and proteins, which are highly susceptible to acid- and enzyme-mediated degradation in the gastrointestinal tract [86]. In this context, the mucosal pellicle serves as a barrier between the epithelial surface and the external environment to shield the mucosa from microorganisms, toxins or proteolytic attack. Thus, the barrier function of the mucosal pellicle, and mucins in particular, can greatly influence the efficiency of drug delivery. Unfortunately, detailed studies on the permeability of the oral mucosal pellicle are not available. The data presented originate from studies on the gastrointestinal tract and animal models. Nevertheless, some general principles apply to all mucin-coated surfaces. Prior to adsorption, the highly viscous mucin layer may simply slow the rate of drug passage or it may loosely bind and concentrate the drug at the epithelial membrane surface which may increase the passive diffusion rate. For instance, the absorption of a series of alkaloids into the blood circulation is correlated to their diffusion coefficients in a mucus layer [87]. Antibiotics such as tetracycline have been shown to complex with mucus and therefore have their transport delayed [88, 89]. Binding of tetracycline was demonstrated to occur with the carbohydrate (sialic acid) as well as the protein moieties of mucin. Mild analgesics such as acetaminophen were impeded in their diffusion through mucin implying the possibility of binding of this drug to the mucosal barrier in a manner similar to some antibiotics bearing nitrogen groups [90]. Several characteristics of mucin may affect drug permeability. For instance, mucin gel is considered to be a weak cationic exchanger due to negatively charged sulfate and sialic acid and thus can reduce the transfer of anionic compounds. Also, the mucin network may act as a molecular sieve. Movement of components with molecular mass greater than 30 kDa is retarded through a mucin network; however, there was no consistent effect between components ranging in size from 340-660 Daltons [91]. Since mucous secretions contain non-glycoprotein constituents such as lipids [92] and proteins [84, 85], these constituents can lead to decomposition or binding of penetrating compounds. For example, hydrogen peroxide is degraded by salivary peroxidase present in the mucin network making the mucosal pellicle almost impermeable for hydrogen peroxide. Recently, cell lines are being developed to secrete mucins which lead to the formation of a mucous pellicle layer. For example, the human intestinal goblet cell line HT29-H was shown to produce a mucin layer that covers the apical cell surface, providing a significant barrier to the absorption of the lipophilic drug testosterone [86]. Further experiments with this type of defined model system will provide more accurate information on mucin's barrier properties and its impact on drug delivery. Once the kinetics and structural interactions between drugs and the mucin barrier are understood, mucin's structure might be biosynthetically or chemically altered to control the dynamics of mucin's barrier function.

B. Drug Delivery

Currently two general classes of compounds are available that can be used to enhance drug delivery through mucin-coated epithelial surfaces. These are bioadhesive polymers and oligosaccharide specific drug carriers.

The capacity of bioadhesive polymers to adhere to the mucin-epithelial surfaces has been used to design drug-delivery systems for application to mucin-rich environments. Similar to mucins, bioadhesive polymers should be water-swellable, long-chain polymers with polar components [93, 94]. These polymers have to meet several physicochemical properties for maximal attachment to the mucin network. The bioadhesion process comprises three main aspects: (i) the establishment of an intimate contact between the bioadhesive system and the oral surface; (ii) the interdiffusion of the bioadhesive polymer chains into the mucin network; and (iii) the formation of bonds. The interdiffusion of chains from the bioadhesive polymer and mucin is first the consequence of the disentanglement of the stretched and twisted molecules of the bioadhesive polymer, and second, of their diffusion into the mucus. Swelling of the polymer in water is a prerequisite for favorable bioadhesion. In addition, the polymer charge can help or hinder interdiffusion [95]. When intimate contact is established, interfacial bond formation can occur consisting of electrostatic forces, van der Waal forces, hydrogen bonds and hydrophobic interactions. Several polymers including cellulose derivatives [96], polyethylene glycol [97] and polyacrylic acids [97] have been described as bioadhesive polymers. In vivo, some of these polymers adhere well for a few hours, although some are mildly irritating to the oral mucosa [98]. However, thermally modified starches show some promise as non-irritant bioadhesion polymers for buccal application [99]. Also, certain polymers have been developed such as poly-L-lysine and methacrylamide that can be designed by attachment of biologically active side groups [100]. These side groups might be used to target drugs to specific cell surface receptors.

The use of bioadhesive polymers has some disadvantages. Since bioadhesion relies partly on physicochemical interactions involving non-specific surface energy thermodynamics, bioadhesive polymers may not be selective for mucosal surfaces. They can also interact with food and other foreign substances before reaching their intended site of adhesion. Besides, biocompatability problems can occur ranging from simple tissue irritation to a more serious immune response. To circumvent these problems, drug carriers can be designed for targeting to specific receptor sites on the mucosal pellicle or the underlying cell surface. These recognition/receptor sites could then serve to bind the drug carrier for the subsequent delivery of the therapeutic agent. The most likely site for targeting is the oligosaccharide units of mucin in the mucosal pellicle and cell surface glycoconjugates. In addition to biocompatability, oligosaccharides from both sites share many structural similarities. Consequently, the drug carrier could attach to both sites, thereby increasing its efficiency. Carriers specifically recognizing these oligosaccharides might be found among antibodies [101], bacterial adhesins [102] and plant lectins [103].

Certain salivary proteins might be used as specific drug-carriers. They offer the advantage of biocompatibility. Our current detailed knowledge of the structure and function of salivary molecules permits us to custom-engineer multifunctional proteins with an antimicrobial (drug) domain and a targeting (carrier) domain. For example, a cystatin/histatin fusion protein has been constructed using recombinant techniques [104]. Such a molecule may have a broadened antimicrobial spectrum (e.g., candidacidal and bactericidal domains). One portion could be a cysteine protease inhibitor (e.g., cystatin) to protect a candidacidal domain from exogenous proteolysis. Another example could be a histatin/proline-rich chimeric protein that has a candidacidal component (e.g., histatin) while the proline-rich protein serves as a substrate for mucosal attachment via an epithelial transglutaminase [105].

C. Artificial Salivas

In the previous sections dealing with mucin's role in barrier function and drug delivery, an intact normal mucosal pellicle is present. In clinical situations where salivary flow is decreased or lacking, this oral mucosal pellicle is severely compromised or lost. Here, restoration of this mucin-like protective barrier is necessary to maintain oral health. In radiated patients, saliva secretion is negligible while it can be markedly decreased in subjects with drug-related oral dryness. Where some residual salivary flow remains, stimulants such as pharmaceutical sialogogues, sugarless candies and chewing gum can be used to restore saliva production [106] and the mucosal pellicle. Alternatively, saliva substitutes or artificial salivas can be used [16, 107]. To be effective, an artificial saliva should provide a mucosal pellicle, be long-lasting, inhibit the overgrowth and colonization of oral microflora and induce rehardening of softened enamel. Previous studies have shown some beneficial effects of artificial salivas that contain carboxymethylcellulose (CMC) or porcine gastric mucin [108-112]. The CMC based substitutes usually were evaluated as equally [113] or more effective than glycerin containing mouthwashes [114]. In one of the studies, the mucin-containing saliva appeared to be superior to the CMC saliva [112].

V. DESIGN AND DEVELOPMENT OF MUCINS: FUTURE PROSPECTS FOR THERAPY

Our current knowledge of the complex structural and functional characteristics of salivary secretions argues for new approaches in the development of oral therapeutics. To date, enough information is available to begin designing mucins or mucin analogs as potential therapeutic agents to enhance mucin's barrier function, promote drug delivery and restore the mucosal pellicle. Two general approaches can be considered. The first is an exogenous approach which involves topical application of substances (e.g., artificial salivas) to replace a function(s) that has been lost or to enhance existing function(s). Exogenous compounds can be divided into those that are natural versus unnatural ones. Natural components such as salivary mucins or their derivatives offer the advantage of biocompatibility. The second approach is an endogenous one and involves the replacement or enhancement of function through modulation of the salivary gland's inherent biosynthetic machinery (e.g., gene therapy).

To fulfil these two approaches, it is essential to have detailed information on the structural features of the molecule under consideration. For example, recent trends in glycobiology have demonstrated that the conformation of mucin glycopeptides (e.g., oligosaccharides and flanking peptide moieties) plays an essential role in biological activity. More precisely, glycopeptide conformation may effect the glycosylation patterns of mucins which in turn impacts on biological activity. Thus, information obtained on the 3D structure of mucin glycopeptides by NMR spectroscopy and/or X-ray crystallography is a prerequisite for the design and synthesis of bioactive mucin analogs. Currently, our laboratory is focusing on both the exogenous and endogenous approaches to replace or enhance salivary mucin function. For example, bioactive glycomimetics can be used as mucin analogs in artificial salivas. In addition, gene therapy protocols can be applied for augmenting mucin expression.

A. Glycomimetic Design

Studies by numerous investigators have shown that salivary mucins can interact with many different microorganisms. The majority of these interactions are stereospecific involving mucin's O-linked carbohydrate chains. For example, the major acidic trisaccharide (SAα2,3Galβ1,3GalNAc) of MG2 is involved in the interaction with *Viridans streptococci* [71, 73]. Additional in vitro studies have demonstrated that modifications of mucin's oligosaccharide chains by bacterial glycosidases can lead to attachment of more pathogenic microorganisms [72, 74]. If this modification occurs while mucins are absorbed to hydroxyapaptite, selected cariogenic or periodontopathic bacteria could now adhere to, or colonize, oral surfaces. Similarly, the degradation of mucin oligosaccharides in solution, could reduce mucin-mediated clearance of potentially harmful bacteria. Thus, the O-linked carbohydrate chains of human salivary mucins are important biological determinants. The stereospecific nature of these interactions implies a conformational requirement for these O-linked units. In order to be used as effective therapeutic agents, mucin oligosaccharides will have to maintain a bioactive conformation. To achieve this goal, several issues must be addressed. First, is the bioactive conformation of mucin O-linked units stabilized by adjacent or flanking peptide sequences? Second, how is this conformation affected when the oligosaccharide or glycopeptide is bound to the microbial adhesion? Third, can peptide analogs (e.g., glycomimetics) be made which mimic the biological activity of the mucin oligosaccharide or glycopeptide? The rationale for developing glycomimetics is based upon their resistance to degradation by bacterial glycosidases and the fact that the synthesis of peptides is technically easier than complex carbohydrates. To technically address these questions, the 3D structure of SAα2,3Galβ 1,3GalNAc with adjacent peptide-flanking regions must be determined. The structural parameters obtained will then be compared for peptide structures present in various protein/peptide structure databases. The designed peptide will then be synthesized and its biological activity tested.

B. Gene Therapy

Gene therapy has received considerable attention in the modern era of medicine [115-118]. Currently, the initial phases of human gene therapy trials are under way for diseases such as adenosine deaminase deficiency, various cancers and AIDS [119-121]. The adenovirus-mediated transfer of the human cystic fibrosis transmembrane conductance regulator gene to airway epithelium of a rodent model suggests that human trials will be forthcoming in the near future [118]. Gene transfer to the salivary glands holds the potential for the therapy of salivary gland disorders and for the delivery of therapeutic proteins to the mouth and upper gastrointestinal tract. For example, transfer of new genes may prevent the destruction of salivary gland tissue, impart secretory function to residual tissue, or confer new secretory characteristics to intact glands. Among the different vectors known to act as transfer vehicles, replication-deficient recombinant adenovirus vectors were found to be the most appealing candidates for this purpose [122]. These vectors have been used to transfer genes efficiently to differentiated cells of a variety of organs of animals in vivo

[115-118] and are also being used in a clinical trial in humans to treat the respiratory manifestations of cystic fibrosis [118]. The acinar cells are responsible for all the salivary fluid secretion and most of the exocrine proteins in the saliva [123]. The ductal epithelial cells serve as a conduit carrying the saliva to the mouth, but they also exhibit considerable ion flux, thus regulating the electrolyte composition of saliva [124]. The adenovirus-mediated gene transfer to the salivary glands was distributed to both cell types which results in maximizing the amount of therapeutic protein produced. This is advantageous where one of the cell types (acinar or ductal) is reduced.

Additional information is still needed regarding genes encoding for human salivary apo-mucin and the glycosyltransferases involved in synthesis of oligosaccharide chains. This will not only contribute to the basic knowledge of the structural organization of the mucin genes, but may yield insights into general mechanism of glycoprotein expression as well as the individual differences involved in tissue-specific expression. When the structure of apo-mucin and glycosyltransferase genes are determined and their regulation of expression fully understood, this knowledge may be applied towards the design and development of endogenous gene therapy protocols for augmenting or enhancing mucin expression in relevant disease states.

The application of gene therapy to control mucin-expression is being considered for airway-associated diseases [36]. Over-expression of mucins is a main problem in these diseases and might be controlled by antisense oligodeoxy nucleotides that are complementary to splice-junctions, the ribosome binding-site and/or the translation start region. Chemically modified analogs that are nuclease-resistant could be used for this purpose. However, over-expression of mucins in saliva is not a main problem in oral diseases. Degenerative disorders, auto-immune disease, radiation damage and side-effects from pharmaceuticals are more common causes of salivary hypofunction leading to severe oral problems. Gene therapy represents a plausible strategy by which protein and fluid secretion could be restored. For example increasing the water permeability of the residual tissue could be accomplished by the expression of water channel and appropriate ion transporters. Initially, decisions have to be made regarding which molecules should be targeted for genetic manipulation even though there are no in vivo studies to demonstrate that the absence of any single salivary molecule results in manifestations of salivary dysfunction. Also, gene therapy protocols can only be employed when vectors are developed that can safely and efficiently be injected directly into patients as drugs like insulin are now. Vectors need to be engineered that will target specific cell types, insert their genetic information into a safe site in the genome and be regulated by normal physiological signals.

VI. CONCLUSIONS

Past and future research efforts will provide the precise structural requirements by which salivary mucins perform their biological functions. Such information can be used to replace or augment mucin's role in barrier function and facilitate drug delivery in individuals with normal salivary flow. In patients with reduced or lost saliva secretion, mucin-based artificial salivas and gene therapy protocols offer potential approaches to alleviate or restore lost function.

VII. ACKNOWLEDGMENTS

The authors research programs are supported by USPHS grants DE07585 and DE08240.

REFERENCES

1. I. D. Mandel, and S. Wotman, The salivary secretions in health and disease, *Oral Sci. Rev. 8*:25 (1976).
2. I. D. Mandel, The functions of saliva, *J. Dent. Res. 66*:623 (1987).
3. M. J. Levine, P. C. Jones, R. E. Loomis, M. S. Reddy, I. Al-Hashimi, E. J. Bergey, S. D. Bradway, R. E. Cohen, and L. A. Tabak, Functions of human saliva and salivary mucins, *Oral Mucosal Diseases: Biology, Etiology, and Therapy* (I. C. MacKenzie, C. A. Squier, and E. Dabelsteen, eds.), Laegeforeningens Forlag, Copenhagen, 1987, p. 24.
4. R. E. Cohen, and M. J. Levine, Salivary glycoproteins, *Human Saliva: Clinical Chemistry and Microbiology* (J. O. Tenovuo, ed.), CRC Press, Boca Raton, 1989, p. 101.
5. L. A. Tabak, M. J. Levine, I. D. Mandel, and S. A. Ellison, Role of salivary mucins in the protection of the oral cavity, *J. Oral Pathol. 11*:1 (1982).
6. I. D. Mandel, Sialochemistry in diseases and clinical situations affecting salivary glands, *Crit. Rev. Clin. Lab. Sci. 12*:321 (1980).
7. D. I. Hay, Human glandular salivary proteins, *Handbook of Experimental Aspects of Oral Biochemistry* (E. P. Lazzari, ed.), CRC Press, Boca Raton, 1983, p. 319.
8. I. L. Shannon, Inorganic components of human saliva, *Handbook of Experimental Aspects of Oral Biochemistry* (E. P. Lazzari, ed.), CRC Press, Boca Raton, 1983, p. 307.

9. M. J. Levine, L. A. Tabak, M. S. Reddy, and I. D. Mandel, Nature of salivary pellicles in microbial adherence; Role of salivary mucins, *Molecular Basis of Oral Microbial Adhesion* (S. E. Mergenhagen, and B. Rosan, eds.), American Society for Microbiology, Washington DC, 1985, p. 125.
10. M. J. Levine, M. S. Reddy, L. A. Tabak, R. E. Loomis, E. J. Bergey, P. C. Jones, R. E. Cohen, M. W. Stinson, and I. Al-Hashimi, Structural aspects of salivary glycoproteins, *J. Dent. Res. 66*:436 (1987).
11. R. E. Loomis, A. Prakobphol, M. J. Levine, M. S. Reddy, and P. C. Jones, Biochemical and biophysical comparison of two mucins from human submandibular-sublingual saliva, *Arch. Biochem. Biophys. 258*:452 (1987).
12. M. S. Reddy, L. A. Bobek, G. G. Haraszthy, A. R. Biesbrock, and M. J. Levine, Structural features of the low-molecular-mass human salivary mucin, *Biochem. J. 287*: 639 (1992).
13. D. P. Dickinson, A. L. Ridall, and M. J. Levine, Human submandibular gland statherin and basic histidine-rich peptide are encoded by highly abundant mRNA's derived from a common ancestral sequence, *Biochem. Biophys. Res. Commun. 149*:784 (1987).
14. M. S. Lamkin, and F. G. Oppenheim, Structural features of salivary function, *Crit. Rev. Oral Biol. Med. 4*:251 (1993).
15. M. J. Levine, Salivary macromolecules: A structure/function synopsis, *Ann. N. Y. Acad. Sci. 694*:11 (1993).
16. M. J. Levine, Development of artificial salivas, *Crit. Rev. Oral Biol. Med. 4*:279 (1993).
17. R. J. Gibbons, D. I. Hay, and D. H. Schlesinger, Delineation of a segment of adsorbed salivary acidic proline-rich proteins which promotes adhesion of *Streptococcus gordonii* to apatitic surfaces, *Infect. Immun. 59*:2948 (1991).
18. R. J. Gibbons, and D. I. Hay, Human salivary acidic proline-rich proteins and statherin promote the attachment of *Actinomyces viscosus* LY7 to apatite surfaces, *Infect. Immun. 55*:439 (1988).
19. P. A. Raj, M. Johnsson, M. J. Levine, and G. H. Nancollas, Salivary statherin: Dependence of sequence, charge, hydrogen bonding potency and helical conformation for adsorption to hydroxyapaptite and inhibition of mineralization, *J. Biol. Chem. 267*:5968 (1991).
20. W. H. Douglas, E. S. Reeh, N. Ramasubbu, K. K. Bhandary, P. A. Raj, and M. J. Levine, Statherin: A major boundary lubricant of human saliva, *Biochem. Biophys. Res. Commun. 180*:91 (1991).
21. P. A. Raj, S. -D. Soni, and M. J. Levine, Membrane-induced helical conformations of an active candidacidal fragment of salivary histatins, *J. Biol. Chem. 269*:9610 (1994).

22. M. Johnson, C. F. Richardson, E. J. Bergey, F. A. Scannapieco, M. J. Levine, and G. H. Nancollas, The influence of salivary proteins on the growth, aggregation, and surface properties of hydroxyapaptite particles, *Mat. Res. Soc. Proc. 174*:81 (1990).
23. F. A. Scannapieco, K. Bhandary, N. Ramasubbu, and M. J. Levine, Structural relationship between the enzymatic and streptococcal binding sites of human salivary α-amylase, *Biochem. Biophys. Res. Commun. 173*:1109 (1990).
24. C. -C. Tseng, F. A. Scannapieco, and M. J. Levine, Use of a replica-plate assay for the rapid assessment of salivary protein-bacterial interactions, *Oral Microbiol. Immunol. 7*:53 (1992).
25. D. I. Hay, The interaction of human parotid salivary proteins with hydroxyapatite, *Arch. Oral. Biol. 18*:1517 (1973).
26. A. Bennick, M. Cannon, and G. Madapallimattam, The nature of the hydroxyapatite-binding site in salivary acidic proline-rich proteins, *Biochem. J. 183*:115 (1979).
27. D. I. Hay, E. R. Carlson, S. K. Schluckebier, E. C. Moreno, and D. H. Schlesinger, Inhibition of calcium phosphate precipitation by human salivary acidic proline-rich proteins: Structure-activity relationships, *Calcif. Tissue Int. 40*:126 (1987).
28. D. I. Hay, and E. C. Moreno, Statherin and acidic proline-rich proteins, *Human Saliva: Clinical Chemistry and Microbiology* (J. O. Tenovuo, ed.), CRC Press, Boca Raton, 1989, p. 131.
29. M. Johnsson, C. F. Richardson, E. J. Bergey, M. J. Levine, and G. H. Nancollas, The effects of human salivary cystatins and statherin on hydroxyapaptite crystallization, *Arch. Oral Biol. 36*:631 (1991).
30. L. A. Bobek, and M. J. Levine, Cystatins - inhibitors of cysteine proteinases, *Crit. Rev. Oral Biol. Med. 3*:307 (1992).
31. J. C. Atkinson, and P. C. Fox, Salivary gland dysfunction, *Clin. Ger. Med. 8*:499 (1992).
32. L. M. Sreebny, and G. Broich, Xerostomia (dry mouth), *The Salivary System* (L. M. Sreebny, ed.), CRC Press, Boca Raton, 1987, p. 179.
33. P. C. Fox, Salivary monitoring in oral diseases, *Ann. N. Y. Acad. Sci. 694*:234 (1993).
34. I. H. Valdez, and P. C. Fox, Diagnosis and management of salivary dysfunction, *Crit. Rev. Oral Biol. Med. 4*:271 (1993).
35. H. A. Waterman, C. Blom, H. J. Holterman, E. J. 's-Gravenmade, and J. Mellema, Rheological properties of human saliva, *Arch. Oral Biol. 33*:589 (1988).
36. M. Verma, and E. A. Davidson, Glycopinion mini-review: Mucin genes: structure, expression and regulation, *Glycoconjugate J. 11*:172 (1994).
37. G. J. Strous, and J. Dekker, Mucin-type glycoproteins, *CRC Rev. Biochem. Mol. Biol. 27*:57 (1992).

38. M. J. L. Ligtenberg, H. L. Vos, A. M. C. Gennissen, and J. Hilkens, Episialin, a carcinoma-associated mucin, is generated by a polymorphic gene encoding splice variants with alternative amino termini, *J. Biol. Chem. 265*:5573 (1990).
39. J. R. Gum Jr., J. W. Hicks, N. W. Toribara, B. Siddiki, and Y. S. Kim, Molecular cloning of human intestinal mucin (MUC2) cDNA. Identification of the amino terminus and overall sequence similarity to prepro-Von Willebrand factor, *J. Biol. Chem. 269*:2440 (1994).
40. J. R. Gum, J. W. Hicks, D. M. Swallow, R. L. Lagace, J. C. Byrd, D. T. A. Lamport, B. Siddiki, and Y. S. Kim, Molecular cloning of cDNAs derived from a novel human intestinal mucin gene, *Biochem. Biophys. Res. Commun. 171*:407 (1990).
41. N. Porchet, V. C. Nguyen, J. Dufosse, J. P. Audie, V. Guyonnet-Duperat, M. S. Gross, C. Denis, P. Degand, A. Bernheim, and J. P. Aubert, Molecular cloning and chromosomal localization of a novel human tracheo-bronchial mucin cDNA containing tandemly repeated sequences of 48 base pairs, *Biochem. Biophys. Res. Commun. 175*:414 (1991).
42. D. Meerzaman, P. Charles, E. Daskal, M. H. Polymeropoulos, B. M. Martin, and M. C. Rose, Cloning and analysis of cDNA encoding a major airway glycoprotein, human tracheobronchial mucin (MUC5), *J. Biol. Chem. 269*:12932 (1994).
43. N. W. Toribara, A. M. Robertson, S. B. Ho, W. -L. Kuo, E. Gum, J. W. Hicks, J. R. Gum, J. C. Byrd, B. Siddiki, and Y. S. Kim, Human gastric mucin. Identification of a unique species by expression cloning, *J. Biol. Chem. 268*:5879 (1993).
44. L. A. Bobek, H. Tsai, A. R. Biesbrock, and M. J. Levine, Molecular cloning, sequence, and specificity of expression of the gene encoding the low molecular weight human salivary mucin (MUC7), *J. Biol. Chem. 268*:20563 (1993).
45. I. B. Wilson, Y. Gavel, and G. von Heijne, Amino acid distributions around O-linked glycosylation sites, *Biochem. J. 275*:529 (1991).
46. M. P. Williamson, The structure and function of proline-rich regions in proteins, *Biochem. J. 297*:249 (1994).
47. J. Dufosse, N. Porchet, J. -P. Audie, V. Guyonnet-Duperat, A. Laine, I. Van-Seuningen, S. Marrakchi, P. Degand, and J. -P. Aubert, Degenerate 87-base-pair tandem repeats create hydrophilic/hydrophobic alternating domains in human mucin peptides mapped to 11p15, *Biochem. J. 293*:329 (1993).
48. J. Dekker, and G. J. Strous, Covalent oligomerization of rat gastric mucin occurs in the rough endoplasmic reticulum, is N-glycosylation-dependent, and precedes initial O-glycosylation, *J. Biol. Chem. 265*:18116 (1990).

49. A. Prakobphol, M. J. Levine, L. A. Tabak, and M. S. Reddy, Purification of a low-molecular-weight, mucin-type glycoprotein from human submandibular-sublingual saliva, *Carbohydr. Res. 108*:111 (1982).
50. R. E. Cohen, A. Aguirre, P. C. Jones, M. S. Reddy, M. E. Neiders, and M. J. Levine, Immunocytochemistry of human salivary mucins, *J. Dent. Res. 66*:302 (1987).
51. M. M. Baig, R. J. Winzler, and O. M. Rennert, Isolation of mucin from human submaxillary secretions, *J. Immunol. 111*:1826 (1973).
52. I. Oemrawsingh, and P. A. Roukema, Composition and biological properties of mucins, isolated from human submandibular glands, *Arch. Oral Biol. 19*:753 (1974).
53. D. R. Green, and G. Embery, Structural studies on a sulphated glycoprotein preparation isolated from human saliva, *Arch. Oral Biol. 30*:859 (1985).
54. B. L. Slomiany, V. L. Murty, A. Slomiany, J. Zielenski, and I. D. Mandel, Mucus glycoprotein of human saliva: differences in the associated and covalently bound lipids with caries, *Biochim. Biophys. Acta 882*:18 (1986).
55. A. Klein, C. Carnoy, J. M. Wieruszeski, G. Strecker, A. M. Strang, H. van Halbeek, P. Roussel, and G. Lamblin, The broad diversity of neutral and sialylated oligosaccharides derived from human salivary mucins, *Biochemistry 31*:6152 (1992).
56. M. S. Reddy, M. J. Levine, and A. Prakobphol, Characterization of oligosaccharides from the lower molecular weight salivary mucin of a normal individual and one with cystic fibrosis, *J. Dent. Res. 64*:33 (1985).
57. N. Ramasubbu, M. S. Reddy, E. J. Bergey, G. G. Haraszthy, S. -D. Soni, and M. J. Levine, Large-scale purification and characterization of the major phosphoproteins and mucins of human submandibular-sublingual saliva, *Biochem. J. 280*:341 (1991).
58. A. M. Wu, G. Csako, and A. Herp, Structure, biosynthesis, and function of salivary mucins, *Mol. Cell. Biochem. 137*:39 (1994).
59. M. N. Hatton, R. E. Loomis, M. J. Levine, and L. A. Tabak, Masticatory lubrication: The role of carbohydrate in the lubricating property of a salivary glycoprotein-albumin complex, *Biochem. J. 230*:817 (1985).
60. E. S. Reeh, A. Aguirre, R. L. Sakaguchi, J. D. Rudney, M. J. Levine, and W. H. Douglas, The relative lubricity of salivary fluids, *Clin. Mater. 6*:151 (1990).
61. A. R. Biesbrock, M. S. Reddy, and M. J. Levine, Interaction of a salivary mucin-secretory immunoglobulin A complex with mucosal pathogens, *Infect. Immun. 59*:3492 (1991).

62. M. P. Hoffman, and C. G. Haidaris, Analysis of *Candida albicans* adhesion to salivary mucin, *Infect. Immun. 61*:1940 (1993).
63. M. E. Edgerton, F. A. Scannapieco, M. S. Reddy, and M. J. Levine, Human submandibular-sublingual saliva promotes adhesion of *Candida albicans* to polymethylmethacrylate, *Infect. Immun. 61*:2644 (1993).
64. M. S. Reddy, M. J. Levine, and W. Paranchych, Low-molecular-mass human salivary mucin, MG2: Structure and binding of *Pseudomonas aeruginosa*, *Crit. Rev. Oral Biol. Med. 4*:315 (1993).
65. M. S. Reddy, A. R. Biesbrock, and M. J. Levine, 1995 (unpublished results).
66. H. M. Koop, M. Valentijn-Benz, A. V. Nieuw Amerongen, P. A. Roukema, and J. de Graaff, Aggregation of oral bacteria by salivary mucins in comparison to salivary and gastric mucins of animal origin, *Antonie van Leeuwenhoek 58*:255 (1990).
67. R. P. Ellen, E. D. Fillery, K. H. Chan, and D. A. Grove, Sialidase-enhanced lectin-like mechanism for *Actinomyces viscosus* and *Actinomyces naeslundii* hemagglutination, *Infect. Immun. 27*:335 (1980).
68. H. T. Sojar, J. -Y. Lee, M. S. Reddy, and R. J. Genco, Isolation and characterization of a lectin-like molecule from the cell surface of *Porphyromonas gingivalis*, *J. Dent. Res. 74*:508 (1995).
69. E. C. I. Veerman, A. J. M. Ligtenberg, L. C. P. M. Schenkels, E. Walgreen-Weterings, and A. V. Nieuw Amerongen, Binding of high molecular weight salivary mucins (MG1) to *Haemophilus parainfluenzae*, *J. Dent. Res. 74*:351 (1995).
70. S. Ebisu, H. Nakae, H. Fukuhara, and H. Okada, The mechanisms of *Eikenella corrodens* aggregation by the salivary glycoprotein and the effect of glycoprotein on oral bacterial aggregation, *J. Periodont. Res. 27*:615 (1992).
71. P. A. Murray, M. J. Levine, L. A. Tabak, and M. S. Reddy, Specificity of salivary-bacterial interactions: II. Evidence for a lectin on *Streptococcus sanguis* with specificity for a NeuAca2,3Galb1,3GalNAc sequence, *Biochem. Biophys. Res. Commun. 106*:390 (1982).
72. R. J. Gibbons, I. Etherden, and E. C. Moreno, Association of neuraminidase-sensitive receptors and putative hydrophobic interactions with high-affinity binding sites for *Streptococcus sanguis* C5 in salivary pellicles, *Infect. Immun. 42*:1006 (1983).
73. P. A. Murray, A. Prakobphol, T. Lee, C. I. Hoover, and S. J. Fischer, Adherence of oral streptococci to salivary glycoproteins, *Infect. Immun. 60*:31 (1992).
74. G. I. Torres, M. S. Reddy, F. A. Scannapieco, and M. J. Levine, Low-molecular weight salivary mucin promotes adhesion of *Streptococcus gordonii* to hydroxyapaptite, *J. Dent. Res. 72*:363 (1993).

75. E. J. Bergey, M. Gu, A. R. Collins, S. D. Bradway, and M. J. Levine, Modulation of *Herpes simplex* virus type 1 replication by human salivary secretions, *Oral Microbiol. Immunol. 8*:89 (1993).
76. E. J. Bergey, M. -I. Cho, M. -L. Hammarskjold, D. Rekosh, M. J. Levine, B. M. Blumberg, and L. G. Epstein, Aggregation of human immunodeficiency virus type 1 by human salivary secretions, *Crit. Rev. Oral Biol. Med. 4*:467 (1993).
77. C. A. Squier, Oral complications of cancer therapies. Mucosal alterations, *NCI Monogr. 9*:169 (1990).
78. B. Jany, and C. B. Basbaum, Mucin in disease. Modification of mucin gene expression in airway disease, *Am. Rev. Respir. Dis. 144*:S38 (1991).
79. P. C. Denny, P. A. Denny, D. K. Klauser, S. H. Hong, M. Navazesh, and L. A. Tabak, Age-related changes in mucins from human whole saliva, *J. Dent. Res. 70*:1320 (1991).
80. M. Rhodes, A. Allen, and T. W. J. Lennard, Mucus glycoprotein biosynthesis in the human gall bladder: inhibition by aspirin, *Gut 33*:1109 (1992).
81. P. L. Devine, and I. F. C. McKenzie, Mucins: structure, function, and associations with malignancy, *Bioessays 14*:619 (1992).
82. E. C. I. Veerman, M. Valentijn-Benz, and A. V. Nieuw Amerongen, Viscosity of human salivary mucins: effect of pH and ionic strength and role of sialic acid, *J. Biol. Buccale 17*:297 (1989).
83. A. Allen, Mucus - a protective secretion of complexity, *TIBS 8*:169 (1983).
84. S. D. Bradway, E. J. Bergey, P. C. Jones, and M. J. Levine, Oral mucosal pellicle. Adsorption and transpeptidation of salivary components to buccal epithelial cells, *Biochem. J. 261*:887 (1989).
85. S. D. Bradway, E. J. Bergey, F. A. Scannapieco, N. Ramasubbu, S. Zawacki, and M. J. Levine, Formation of salivary-mucosal pellicle: the role of transglutaminase, *Biochem. J. 284*:557 (1992).
86. A. Wikman, J. Karlsson, I. Carlstedt, and P. Artursson, A drug absorption model based on the mucus layer producing human intestinal goblet cell line HT29-H, *Pharm. Res. 10*:843 (1993).
87. F. Nimmerfall, and J. Rosenthaler, Significance of the goblet-cell mucin layer, the outermost luminal barrier to passage through the gut wall, *Biochem. Biophys. Res. Commun. 94*:960 (1980).
88. M. P. Baybrooks, B. W. Barry, and E. T. Abbs, The effect of mucin on the bioavailability of tetracycline from the gastrointestinal tract; in vivo, in vitro correlation, *J. Pharm. Pharmacol. 27*:508 (1975).
89. P. Kearney, and C. Marriott, The effect of an endogenous mucus layer on tetracycline absorption. *J. Pharm. Pharmacol. 34*:71P (1982).

90. J. -J. Niibuchi, Y. Aramaki, and S. Tsuchiya, Binding of antibiotics to rat intestinal mucin, *Int. J. Pharm. 30*:181 (1986).
91. M. A. Desai, C. V. Nicholas, and P. Vadgama, Electrochemical determination of the permeability of porcine mucus to model solute compounds, *J. Pharm. Pharmacol. 43*:124 (1991).
92. J. Sarosiek, A. Slomiany, A. Takagi, and B. L. Slomiany, Hydrogen ion diffusion in dog gastric mucus glycoprotein: effect of associated lipids and covalently bound fatty acids, *Biochem. Biophys. Res. Commun. 118*:523 (1984).
93. D. Harris, and J. R. Robinson, Bioadhesive polymers in peptide drug delivery, *Biomaterials 11*:652 (1990).
94. M. A. Longer, and J. R. Robinson, Fundamental aspects of bioadhesion, *Pharm. Int. 7*:114 (1987).
95. D. Duchene, and G. Ponchel, A new pharmacotechnical method for improving therapeutic efficiency, *STP Pharma 5*:830 (1989).
96. R. Gurny, J. M. Meyer, and N. A. Peppas, Bioadhesive intraoral release systems: design, testing and analysis, *Biomaterials 5*:336 (1984).
97. J. L. Chen, and G. N. Cyr, Compositions producing adhesion through hydration, *Adhesion in Biological Systems* (R. S. Marly, ed.), Academic Press, New York and London, 1970, p. 163.
98. G. Ponchel, F. Touchard, D. Duchene, and N. A. Peppas, Bioadhesive analysis of controlled-release systems. I. Fracture and interpenetration analysis in poly(acrylic acid)-containing systems, *J. Control. Rel. 5*:129 (1987).
99. P. Bottenberg, R. Cleymaet, C. de Muynck, J. P. Remon, D. Coomans, Y. Michotte, and D. Slop, Development and testing of bioadhesive, fluoride-containing slow-release tablets for oral use, *J. Pharm. Pharmacol. 43*:457 (1991).
100. J. F. Bridges, J. F. Woodley, R. Duncan, and J. Kopecek, Soluble N-(2-hydroxypropyl) methacrylamide copolymers as a potential oral, controlled-release, drug delivery system: I. Bioadhesion to the rat intestine in vitro, *Int. J. Pharm. 44*:213 (1988).
101. G. Molema, and D. K. F. Meijer, Targeting of drugs to various blood cell types using (neo-)glycoproteins, antibodies and other protein carriers, *Adv. Drug Del. Rev. 14*:25 (1994).
102. A. J. Caston, S. S. Davis, and P. Williams, The potential of fimbrial proteins for delaying intestinal transit of drug delivery systems, *Proc. Int. Symp. Control Rel. Bioact. Mater. 17*:313 (1990).
103. C. -M. Lehr, J. A. Bouwstra, W. Kok, A. B. J. Noach, A. G. de Boer, and H. E. Junginger, Bioadhesion by means of specific binding of tomato lectin, *Pharm. Res. 9*:547 (1992).

104. L. A. Bobek, H. Tsai, and M. J. Levine, Expression of human salivary histatin and cystatin/histatin chimeric cDNAs in *Escherichia coli*, *Crit. Rev. Oral Biol. Med.* *4*:581 (1993).
105. S. D. Bradway, and M. J. Levine, Do proline-rich proteins modulate a transglutaminase catalyzed mechanism of candidal adhesion?, *Crit. Rev. Oral Biol. Med.* *4*:293 (1993).
106. P. C. Fox, P. F. van der Ven, B. C. Sonies, J. M. Weiffenbach, and B. J. Baum, Xerostomia: evaluation of a symptom with increasing significance, *J. Am. Dent. Assoc.* *110*:519 (1985).
107. M. J. Levine, A. Aguirre, M. N. Hatton, and L. A. Tabak, Artificial salivas: Present and future, *J. Dent. Res.* *66*:693 (1987).
108. I. L. Shannon, B. R. McCrary, and E. N. Starcke, A saliva substitute for use by xerostomic patients undergoing radiotherapy to the head and neck, *Oral Surg. Oral Med. Oral Pathol.* *44*:656 (1977).
109. O. Donatsky, T. Johnsen, P. Holmstrup, and U. Bertram, Effect of Saliment on parotid salivary gland secretion and on xerostomia caused by Sjögren's syndrome, *Scand. J. Dent. Res.* *90*:157 (1982).
110. A. Vissink, E. J. 's-Gravenmade, A. K. Panders, A. Vermey, J. K. Petersen, L. L. Visch, and R. M. H. Schaub, A clinical comparison between commercially available mucin- and CMC-containing saliva substitutes, *Int. J. Oral Surg.* *12*:232 (1983).
111. A. J. Duxbury, N. F. Hayes, and N. S. Thakkar, Clinical trial of a mucin-containing artificial saliva, *IRCS Med. Sci.* *13*:1193 (1985).
112. A. Vissink, R. M. H. Schaub, L. J. van Rijn, E. J. 's-Gravenmade, A. K. Panders, and A. Vermey, The efficacy of mucin-containing artificial saliva in alleviating symptoms of xerostomia, *Gerodontology* *6*:95 (1987).
113. D. Wiesenfeld, A. M. Stewart, and D. K. Mason, A critical assessment of oral lubrication in patients with xerostomia, *Br. Dent. J.* *155*:155 (1983).
114. A. C. Klestov, J. Webb, D. Latt, G. Schiller, K. McNamara, D. Y. Young, J. Hobbes, and J. Fetherston, Treatment of xerostomia: A double blind trial in 108 patients with Sjögren's syndrome, *Oral Surg. Oral Med. Oral Pathol.* *51*:594 (1981).
115. G. Bajocchi, S. Feldman, R. G. Crystal, and A. Mastrangeli, Direct in vivo gene transfer to ependymal cells in the central nervous system using recombinant adenovirus vectors, *Nat. Genet.* *3*:229 (1993).
116. P. Lemarchand, H. A. Jaffe, C. Danel, M. C. Cid, H. K. Kleinman, L. D. Stratford-Perricaudet, M. Perricaudet, A. Pavirani, J. -P. Lecocq, and R. G. Crystal, Adenovirus-mediated transfer of a recombinant human α_1-antitrypsin cDNA to human endothelial cells, *Proc. Natl. Acad. Sci. USA* *89*:6482 (1992).

117. A. Mastrangeli, C. Danel, M. A. Rosenfeld, L. D. Stratford-Perricaudet, M. Perricaudet, A. Pavirani, J. -P. Lecocq, and R. G. Crystal, Diversity of airway epithelial cell targets for in vivo recombinant adenovirus-mediated gene transfer, *J. Clin. Invest. 91*:225 (1993).
118. M. A. Rosenfeld, K. Yoshimura, B. C. Trapnell, K. Yoneyama, E. R. Rosenthal, W. Dalemans, M. Fukayama, J. Bargon, L. E. Stier, L. D. Stratford-Perricaudet, M. Perricaudet, W. B. Guiggno, A. Pavirani, J. -P. Lecoq, and R. G. Crystal, In vivo transfer of the human cystic fibrosis transmembrane conductance regulator gene to the airway epithelium, *Cell 68*:143 (1992).
119. L. Thompson, At age 2, gene therapy enters a growth phase, *Science 258*:744 (1992).
120. R. A. Morgan, and W. F. Anderson, Human gene therapy, *Ann. Rev. Biochem. 62*:191 (1993).
121. J. S. Cohen, and M. E. Hogan, The new genetic medicines, *Scientific American 271*:76 (1994).
122. A. Mastrangeli, B. O'Connell, W. Aladib, P. C. Fox, B. J. Baum, and R. G. Crystal, Direct in vivo adenovirus-mediated gene transfer to salivary glands, *Am. J. Physiol. 266*:G1146 (1994).
123. J. A. Young, and E. W. van Lennep, Transport in salivary and salt glands, *Transport Organs* (G. Giebisch, ed.), Springer-Verlag, New York, 1979, p. 563.
124. J. H. Thaysen, N. A. Thorn, and I. L. Schwartz, Excretion of sodium, potassium, chloride and carbon dioxide in human parotid saliva, *Am. J. Physiol. 178*:155 (1954).

10

Mucoadhesive Hydrogels for Buccal Delivery

Ian W. Kellaway
The Welsh School of Pharmacy, Wales

Simon J. Warren
Cardiff Scintigraphics Ltd., Wales

I. INTRODUCTION

An effective buccal mucosa delivery device must establish and maintain intimate contact with the mucus layer overlying the epithelial tissue. At present much effort is being channeled into the study of a class of polymeric compounds with apparent mucoadhesive properties. Devices fabricated from such materials must reversibly adhere to the mucosal surface without causing tissue damage or discomfort to the patient. Ideally drug release should be unidirectional and the rate of release should be controlled by the properties of the device independently of the environmental conditions.

Mucoadhesive polymers have been utilized in many different dosage forms in efforts to achieve systemic delivery of drugs through the buccal mucosa [1]. Formulations include tablets, patches, tapes, films, semisolids (ointments and gels) and powders. The focus of this chapter will be hydrogels formulated from mucoadhesive polymers. In the examples illustrated the mucoadhesive hydrogel may function purely as an anchor to maintain the device at the desired location or alternatively it may also serve as a reservoir containing the active agent and so determine the drug release profile. Before detailing literature reports of mucoadhesive hydrogels in the context of buccal drug delivery it is appropriate to review some of the salient features of mucoadhesive polymers, and the nature of the polymer-substrate interaction. Similarly the principal features of hydrogels which may influence drug release will be discussed.

II. MUCOADHESIVE POLYMERS AND MECHANISMS OF MUCOADHESION

Bioadhesion is the term that describes the adhesion of a polymer to a biological substrate whilst mucoadhesion relates to mucus or a mucosal membrane as the substrate. Many research groups are currently investigating the physicochemical properties of such polymers. A general consensus of the most important physicochemical features of such mucoadhesive has been reached, and these may be summarized as follows [2, 3]:

1. Generally hydrophilic molecules that contain numerous hydrogen bond forming groups.
2. Surface tension characteristics suitable for wetting mucus/mucosal tissue surfaces.
3. The polymers are predominantly anionic in nature containing many carboxyl groups.
4. Usually have a high molecular weight i.e., > 100 000.
5. Sufficient flexibility to penetrate the mucus network or tissue crevices.

Several mechanisms of the polymer/substrate interaction in mucoadhesive bond formation have been suggested, namely, the electronic, adsorption, wetting, diffusion, and fracture theories [4]. If however, mucoadhesion is considered in terms of three stages, wetting, interpenetration and interaction of substrate and polymer, then the relevance of the physicochemical properties listed above becomes evident.

To develop an intimate contact between the interacting molecules the mucoadhesive must "wet" the substrate. Since mucoadhesive interactions occur in the presence of water (mucus consists of 95% water [5], then the importance of the hydrophilic properties of the polymer can be appreciated. A low water polymer contact angle will encourage hydration of the polymer chains, and increased segmental mobility; spreading of the polymer over the mucus also occurs promoting an intimate contact. Thereafter it is important that the polymer chains are able to diffuse into the mucus network so that interdigitation between the interacting species may occur [2]. Thus the polymer must have a sufficient linear chain length (molecular weight consideration) to ensure interpenetration can occur [6]. The segmental mobility of the polymer chain is of great importance to encourage entanglement between the interacting molecules. Early studies investigating the mechanism of adhesion of hydrocolloids [7] proposed that upon hydration the synthetic polymer molecules became more freely mobile and were able to orientate adhesive sites favorably with those of the substrate. As the level of hydration increased, adhesive properties were found to be reduced since mucoadhesive bonds became over extended.

Hunt [8] stated that based on estimates of the rate of polymer diffusion through mucus networks and the depth of penetration required for mucoadhesion [2] that it was unlikely that interdigitation alone could account for the mucoadhesive interaction because of the time dependency of the process. Therefore the establishment of secondary bond formation i.e., van der Waals interactions, assumes significance [6]. It is proposed that the hydrogen bond forming capacity of the polymer is important in this effect, and may explain the well documented mucoadhesive properties of polymers possessing numerous carboxyl groups such as Carbopol and polycarbophil. A systematic investigation of this property was carried out by Park and Robinson [5]. The study demonstrated that the in vitro mucoadhesive properties of custom synthesized polycarbophil hydrogels were modified as a function of pH. At pH values above the pKa of the polymer the strength of the interaction was progressively reduced as a greater proportion of the carboxyl groups were ionized and thus precluded from hydrogen bond formation. Also the greater swelling of the polymer as the degree of ionization increased lead to a reduction in mechanical strength and a concomitant reduction in mucoadhesive properties [5]. However, recently reported studies by Bouckaert and Remon [9] challenge the importance of hydrogen bonding between the mucoadhesive and the glycoprotein. These workers found, using a method described by Ponchel et al [10], that the in vitro work of adhesion in separating Carbopol 907 tablets from porcine gingiva was equivalent at pH 5 and pH 7.4. Over this pH range the number of ionized carboxylic groups (pKa = 4.75) increased from 9 to 96% [9]. It may be deduced that the physical mechanisms of mucoadhesion, i.e., interpenetration and entanglement, therefore are of greater importance than secondary bond interactions.

Overall it may be concluded that the most efficient mucoadhesive polymers have physicochemical properties that are closely related to those of the mucus substrate. It is widely recognized that the mucus layer is composed of an entangled, hydrated network of high molecular glycoprotein molecules [11, 12]. The glycoprotein is commonly referred to as having a bottle brush structure, that is an amino acid backbone with numerous carbohydrate side chains. The terminal groups of the side chains are often sialic acid residues (pKa < 3), or frequently sulfated galactose or N-acetyl glucosamine [13]. The linkage of the side chain to the back bone is usually via an O-glycosidic bond between C1 in N-acetyl galactosamine and the hydroxyl group of either serine or threonine. Thus under appropriate pH conditions i.e., the pH of saliva generally lies in the range 5.8-7.4 [14], the terminal groups confer upon the glycoprotein an overall negative charge [15]. The structural similarities of the two polymers i.e., salivary glycoprotein and mucoadhesive, would suggest a small interfacial tension exists upon mixing which promotes interaction and the development of a mucoadhesive bond.

III. MUCOADHESIVE TESTING

An integral facet of the development of a mucoadhesive drug delivery device is an assessment of its adhesive properties. During development rapid in vitro screening of such materials is desirable and several suitable techniques have been reported in the literature. Kellaway [16] classified these methods into (i) mechanical and (ii) spectroscopic techniques.

Mechanical testing methods include tensile tests, and shear and peel testing. Such methods have been widely reviewed e.g., Park and Park [17] and Helliwell [18]. Other mechanical characteristics such as the change of rheological properties of mucus in the presence of mucoadhesive polymers may be assessed using these methods e.g., Allen [19].

Spectroscopic methods including the fluorescent probe technique reported by Park and Robinson [20], electron spin resonance [21] and nuclear magnetic resonance experiments [16] may also be undertaken. Photon correlation spectroscopy (dynamic light scattering) has also been utilized to study the interactions of mucoadhesives and mucus glycoproteins [16].

In vivo aspects of mucoadhesion testing were recently reviewed by Helliwell [18], the three commonly performed methods i.e., gamma scintigraphy, perfused intestinal loop and radiolabeled transit studies were discussed.

IV. MUCOADHESION IN THE BUCCAL CAVITY

The environmental factors which may influence mucoadhesion to the buccal tissue are very different to those encountered at other mucosal sites which may be considered candidates for mucoadhesive agents e.g., oral, nasal, rectal and vaginal. In contrast to the latter regions, the mucus layer overlying the buccal tissue is very thin; Collins and Dawes [22] calculated the average saliva film thickness in the mouth as a whole to be 70-100 μm. Also since the minor salivary glands, which secrete up to 70% of the total mucin [11], are sparsely distributed throughout the oral cavity the build up of a diffusion limiting mucus barrier under the device is very unlikely.

As described above hydration of the mucoadhesive polymer is essential to initiate the mucoadhesive bonding process. In the case of formulations applied in the non-hydrated state, which is the most convenient (i.e., from the point of view of drug stability and convenience to the patient), it is essential that sufficient water is available so that rapid hydration to a flexible rubbery state occurs. The capillary attraction forces arising when water from the space between the mucosa and the polymer is taken up by a dry system may be considerable [23]. It is of great importance that the mucoadhesive material will develop a bond with only the minimum of applied force for a practical length of time i.e., finger pressure for a few seconds. On the other hand provided that the bond can be successfully established, the reduction in the rate of swelling, due to water uptake from the tissue surface only, may prolong the association of the device with the mucosa as suggested by Chen and Cyr [7]. It has been speculated by Smart et al [24] that removal of water from the underlying mucus layer by the hydrating polymer may increase the cohesive properties of the mucus and thus play a vital role in the establishment of an effective mucoadhesive bond. An additional consideration arises should the mucoadhesive polymer function both as the matrix from which the drug is released, and the adhesive. In these instances the rate of drug release may be greatly influenced by the rate of hydration, this eventuality will be examined at length in the discussion of hydrogels.

The efficacy of the device may be enhanced by ensuring unidirectional drug release, this may be achieved by the inclusion of a non-permeable backing membrane. Furthermore, if the backing is non-adhesive the device may be easily and accurately applied and the possibility of attachment to non-target tissues is reduced. The inclusion of a backing membrane on the device may greatly complicate the manufacturing process, however, several reports of such devices can be found in the literature. Unfortunately problems have been encountered due to the development of swelling stresses within the device at the interface of the mucoadhesive polymer and the non-hydrating, or more slowly hydrating backing film. The consequence of this process is the device may separate into its component parts, therefore the bonding at the interface of the two elements should be carefully considered.

V. HYDROGELS

Hydrogels are characterized by hydrophilic polymeric networks that in the presence of water hydrate and swell, however dissolution is prevented by chemical crosslinks between the polymer chains. The extent of hydration and swelling is often great, such that the amount of water absorbed is several times the dry weight of the hydrogel. This feature is of particular significance since it contributes to the high degree of biocompatibility associated with hydrogels [25]. In the instance of synthetic hydrogels the method of preparation should be carefully monitored to ensure the biocompatibility properties are not compromised. This commonly occurs during the polymerization reaction, as a consequence of the use of initiators and the presence of free radicals which may contaminate the end product. Likewise unreacted monomer and/or crosslinking compounds must be removed. These problems may be circumvented by crosslinking pre-polymerized compounds with agents of known biocompatibility. Examples of this approach have been demonstrated by Hunt and Kellaway [26] and Warren et al [27], where Carbopol 907 was crosslinked, via an esterification reaction with glycerol, Caradol or sucrose to form hydrogel materials.

A. Hydrogel Swelling and Mucoadhesion

It is evident from the preceding discussion that the physicochemical properties of mucoadhesive polymers are ideal for the synthesis of hydrogels and thus the concept of mucoadhesive hydrogels may be realized. Equally it may be deduced that hydrogels formulated from mucoadhesive polymers will in the main be anionic in nature, a property that will have a profound effect on the swelling characteristics of the hydrogels. The discussion of mucoadhesive interactions stressed the importance of the mobility of polymer chains to facilitate interpenetration into the mucus layer and favorable alignment of sites contributing to the formation of the mucoadhesive bond. Water sorption and swelling of hydrogels is a complex process, that can be strongly influence by the local environment. In the instance of ionic gels, pH and ionic strength, as well as water availability, will affect the extent of swelling [28].

The influence of the swelling process on the adhesion of a hydrogel to the buccal mucosa will be examined. For most applications the hydrogel will be applied to the mucosa in the non-hydrated, glassy state. Water sorption reduces the glass transition temperature (Tg) below ambient conditions and the xerogel becomes progressively rubbery. The glassy-rubbery transition provides macroscopic evidence of the plasticization of the hydrogel by water and the subsequent increased mobility of the polymer chains. Thus for effective mucoadhesion it is imperative that the hydrogel material in contact with the mucosal layer swells rapidly, at the point of contact, to promote suitable interactions with mucus glycoproteins.

Swelling in the case of nonionic gels is the product of the solvent/polymer interaction which, if favorable, promotes water absorption, and the elasticity of the crosslinked network which tends to oppose swelling [29]. Swelling of anionic gels, will, additionally be influenced by the ionic content of the polymer network, pH and the ionic strength of the hydrating medium. Under pH conditions greater than the pKa of anionic hydrogels, swelling will be greatest and the density of, for example carboxyl groups, will further affect the process. As water diffuses into the matrix the degree of ionization increases forming a concentrated ionic solution within the hydrogel. The counter ions tend to diffuse out of this concentrated region while external water molecules will be driven in to dilute the ionic solution within the matrix. Dissolution of the hydrogel is prevented by the crosslinks, but swelling remains as a consequence of the difference in concentration between the internal and external solutions. The swelling pressure is the product of the opposing tendencies of dilution and the elasticity of the polymer network preventing dilution, with the situation analogous to osmotic equilibrium [30].

B. Drug Release from Hydrogels

In addition to the importance of the swelling process on the adhesion of a xerogel to the mucosal surface, the influence of swelling on the drug release process should be considered. As stated previously two roles for the mucoadhesive hydrogel in buccal drug delivery can be defined.

In the first instance the mucoadhesive material may simply function as an adhesive and serve solely to anchor a drug containing matrix to the target mucosa (Figure 1a) e.g., Ishida et al, [31]. Alternatively, the mucoadhesive

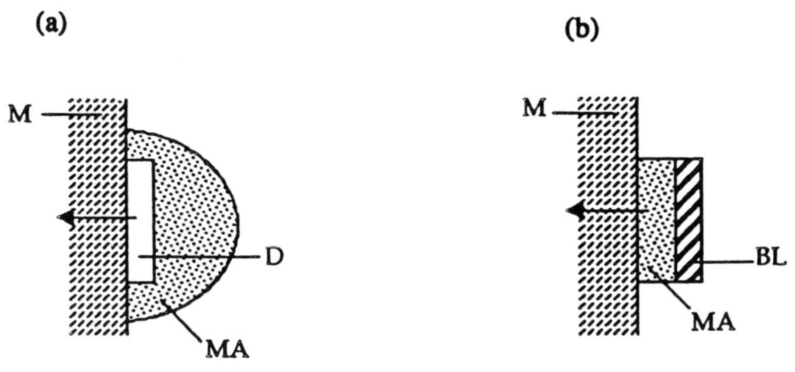

Figure 1. Schematic view of two different types of mucoadhesive device for buccal drug delivery. Case (a) mucoadhesive material (MA) ensures intimate and prolonged contact of the drug containing core (D) with the absorbing mucosa (M). Case (b) the drug is incorporated within the mucoadhesive material (MA) and the release of the active agent is therefore influenced by swelling induced changes of the mucoadhesive material. The presence of an impermeable backing layer (BL) ensures unidirectional drug release and may prolong mucoadhesion.

matrix may be loaded with the drug and thus determine its availability for absorption as well as anchoring the device at the selected mucosal site (Figure 1b) e.g., Nagai and Konishi [32].

Examples of each of these systems will be considered later in this chapter. Firstly, the mechanisms of drug release through hydrogel systems will be considered. In the discussion of mucoadhesive processes it was noted that the mucoadhesive systems may be applied in a hydrated or nonhydrated state, for convenience the latter strategy is preferable. Thus drug transport phenomenon through preswollen matrices and actively swelling networks may occur depending upon the design of the device.

1. Drug release from prehydrated hydrogels

From a theoretical point of view transport through swollen matrices is a diffusion controlled process. The active agent may be incorporated by equilibrating the hydrogel in a drug solution of known concentration, and provided the exposure time is sufficient the active agent will be uniformly distributed throughout the matrix [33]. The drug release profiles can be measured using standard dissolution testing procedures e.g., [34, 35]. The amount of drug diffused typically shows a square root time dependence. The increasing diffusional pathlength of the drug with time precludes the possibility of constant solute release rates, at least from systems with simple planar geometry [36].

It has been the goal of many researchers to achieve constant, or zero-order release from such systems. Several approaches have been investigated, including nonuniform drug distribution, increasing the degree of crosslinking at the surface of the matrix, or varying the geometry of the device [36, 37, 38].

2. Drug release from swelling hydrogels

Drug release from dynamically swelling hydrogels may occur if the matrix is applied in the nonhydrated state and is a far more complex phenomenon. Many research groups have concentrated efforts on such solvent activated systems as a possible means of overcoming the poor release characteristics of the systems described above i.e., to achieve zero-order release kinetics [39]. Drug loading of such devices can in itself be problematic since unless the drug can be incorporated during the synthesis process, a convoluted procedure of swelling in drug solution and drying must be undertaken to produce the solvent free, glassy hydrogel loaded with drug.

In much the same way that mucoadhesive interactions will not be initiated until the xerogel imbibes water the same is true of drug release. Before water

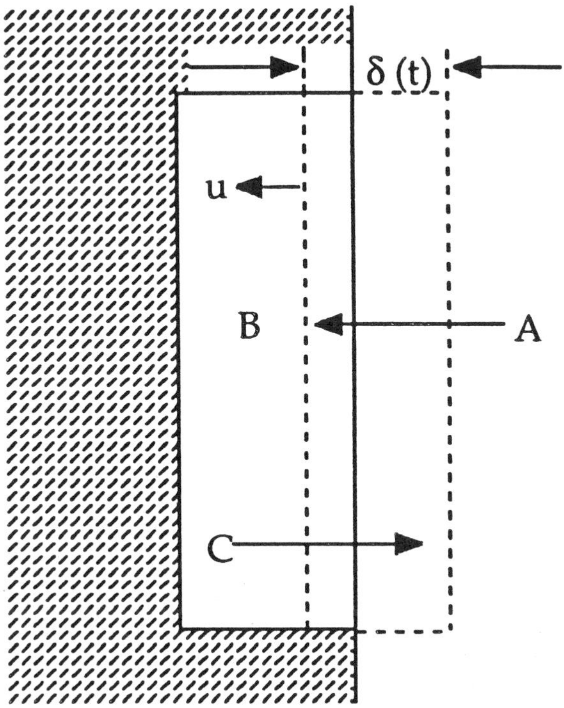

Figure 2. Schematic representation of swelling-controlled release system. As the penetrant A enters the glassy polymer B, bioactive agent C is released through the gel phase of thickness d(t). (From Langer and Peppas [36] with permission).

penetrates the glassy xerogel the dispersed drug is fixed within the matrix. If the polymer is thermodynamically compatible with the dissolution media then the Tg will be lowered and the glassy to rubbery transition occurs [37]. The plasticization of the network by the penetrant leads to considerable volume expansion.

The molecular rearrangements taking place in a swelling hydrogel are shown schematically in Figure 2 [36]. Two interfaces or fronts exist: the swelling interface between the glassy core of the matrix and the rubbery region which advances into the core as water or biological fluid is imbibed; and the front separating the advancing swollen region from the swelling medium. Drug release under these circumstances may be affected by both the rate of polymer relaxation and diffusion of penetrant, and consequently may be Fickian or non-Fickian in nature [29, 39].

In systems, in which certain parameters are defined, the relative importance of the rate of penetrant diffusion and polymer relaxation can be determined by calculating the Deborah number (D_e). This is expressed as the ratio of the polymer relaxation time (τ) to the diffusion time (θ) as follows:

$$D_e = \frac{\tau}{\theta} \quad (1)$$

where

$$\theta = \frac{L^2}{D_{wp}} \quad (2)$$

where L is the characteristic length of the device and D_{wp} is the water diffusion coefficient [37]. A value of $D_e \ll 1$ indicates that the polymer relaxation time is effectively infinite and therefore water ingression occurs through an essentially unchanging matrix, by a Fickian mechanism. If $D_e \gg 1$ then molecular relaxation is extremely rapid compared to water ingression and again penetrant uptake occurs by a Fickian mechanism in the rubbery state. Both of these processes are characterized by the linear relationship between penetrant uptake and the square root of swelling time. The third possibility, that $D_e \approx 1$, indicates that diffusion and relaxation occur on the same time scale, thus both influence transport, a phenomenon referred to as non-Fickian or anomalous transport. In systems where polymer relaxation occurs it is possible that solvent uptake is limited by the movement of the swelling front into the glassy hydrogel i.e., relaxation of the polymer molecules. In some instances the rate of this process may occur with a linear dependence on time, such zero-order phenomenon are referred to as Case II kinetics [37].

Concurrent to the penetrant uptake processes drug transport will be occurring in a countercurrent manner. The relative rates of penetrant uptake and drug diffusion have profound effects on the underlying mechanisms of drug release [40]. In one extreme, drug diffusion through the swollen gel matrix may be very slow compared to sorption of the dissolution medium, in this instance Fickian diffusion may occur. Conversely, if drug diffusion is rapid then the process may be limited by the rate of polymer relaxation, i.e., the movement of the swelling front into the glassy polymer for the release of drug. In such instances if penetrant uptake is linear with respect to time then drug release may also be constant with time. In accordance with the situation described above drug release may then be regarded as zero-order, i.e., an example of Case II kinetics.

VI. MUCOADHESIVE HYDROGEL SYSTEMS FOR BUCCAL DRUG DELIVERY

The foregoing discussion has explained the concept of mucoadhesion and described the important physicochemical properties of mucoadhesive polymers. It was stressed that such materials would be ideally suited as components of mucoadhesive hydrogels. The salient features of hydrogels were considered in the context of adhesive interactions with mucus glycoproteins and also with regard to drug release processes. In this final section examples of delivery systems, used for both local and systemic effects in vivo will be reviewed. As indicated previously two roles for mucoadhesive hydrogels can be identified, i.e., functioning solely as an adhesive or alternatively both as an adhesive and as a barrier (possibly rate controlling) through which the active agent must diffuse en route to the mucosa. The dosage forms considered in this section are all formulated from hydrocolloid materials, however, due to the absence of crosslinking in some cases, these materials are not strictly hydrogels. Consequently devices have been classified as: (i) swellable or (ii) hydrogel systems.

A. Mucoadhesive Swellable Systems

1. Tablets formulated by direct compression

Buccal tablets, formulated by direct compression of blends of mucoadhesive hydrophilic polymers, incorporating active agents have been studied in some depth. An attractive feature of such a device is the ease of fabrication, however, this is countered by several disadvantages. In most cases drug diffusion is not unidirectional and the manufacturing process would be greatly complicated by the incorporation of a non-permeable backing layer. Also the absence of crosslinking means that dissolution and/or erosion processes will occur as the device absorbs water.

Ishida et al [31] examined the possibility of buccal delivery of insulin using a novel mucoadhesive dosage form. Insulin was incorporated into a core material of cocao butter and sodium glycocholate, and a mixture (2:1) of Carbopol 934 (CP) and hydroxypropyl cellulose (HCP) was compressed around the core. Systemic insulin absorption was measured in beagle dogs although the percentage absorbed was low, approximately 0.5% compared to intramuscular injection. Mucoadhesive properties however were satisfactory with the devices adhering for up to 6 hours. Ishida and co-workers [41] improved the design of the device by adding an impermeable backing layer comprised of magnesium stearate. In this instance the device was developed to deliver a sustained level of the local anesthetic lidocaine for the treatment of toothache.

Tablets of similar design, i.e., mucoadhesive layer (CP:HCP) containing the active agent and a supporting non-adhesive layer of lactose were reported by Nagai [42]. The formulation contained triamcinolone acetonide and proved effective in the treatment of apthous stomatitis, an infection of the mouth. The formulation was subsequently marketed in Japan under the brand name "Aftach".

Recently a mucoadhesive tablet containing 5% polyacrylic acid (either Carbopol 907, 910 or 934/934P) and 95% drum dried waxy maize starch was reported by Bouckaert et al [43]. The formulation containing Carbopol 907 was found to adhere for up to 13.5 hours in volunteers (subjects were permitted to eat and drink), and at the end of this period the tablet was completely eroded [43]. It may be assumed that the waxy starch component of the formulation reduced the rate of swelling and prolonged the mucoadhesive interaction. The devices were used to provide a constant level of miconazole in the saliva bathing the mouth for the topical treatment of fungal infections.

A commercially available buccal tablet formulation is produced by Forest Laboratories. The transmucosal tablet contains nitroglycerin, for the treatment of angina, prepared in a matrix of hydroxypropyl cellulose known as "Synchron". Gamma scintigraphy has been utilized to show that this formulation adheres to the buccal mucosa for several hours, an association which provides clinical activity over a period of 5-6 hours. During this time the tablet swells to form a gel layer and swelling and erosion processes combine to produce zero-order release kinetics of the drug [44]. The absence of crosslinking ensures that ultimately the device is completely eroded.

Deasy and O' Neill [45] reported a more sophisticated formulation for the systemic delivery of timolol maleate. Once again the mucoadhesive device was formed by direct compression with no crosslinking of the polymers used, in this instance sodium carboxymethyl cellulose (NaCMC), Carbopol 934 or hydroxypropyl cellulose were investigated. The drug was contained within a core, which was coated with mucoadhesive material such that the core was exposed on a single planar face of the device. The opposite face was coated with a non-swelling, impermeable layer of magnesium stearate. During in vitro swelling studies of the compact it was found that the cap occasionally cracked, due to differential expansion, thus allowing unwanted diffusion of the drug. The lower swelling rate of HPC, prevented cracking of the cap but displayed unacceptable mucoadhesion properties in vivo. A 2:1 mixture of HPC:CP provided adequate mucoadhesion without premature cracking of the cap. Drug absorption was based on residual assay determination, and in humans a mean of 34% was absorbed over a 3 hour period. The inclusion of a permeation enhancer sodium lauryl sulfate (0.01%) increased this level to 61%.

Another recent example of mucoadhesive tablets formulated by direct compression was reported by Anlar et al [46]. In this instance hydroxypropyl methylcellulose (HPMC) and Carbopol 910 blends 20:80 w/w were examined in vivo in volunteers, for their effectiveness to deliver morphine sulfate. To ensure unidirectional drug release the devices were manually coated, on all sides except one, with a solution of the water impermeable polymer Eudragit RSPM. Drug absorption was estimated by assay of the residual drug remaining in the tablet after predetermined exposure times to the mucosa.

2. *Polymer films*

Sustained local delivery of prostaglandins to the gingiva for the purpose of accelerating orthodontic tooth movement, was achieved by Nagai and Konishi [32] by means of an adhesive plaster. The device consisted of two layers, a water impermeable non-adhesive backing and a water activated adhesive layer containing the bioactive agent. The exact composition and proportions of the materials constituting the mucoadhesive layer were not detailed although carboxymethyl cellulose, a proven mucoadhesive [47] was included. The plaster was found to adhere during eating and drinking, the impermeable backing membrane reduced the rate of hydration, and adhesion for periods of 8 hours were recorded in primates. Clinical evaluations were undertaken in human volunteers and the patch was well tolerated with no adverse effects during chronic applications of two months. The efficacy observed during the trial was sufficient to warrant further investigations.

A patch of quite complex design was detailed by Veillard et al [48], with unidirectional drug release assured by the presence of an impermeable backing membrane. The drug was incorporated into a rate limiting membrane sandwiched between the backing film and a mucoadhesive film prepared from polycarbophil. Details of the materials used in the fabrication of the patch were not published, however the device was observed to adhere to the mucosa of volunteers, with food and water permitted, for approximately 17 hours. The authors stated that the water swollen polycarbophil allowed some movement of the buccal membrane and thus provided comfort to the patient.

Anders and Merkle [49] reported the fabrication of mucoadhesive two-ply laminate films. The backing layer, Multiphor sheet (commonly used as a backing layer for gel chromatography) faced into the oral cavity and was impermeable to the drug. An aqueous solution of a mucoadhesive hydrocolloid, hydroxyethyl cellulose (HEC), and the drug was cast onto the sheet, and dried to form a laminate. The presence of an agarose graft on one surface of the Multiphor sheet ensured that the binding between the HEC and the backing film was stable even in the hydrated state. The devices, up to 12 cm^2 in area and loaded with protirelin, were applied to the buccal mucosa of healthy volunteers. Adhesion to the buccal mucosa was observed for periods up to 30 minutes. In these studies drug absorption was not measured, the authors reported only the amount of drug remaining within the patches after 30 minutes exposure to the buccal mucosa. It was demonstrated that by increasing the viscosity grade of the mucoadhesive a greater fraction of drug remained within the patch.

3. *Hydrogels*

Cassidy et al [34] investigated the transbuccal absorption of diclofenac sodium from a hydrogel formulated from 80:20 w/w hydroxyethyl methacrylate (HEMA) and a hydrophobic difunctional macromolecular crosslinker. The device however possessed no inherent mucoadhesive properties and was anchored to the mucosa of human volunteers by a rim of dental adhesive and covered with a backing of non-permeable Surlyn. A high loading of the drug within the hydrogel was achieved and the gel was applied in the hydrated state. As would be expected for a dispersed monolith the dissolution of drug from the hydrated disc was linear with the square root of time over 4 hours. Measurable levels of diclofenac sodium were found in the plasma 0.5 hours after the application of the hydrogel, the results indicate that ionized species may be absorbed across the buccal mucosa. It seems probable that the drug diffuses along an aqueous pathway between the cells, i.e., by the paracellular route, rather than partitioning into the cells. The steady state flux of the drug across the buccal mucosa was 1000 fold greater than that observed across human skin in vitro [50].

The same hydrogel formulations and method of application were used to investigate the absorption of buprenorphine across the buccal mucosa of beagle dogs [51]. The hydrogels were applied for 3-4 hours and apparent steady-state plasma levels were attained in this period. Following removal of the devices a slow decline in plasma concentration was observed, leading the authors to speculate on the presence of a depot in the buccal mucosa.

Warren et al [27, 52] reported in vitro findings of peptide release from Carbopol 907 hydrogels crosslinked with sucrose. To promote unidirectional drug delivery the mucoadhesive Carbopol 907 film was backed by a less hydrophilic hydrogel. The backing membrane was composed of Carbopol crosslinked with Caradol [26]. Since this film was swellable, although to a lesser degree than the mucoadhesive layer, problems caused by differential swelling were overcome. In vivo studies showed that the laminate patches adhered in excess of 6 hours in contrast with Carbopol/sucrose hydrogels which swelled rapidly due to saliva uptake and adhered for a maximum of 45 minutes. The absorption of a model nonapeptide, oxytocin, from the patches was compared with that from a peptide solution maintained on the mucosa for a two hour period. Onset of absorption was much more rapid and higher plasma levels were recorded from solution compared to the patches. However, in both cases apparent zero-order absorption profiles were observed with approximate mean plasma levels of 2.00 ng mL^{-1} (solution) and 0.05 ng mL^{-1} (patch) [53].

VII. SUMMARY

A review of the literature has shown that very few investigations of drug delivery from mucoadhesive hydrogels applied to the buccal mucosa have been undertaken. When applied to this site mucoadhesive materials have most commonly been utilized as components of directly compressed tablets. The examples listed above provide evidence that such devices can adhere to the mucosal tissue over prolonged periods, thus making them candidates for sustained or controlled delivery of drugs to the systemic circulation.

Two roles for the mucoadhesive hydrogel in drug delivery to the buccal mucosa have been defined. The least complex is to function solely as a mucoadhesive and have no influence over the drug delivery process. In this way the degree of hydration of the mucoadhesive polymer effects only the duration of adhesion.

Alternatively both the adhesive and drug release properties of the device may be attributed to the mucoadhesive polymer. From the point of view of drug stability and duration of adhesion, such devices must be applied in the non-hydrated state. In this case the formulation scientist is confronted by several problems. The greatest is the conflicting need for rapid hydration of the hydrogel upon contact with the mucosa to ensure drug is available for absorption, whereas in contrast, a slow rate of hydration is necessary to ensure a prolonged period of adhesion. The requirement that the device should demonstrate undirectional drug release and adhere only to the target tissue dictates that a non-adhesive drug impermeable backing layer be a component of the device. The presence of an impermeable backing membrane creates further problems since during hydration, stress develops at the junction between the swelling and non-swelling components. This may lead to buckling of the device and the failure of the mucoadhesive joint or disruption of the laminate. Such difficulties may be overcome by modifying the hydrogel membrane such that there is a gradient in hydrophilicity from one face to the other [54].

It may be concluded, that the paucity of literature reports on buccal drug delivery from mucoadhesive hydrogels, can be attributed to the constraints placed upon the formulation scientist. The ideal drug loaded hydrogel device must have the following properties: application in the non-hydrated state; exhibit undirectional drug release; swell sufficiently rapidly to provide a high concentration of drug for absorption; drug release and mucoadhesive properties appropriate for single daily dosing. Such features may only be conferred upon the device following elaborate mucoadhesive synthesis and/or complicated delivery system manufacturing methods.

REFERENCES

1. M. E. deVries, H. E. Boddé, J. C. Verhoef, and H. E. Junginger, Developments in buccal drug delivery, *Crit. Rev. Ther. Carrier Syst. 8*:271 (1991).
2. N. A. Peppas, and P. A. Buri, Surface, interfacial and molecular aspects of polymer bioadhesion on soft tissues, *J. Control. Rel. 2*:257 (1985).
3. G. Hunt, P. Kearney, and I. W. Kellaway, Mucoadhesive polymers in drug delivery systems, *Drug Delivery Systems: Fundamentals and Techniques* (P. Johnson, and J. G. Lloyd-Jones, eds.), Ellis Horwood, Chichester, 1987, p. 180.
4. J. -M. Gu, J. R. Robinson, and S. -H. S. Leung, Binding of acrylic polymers to mucin/epithelial surfaces: Structure-property relationships, *Crit. Rev. Ther. Drug Carrier Syst. 5*:21 (1988).
5. H. Park, and J. R. Robinson, Physico-chemical properties of water insoluble polymers important to mucin/epithelial adhesion, *J. Control. Rel. 2*:47 (1985).
6. M. A. Longer, and J. R. Robinson, Fundamental aspects of bioadhesion, *Pharm. Int. 5*:114 (1986).
7. J. L. Chen, and G. N. Cyr, Compositions producing adhesion through hydration, *Adhesion in Biological Systems* (R. S. Manly, ed.), Academic Press, London, 1970, p. 163.
8. G. Hunt, Mucoadhesive materials for drug delivery. Ph. D. Thesis. UWIST, Cardiff, 1988.
9. S. Bouckaert, and J. -P. Remon, In vitro bioadhesion of a buccal, miconazole slow release tablet, *J. Pharm. Pharmacol. 45*:504 (1993).
10. G. Ponchel, D. Duchene, and N. A. Peppas, Fracture analysis of the bioadhesive interactions between surface swollen, poly(acrylic acid) containing tablets and the bovine sublingual tissue, *Proc. Int. Symp. Control. Rel. Bioact. Mater. 14*:8 (1987).
11. L. A. Tabak, M. J. Levine, I. D. Mandel, and J. A. Ellison, Role of salivary mucins in the protection of the oral cavity, *J. Oral Pathol. 11*:1 (1982).
12. M. J. Levine, M. S. Reddy, L. A. Tabak, R. E. Loomis, E. J. Bergey, P. C. Jones, R. E. Cohen, M. W. Stinson, and I. Al-Hashim, Structural aspects of salivary glycoproteins, *J. Dent. Res. 66*:436 (1987).
13. A. Allen, Structure of gastrointestinal mucus glycoproteins and the viscous and gel-forming properties of mucus, *Br. Med. Bull. 34*:28 (1978).

14. M. M. Veillard, Buccal and gastrointestinal drug delivery systems, *Bioadhesion: Possibilities and Future Trends* (R. Gurny, and H. E. Junginger, eds.), Stuttgart, 1990, p. 124.
15. H. S. Ch'ng, H. Park, P. Kelly, and J. R. Robinson, Bioadhesive polymers as platforms for oral controlled drug delivery II. Synthesis and evaluation of some swelling water insoluble bioadhesive polymers, *J. Pharm. Sci. 74*:399 (1985).
16. I. W. Kellaway, In vitro test methods for the measurement of mucoadhesion, *Bioadhesion: Possibilities and Future Trends* (R. Gurny, and H. E. Junginger, eds.), Stuttgart, 1990, p. 86.
17. K. Park, and H. Park, Test methods of bioadhesion, *Bioadhesive Drug Delivery Systems* (V. Lenaerts, and R. Gurny, eds.), CRC Press, Boca Raton, Florida, 1990, p. 43.
18. M. Helliwell, The use of bioadhesives in targeted delivery within the gastrointestinal tract, *Adv. Drug Del. Rev. 11*:221 (1993).
19. A. Allen, S. N. E. Foster, and J. P. Pearson, Interaction of polyacrylate, carbomer, with gastric mucus and pepsin, *Br. J. Pharmacol. 87*:126P (1986).
20. K. Park, and J. R. Robinson, Bioadhesive platforms for oral controlled drug delivery: method to study bioadhesion, *Int. J. Pharm. 19*:107 (1984).
21. P. Kearney, I. W. Kellaway, J. C. Evans, and C. Rowlands, Probing the mucus barrier with spin labels, *J. Pharm. Pharmacol. 36*:26 (1984).
22. L. M. C. Collins, and C. Dawes, The surface area of the adult human mouth and the thickness of the salivary film covering the teeth and the oral mucosa, *J. Dent. Res. 66*:1300 (1987).
23. C. -M. Lehr, J. A. Bouwstra, H. E. Boddé, and H. E. Junginger, A surface energy analysis of mucoadhesion: Contact angle measurements on polycarbophil and pig intestinal mucosa in physiologically relevant fluids, *Pharm. Res. 9*:70 (1992).
24. J. D. Smart, B. Carpenter, and S. A. Mortazavi, Is mucus dehydration an important factor in mucoadhesion? *Proc. Int. Symp. Control. Rel. Bioact. Mater. 18*:629 (1991).
25. B. D. Ratner, Biomedical applications of hydrogels: Review and critical appraisal, *Biocompatibility of Clinical Implant Materials* (D. F. Williams, ed.) Volume II, CRS Press, Boca Raton, 1981, p. 145.
26. G. Hunt and I. W. Kellaway, The evaluation of swelling and solute transport in modified poly (acrylic acid) for mucoadhesive controlled release applications, *J. Pharm. Pharmacol. 38*:22P (1986).
27. S. J. Warren I. W. Kellaway, and P. Timmins, Mucoadhesive hydrogels for buccal delivery of peptides, *Proc. Int. Symp. Control. Rel. Bioact. Mater. 16*:402 (1989).

28. H. F. Mark, N. M. Bikales, C. G. Overberger, and G. Menges, eds. *Encyclopedia of Polymer Science and Engineering*, 2nd edn., Wiley and Sons, Chichester, 1987.
29. N. A. Peppas and A. R. Khare, Preparation and properties of hydrogels, *Adv. Drug Del. Rev. 11*:1 (1993).
30. R. Paterson, *An Introduction to Ion Exchange*, London, UK. 1970.
31. M. Ishida, Y. Machida, N. Nambu, and T. Nagai, New mucosal dosage form of insulin, *Chem. Pharm. Bull. 23*:810 (1981).
32. T. Nagai, and R. Konishi, Buccal/Gingival drug delivery systems, *J. Control. Rel. 6*:353 (1987).
33. F. Forni, G. Coppi, V. Iannuccelli, M. A. Vandelli, and M. T. Bernabei, Distribution of drugs polymers loaded by swelling, *J. Pharm. Sci. 78*:25 (1989).
34. J. Cassidy, B. Berner, K. Chan, V. John, S. Toon, B. Holt, and M. Rowland, Human transbuccal absorption of diclofenac sodium from a prototype hydrogel delivery device, *Pharm. Res. 10*:126 (1993).
35. R. W. Korsmeyer, and N. A. Peppas, Effect of the morphology of hydrophilic polymeric matrices on the diffusion and release of water soluble drugs, *J. Memb. Sci. 9*:211 (1981).
36. R. Langer, and N. A. Peppas, Chemical and physical structure of polymers as carriers for controlled release of bioactive agents: A review, *JMS-Rev. Macromol. Chem. Phys. C 23*:61 (1983).
37. P. I. Lee, Kinetics of drug release from hydrogel matrices, *J. Control. Rel. 2*:277 (1985).
38. E. S. Lee, S. W. Kim, S. H. Kim, J. R. Cardinal, and H. Jacobs, Drug release from hydrogel devices with rate controlling barriers, *J. Memb. Sci. 7*:293(1980).
39. R. W. Korsmeyer, and N. A. Peppas, Solute and penetrant diffusion in swellable polymers III. Drug release from glassy poly(HEMA-co-NVP) copolymers, *J. Control. Rel. 1*:89 (1984).
40. H. B. Hopfenberg, A. Apicella, and D. E. Saleeby, Factors affecting water sorption in and solute release from glassy ethylene-vinyl alcohol copolymers, *J. Memb. Sci. 8*:273 (1981).
41. M. Ishida, N. Nambu, and T. Nagai, Mucosal dosage form of lidocaine for toothache using hydroxypropyl cellulose and Carbopol, *Chem. Pharm. Bull. 30*:980 (1982).
42. T. Nagai, Adhesive topical drug delivery system, *J. Control. Rel. 2*:121 (1985).
43. S. Bouckaert, R. A. Lefebvre, and J-P. Remon, In vitro/in vivo correlation of the bioadhesive properties of a buccal bioadhesive miconazole slow release tablet, *Pharm. Res. 10*:853 (1993).

44. J. M. Schor, S. S. Davis, A. Nigalaye, and S. Bolton, Susadrin transmucosal tablets (Nitroglycerin in "Synchron" controlled release base), *Drug Dev. Ind. Pharm. 9*:1359 (1983).
45. P. B. Deasy, and C. T. O' Neill, Bioadhesive dosage form for peroral administration of timolol base, *Pharm. Acta Helv. 64*:231 (1989).
46. S. Anlar, Y. Capan, O. Guven, A. Gogus, T. Dalkara, and A. A. Hincal, Formulation and *in vitro–in vivo* evaluation of buccoadhesive morphine sulphate tablets, *Pharm. Res. 11(2)*:231 (1994).
47. J. D. Smart, I. W. Kellaway, and H. E. C. Worthington, An in-vitro investigation of mucosa-adhesive materials for use in controlled drug delivery, *J. Pharm. Pharmacol. 36*:295 (1984).
48. M. M. Veillard, M. A. Longer, T. W. Martens, and J. R. Robinson, Preliminary studies of oral mucosal delivery of peptide drugs, *J. Control. Rel. 6*:123 (1987).
49. R. Anders, and H. P. Merkle, Evaluation of laminated mucoadhesive patches for buccal drug delivery, *Int. J. Pharm. 49*:231 (1989).
50. G. C. Mazzenga, S. M. Dinh, B. Berner, and J. D. DeNuzzio, Iontophoretic delivery of diclofenac-Na ("Voltaren") in vitro, *Proc. Int. Symp. Control. Rel. Bioact. Mater. 17*:433 (1990).
51. J. P. Cassidy, N. M. Landzert, and E. Quadros, Controlled buccal delivery of buprenorphine, *J. Control. Rel. 25*:21 (1993).
52. S. J. Warren, I. W. Kellaway, and P. Timmins, The in vitro characterization of mucoadhesive hydrogel materials for the buccal delivery of peptides, *J. Pharm. Pharmacol. 42*:140P (1990).
53. I. W. Kellaway, S. J. Warren, and P. Timmins, Hydrogels for buccal application, *Buccal and Nasal Administration as an Alternative to Parenteral Administration* (D. Duchene, ed.), European Symposium, Paris, 1991.
54. C. E. Rogers, Transport through polymer membranes with a gradient of inhomogeneity, *J. Polym. Sci. 10*:93 (1965).

11

Systemic Oral Mucosal Drug Delivery and Delivery Systems

Michael J. Rathbone
InterAg, New Zealand

Gilles Ponchel
University of Paris, France

Firoz A. Ghazali
University of Otago, New Zealand

I. INTRODUCTION

The formulation of a drug into a delivery system designed for peroral administration e.g., tablet, capsule, etc., has been the traditional way to systemically administer drugs for centuries. However, not all drugs administered in this way exhibit optimal bioavailability either because of the inherent properties of the drug e.g., acid labile or extensively metabolized by the liver, or limitations associated with the gastrointestinal tract e.g., chemically hostile environment, hepatic first-pass effect or variable absorption characteristics. The inherent problems associated with the drug can, in some cases, be solved by modifying the formulation, e.g., reduction of gastric irritation by application of an enteric coating. On the other hand, poor

Table 1. Comparison of Some Routes for Systemic Drug Delivery Available to the Formulation Scientist.

	Gastro-intestinal	Dermal	Nasal	Oral mucosal	Vaginal
Accessibility	+	+++	++	++	+
Surface area	+++	+++	+	++	+++
Surface environment	+	++	++	+++	+
Permeability	+++	+	+++	++	+++
Reactivity	++	++	+	+++	++
Vascular drainage	+++	+	+++	++	+++
First-pass clearance	+	+++	+++	+++	+
Patient acceptability	++	+++	++	+++	++

+ poor; +++ excellent

bioavailability associated with the limitations of the peroral route can often only be improved by reformulating the drug for delivery via a different route, often referred to as an alternative route for drug delivery. Table 1 compares some of the alternative routes for drug delivery available to the formulation scientist.

Table 1 suggests that as a site for drug delivery the oral cavity offers several advantages over the gastrointestinal route and other alternative routes of drug administration. The membranes that line the oral cavity are readily accessible [1-3], robust [1, 2, 4] and exhibit fast cellular recovery following local stress or damage [4, 5]. Oral mucosal drug delivery systems are easy and painless to administer and well accepted by the patient [1, 3-5]. Precise dosage form localization is possible and there is the ability to terminate delivery when required [1, 2, 5], thus patients could conceivably control the period of administration. For patients suffering with nausea or vomiting, or in a state of unconsciousness, with an upper gastrointestinal tract disease or surgery which affects oral drug absorption, or those who have difficulty swallowing peroral medications, the oral cavity may be a useful site for drug delivery. From a formulation point of view the thin mucin film that exists on the surface of the oral cavity provides the pharmaceutical scientist with the opportunity to retain delivery systems in contact with the mucosa for prolonged periods with the help of mucoadhesive compounds [5].

The presence of up to 32 teeth in the adult mouth creates both advantages and disadvantages for oral mucosal drug delivery. Tooth surfaces provide an extensive hard surface onto which there is the potential to attach delivery devices. However, the masticatory function of teeth needs to be acknowledged in the design of any such system as will the appearance of the device on the tooth. Any system designed to be attached to the surface of the teeth will require robustness and will have to conform to severe size limitations because of the size of tooth surfaces.

The buccal membrane is sufficiently large to allow a delivery system to be placed at different sites on the same membrane on different occasions. This may be advantageous if the drug, components of the delivery system, or other excipients included in the formulation reversibly damage or irritate the mucosa.

The oral cavity appears therefore to be a potential site for the delivery of drugs to the systemic circulation.

There is currently a wide interest in the possibility of exploiting the oral mucosa for systemic drug delivery. A large amount of data has been published on the oral mucosal absorption of drugs from solutions. Such studies have been interpreted as indicating that the oral mucosa is readily permeable. The fact that systemic oral mucosal drug delivery only occupies a minor place in clinical practice attests to the fact that this is not true. Indeed, the success of currently marketed oral mucosal drug delivery systems is attributable to the inherent properties of the drug rather than the ready permeability of the oral mucosa. The lack of preponderance of such systems is also due to the fact that the environment of the oral cavity is not conducive to drug delivery (e.g., the secretion and swallowing of saliva, area available, retention) and that (until recently) formulation scientists have failed to optimize their oral mucosal drug delivery systems to overcome these problems.

A rational approach to formulation must be adopted in the development of any oral mucosal drug delivery system. This must include a knowledge of the anatomy and physiology of the oral cavity, a critical evaluation of the prevailing environmental conditions, attention to patient acceptability and a consideration of the possibilities and limitations of the site of delivery. It is the purpose of this chapter to highlight and discuss these characteristics as they relate to the systemic delivery of drugs via oral mucosa.

II. THE ORAL CAVITY AS A SITE FOR DRUG DELIVERY

A. Physical Description of Oral Cavity

The oral cavity can be divided into two regions; the outer oral vestibule which is bounded by the lips and cheeks and the oral cavity itself, the borders being formed by the hard and soft palates, the floor of the mouth and the pillars of the fauces and tonsils. The primary functions of the mouth are eating, drinking, breathing and speaking and the anatomical and physiological features of the mouth reflect these functions. Such functions dictate delivery system design, influence the release of the drug from the system, or may lead to termination of delivery particularly if delivery systems need to be removed to allow one or more of these function to be performed (e.g., eating or drinking).

The digestion of solid food begins with mastication by the teeth (up to 32 in the adult) together with the secretion of saliva from three pairs of glands; parotid, sublingual and submandibular (submaxillary). The presence of teeth may be used to advantage by the formulation scientist as it presents the opportunity to physically attach delivery systems using dental adhesives [2]. The tongue projects the food mass posteriorly into the back of the throat towards the epiglottis. The dorsal surface of the tongue is a muscular structure which is covered anteriorly with papillae, amongst which are scattered sensory receptors called taste buds. These taste buds may limit the use of certain drugs or excipients if their taste is unacceptable to the patient. It is unlikely that the dorsal surface of the tongue would ever be used as portal for drug entry. The sides and underside of the tongue are smooth and richly supplied with blood vessels. Also present in the mouth are the uvula, which hangs in the middle of the throat, the palatine tonsils, which are between the anterior and posterior tonsillar arches, and the lingual tonsil. The presence of these three lymphoid tissues could mean that drugs administered to the oral cavity could be taken up directly into the lymphatic circulation.

Virtually all of the membranes that line the oral cavity could potentially be used for systemic drug delivery, however, each region possesses different properties and characteristics [6-13], and therefore requires different approaches in the design and formulation of suitable delivery systems.

B. Regional Variations in the Composition of Oral Mucosa Pertinent to Systemic Drug Delivery

Several membranes line the oral cavity and each offers different problems for its utilization as a portal for drug entry to the systemic circulation. The membranes that line the oral cavity have a total area of approximately 200 cm^2 [10] and show differences in structure, thickness and blood flow, depending on their location [7, 11, 13]. Both keratinized and nonkeratinized tissues of varying thickness and composition are found in the oral cavity [7]. Keratinized and nonkeratinized tissue occupy about 50% and 30%, respectively, of the total surface area of the mouth [10]. In general, nonkeratinized tissue is considerably thicker than keratinized tissue but the nonkeratinized floor of the mouth is very thin (approximately 100 μm) [11, 12]. The keratinized layers of the oral mucosa epithelia form a protective surface which is mechanically tough and resistant to physical insult and penetration by any foreign substances. In keratinized tissue the outer layer comprises up to 20 rows of flattened, hexagonal shaped cells termed squames which are filled with a dense crystalline protein called keratin, arranged in interconnecting fibers through the cell [2]. The nonkeratinized mucosa is more mobile and found in regions of the oral cavity where a more flexible mucosa is required for functional purposes e.g., in the buccal and sublingual regions where mastication is predominant.

Probably the two most useful mucosa for systemic drug delivery in the oral cavity are the buccal and sublingual membranes [6]. The total area of the these are 50.2 cm^2 and 26.5 cm^2 [10], with thickness of 500-600 μm and 100-200 μm, respectively [11]. Both these regions are nonkeratinized. The other possible membranes that may have a future role in oral mucosal drug delivery are the gingival and palatal mucosa. Both of these mucosae are keratinized and have thicknesses of 200 μm and 250 μm, respectively [11].

C. Blood Supply to the Oral Mucosa

The blood supply to the oral cavity tissues is delivered via the external carotid artery, which branches into the maxillary, lingual, and facial arteries. Supply of blood to the tongue, sublingual and gingival areas are via the lingual artery, whereas the facial artery supplies blood to the soft palate and lips. The maxillary artery supplies blood to the hard palate and cheeks. Blood from the capillary beds is collected by three main veins that finally flow into the internal jugular vein [1, 5]. Thus delivery of drugs via the oral mucosa drains directly into the systemic circulation and thus avoids first-pass metabolism in the liver. Although blood flow through oral mucosa of humans has not been reported, Squier et al have documented values for blood flow through the oral mucosa of Rhesus monkey as: buccal (2.40 mL/minute/cm^2), sublingual (0.97 mL/minute/cm^2), gingival (1.47 mL/minute/cm^2) and palatal (0.89 mL/minute/cm^2) [13]. It is generally considered that blood flow through human oral mucosa, even during disease, is sufficiently fast as not to be a rate-limiting factor in the absorption of drugs via the oral mucosa.

D. Saliva

A comprehensive and detailed review of the pertinent features of saliva in drug delivery has been given by Rathbone et al [5]. There are three major glands supplying saliva to the oral cavity; parotid, sublingual and submandibular (submaxillary) which lie outside of the oral cavity, and minor salivary glands situated in the tissues lining most of the oral cavity. Saliva functions to moisten the oral cavity, aid the digestion of food, and lubricate the food for mastication and swallowing [14]. Saliva also provides protection to the tissues of the oral cavity by preventing the oral tissues from dehydrating and protecting them from abrasion by rough materials that may enter the mouth [15]. It also plays an important role in either aiding or preventing the attachment of bacteria to the surfaces of the oral cavity [15].

The parotid salivary glands are located anterior and inferior to the external ear and their ducts open into the oral cavity on the cheek opposite the upper first or second molar. Openings to the sublingual and submandibular glands are found on the floor of the mouth on either side of the frenulum (fold of membrane and connective tissue connecting the tongue to the floor of the mouth at the midline anteriorly). The sublingual glands run on either side underneath the tongue; the sublingual and submandibular glands share a common duct opening at the frenulum. Parotid glands secrete serous saliva whereas the mandibular and sublingual glands produce a mucous secretion. Clearly it would be unwise to locate a delivery system over the top of the opening of a major salivary gland duct. In addition different release rates from the same delivery system may be observed if it were to be located close to a duct opening as opposed to some distance away.

Saliva is composed of 99% water and is a complex fluid containing organic and inorganic materials [16]. A detailed account of the composition of saliva is given by Tenovuo [17]. There is considerable variation in the flow rate of saliva between individuals, with time of day and during disease conditions [14]. Secretion is highest during waking hours and lowest during sleep when it is almost undetectable. The amount of saliva produced throughout the day is 1-1.5 L, but this value is variable with some researchers reporting the total production of saliva to be as low as 0.5-0.6 L per day [18]. Such variable salivary flow characteristics may effect the in vivo release profiles of delivery systems designed for prolonged controlled release particularly those that are highly dependent upon saliva for release. The large variability in salivary flow rate particularly between sleeping and wakening hours could result in variations in the amount of drug released during these times. This could result in the need to design removable delivery systems with replacements of differing delivery rates [19].

Saliva is mainly produced by the three pairs of major salivary glands, however, additional small amounts of saliva are secreted into the oral cavity from minor glands on the tongue, buccal, sublingual, retromolar and palatal mucosa. Whole saliva is principally secreted by the parotid (25%) and the submandibular (71%) [18]. The minor salivary glands and the sublingual glands contribute 3% to 4%. Saliva secretion can be stimulated in several ways including mechanical (pressure), chemical (smell, taste) and/or psychic stimuli. Acid stimuli can increase saliva secretion up to 2.5 to 3 fold its normal rate [1].

This may be an important consideration when selecting formulation excipients which are acidic in nature.

Saliva has traditionally been viewed as a bulk volume however recent studies have shown that once secreted into the oral cavity it exists as a thin film between 0.07 and 0.1 mm in thickness [10].

The pH of saliva ranges from 5.8 to 7.4 [14, 16]. The saliva of the oral cavity has a low buffering capacity (principle buffer of saliva being bicarbonate). This may allow local regions to be readily modified through formulation to promote the existence of optimal pH for the absorptive, nonionized, drug species.

Saliva is low in enzyme content [20-26] and its other components such as potassium, calcium, and proteins do not appear to adversely affect drug delivery.

The fact that saliva is continually secreted into the oral cavity means, on the one hand, that there is an ample supply of solvent to dissolve drugs prior to absorption, however, involuntary swallowing of saliva may result in a major part of the dissolved or suspended released drug being removed from the site of absorption. There is also the risk that the delivery system itself could be swallowed. Saliva secretion is a particular problem for the sublingual route where the oral fluids pool under the tongue before swallowing and two major salivary ducts enter the area. As a consequence high concentrations of drug in contact with the sublingual mucosa are sustained for a relatively short period of time and both drug and delivery system are rapidly flushed away by the saliva.

There are no mucous secreting goblet cells in the oral mucosa, however, mucins are found in human saliva [15]. These mucins are water soluble, highly active gelling agents and form a coherent film 10-200 μm thick on oral epithelia [27]. Up to 70% of the total mucin found in saliva is contributed by the minor salivary glands [15] with the remainder being produced almost exclusively by the sublingual glands. The thin film of mucous that lines the oral cavity membranes can be advantageous for the application of mucoadhesive preparations, however, the continuous and copious volumes of saliva that are secreted during the administration period may promote dissolution of such mucoadhesives and terminate their retentive properties.

III. POTENTIAL OF THE ORAL CAVITY AS A SITE FOR SYSTEMIC DRUG DELIVERY

The unique environment of the oral cavity dictates its potential as a site for drug delivery. Because of the rich blood supply and direct access to the systemic circulation the oral mucosal route is suitable for drugs which are susceptible to acid hydrolysis in the stomach or which are extensively metabolized in the liver (first-pass effect) [1-6]. The continual secretion of saliva results in rapid removal of released drug and this may dictate that the oral cavity should be restricted to the delivery of drugs which have a short systemic action. In this respect such formulations would be limited to drugs with suitable inherent characteristics e.g., nitroglycerin. Conversely the thin mucin film which exists on the surface of the oral mucosa provides the pharmaceutical scientist with an opportunity to retain a delivery system in contact with the mucosa for prolonged periods by incorporating mucoadhesive compounds in the formulation. Such a system would be in close contact with the absorbing membrane, thus optimizing the drug concentration gradient across the biological membrane and reducing the diffusional pathway. Therefore, the oral mucosa may be a potential site for controlled or sustained systemic delivery. In this respect the buccal and gingival areas are associated with a smaller flow of saliva, when compared to the sublingual region, thus the duration of adhesion of the delivery system would be longer at these areas than at the sublingual region. Therefore, the buccal or gingival membranes, with their accessible, smooth surfaces, offer a platform for localizing drug delivery systems for prolonged systemic delivery. The dimensions of the oral cavity restrict the size of the delivery system and the permeability of the oral mucosa is low, thus the oral mucosal route would be limited to potent drugs requiring small doses. The environment of the oral cavity, with its continuous secretion of saliva, its mobile tissues and activities such as chewing, eating and swallowing limit the use of the oral cavity as a site for drug delivery and such problems must be considered and overcome when attempting to deliver a drug systemically via this route. Overall, however, the oral cavity appears to be an attractive site for systemic drug delivery assuming that appropriate and optimized oral mucosal drug delivery systems can be formulated and methods for overcoming the low permeability of the oral mucosa to drugs is forthcoming.

IV. FACTORS AFFECTING ORAL MUCOSAL DRUG DELIVERY SYSTEM DESIGN

Many factors affect the successful delivery of a drug molecule to the systemic circulation via oral mucosa (Table 2). Many of these factors are interrelated through a complex, and as yet poorly understood relationship. In general, the approach taken in the development of an oral mucosal drug delivery system is to identify suitable drug candidates based on both their physicochemical properties and ability to penetrate the oral mucosa, and to optimize their delivery through rational drug delivery system design.

Table 2. Drug and Formulation Factors Affecting Systemic Absorption of Drugs Via the Oral Mucosa.

Factors
Biological factors
Area
Thickness (effective diffusional pathlength)
Composition of oral mucosa
Structure of oral mucosa
pH of environment
Saliva flow rates
Composition of saliva
Drug factors
Taste
Discoloration of teeth
Solubility
Partition coefficient
pKa
Biological half-life
Retention
Rate of absorption
Irritation potential
Allergenicity
Diffusion coefficient in the epithelium
Drug stability
Delivery system factors
Feel of delivery system
Taste, color, staining etc., of excipients
Visibility
Release characteristics
Retentive properties
Protection from saliva
Mobility of backing layer or delivery system
Size
Shape
Texture
Irritation potential
Allergenicity

A. Drug Characteristics

The penetration of drugs or other chemicals into or through the oral mucosa depends on a number of factors. These include the physicochemical properties of the drug, the condition of oral mucosa, the composition and thickness of the oral mucosa, the presence of other chemicals (e.g., penetration enhancers) and external conditions impelled by the oral fluids such as pH, amongst others. Under most conditions, the factors with perhaps the greatest influence on the rate and extent of oral mucosal drug absorption are the physicochemical properties of the drug. The physicochemical properties of the drug should be assessed at an early stage in the development of an oral mucosal drug delivery system as they will provide an indication of the feasibility of delivering such a drug via the oral mucosa and may provide information that will assist in defining the strategies that will be required in the formulation of the oral mucosal drug delivery system. The physicochemical properties of a drug influence the rates of diffusion and partitioning within the delivery system and oral mucosa by affecting the:

- drugs physical state in the dosage form e.g., dissolved or suspended
- release rate of the drug from the delivery system
- concentration of released drug in the saliva film
- percentage of absorbable nonionized species at the site of absorption
- drugs ability to partition into the superficial layers of the epithelium
- concentration of drug in the superficial layers of the epithelium
- diffusion rate through the membrane

To appreciate which physicochemical properties of a drug are important in oral mucosal drug delivery, a basic knowledge of the transfer processes from the device and into and through the oral mucosa is required. The steps involved in the transport of drugs through oral mucosa from a delivery system are:

- drug release from the formulation into the salivary film
- drug dissolution in the salivary film
- partitioning into the superficial layers of the epithelial layer
- diffusion through the epithelial layer
- partitioning into and out of the basal lamina
- diffusion through the lamina propria to the blood vessels
- partitioning into, and transport away by, the blood

1. Drug Release from the Formulation

When designing an oral mucosal drug delivery system there are two options available for the formulation scientist. Firstly, the design of a delivery system whose rate of release from the delivery system is slower than the rate of transport through the oral mucosa. In such a case the drug plasma profiles would be controlled by the release characteristics of the delivery system. Second, the design of a drug delivery system whose rate of release from the formulation into the salivary film is faster than drug transport across the epithelial layer. In such a case the drug plasma profiles would be controlled by the penetration rate of the drug through oral mucosa. In either case the rate of release from a formulation would be dependent upon the drug (its physicochemical properties) and the delivery system (its ingredients and formulation). It is the latter that a formulation scientist can modify to control the release of the drug from the delivery system.

2. Drug Solubility in the Salivary Film

The driving force for transport across oral mucosa is the chemical potential gradient (which, within a single phase, reduces to the concentration gradient). To create this gradient within the oral mucosa, released drug becomes dissolved in saliva and establishes a certain concentration of drug in the outer surface of the oral epithelium. This occurs because the drug has an affinity for both the saliva and the oral epithelium. In infinitely diluted solutions (ideal solutions) the thermodynamic activity of a drug is directly related to its concentration. At higher concentrations, as in the case of released drug dissolved in the salivary film, there is a deviation from this ideal behavior due to solute-solute and solute-solvent (saliva) interactions. The extent of this deviation is expressed in the activity coefficient. The activity of the drug in the salivary film, a_S, is the product of the concentration of the drug in the salivary film, C_S, and its activity coefficient in saliva γ_S:

$$a_S = \gamma_S C_S \tag{1}$$

At steady state, since the thermodynamic activity of the drug is continuous across the saliva/epithelium phase boundary, the rate of penetration of the drug, $\frac{dM}{dt}$, through the oral epithelium would be directly proportional to a_S according to the relationship shown in Equation 2

$$\frac{dM}{dt} = A\frac{a_S D}{\gamma_e h} \tag{2}$$

Where γ_e is the effective activity coefficient of the drug in the epithelial layer, D is the diffusion coefficient of the drug in the epithelium, A is the area across which transport is occurring and h is the effective diffusional pathlength of the epithelium. For any given drug transporting across a defined oral cavity membrane D, γ_e and h may be regarded as constant. Thus equation 2 shows that the formulator can modify the rate of penetration of drug by manipulating the concentration of the drug in saliva up to the level of the solubility of the drug. Indeed, to obtain maximal flux of drug through the oral mucosa the formulator must ensure the highest achievable themodynamic activity in the saliva, a_s. This implies maximal values are required for γ_S and C_S, which are obtained at saturation point of the drug in the salivary film. Thus, if the delivery system is designed such that release of drug does not control blood levels, i.e., passage of drug through the membrane is the determinant of drug plasma profiles, to ensure maximal absorption rates the drug should exist in the salivary film at its solubility limit. The concentration of a drug in the salivary film is dependent upon the rate of release and the amount of drug incorporated into the delivery system. However, the concentration of drug in the salivary film can be modified by the addition of suitable formulation components to the delivery system e.g., buffering agents. Such additions must be considered in relation to the processes that influence the absorption. For example, addition of a buffering agent that alters the salivary pH to ensure a high percentage of ionized species may increase the saturation solubility of the drug in the oral fluids but will lead to a larger proportion of the drug having a lower affinity for the membrane and therefore result in a decreased steady-state flux.

3. Partitioning into the Superficial Layers of the Epithelium

As mentioned above, the thermodynamic activity of a drug is continuous across the saliva/epithelium phase boundary, however concentration is not. Such discontinuities in concentration are accounted for by the epithelium:saliva partition coefficient. The partition coefficient is usually assumed to be concentration independent, and can be determined from knowledge of the concentrations of the drug at equilibrium in each phase. Clearly, such a value is difficult to determine experimentally and often the partition coefficient of the drug between a suitable buffered aqueous solution (which mimics the saliva) and an organic solvent such as octanol (which mimics the lipid properties of the epithelium) is used. Although such an approach may allow an investigator to rank the relative affinities of various drugs and relate such values to the absorption process, the limitations of such an approach must be realized in drug candidate selection. The lipid epithelium is a mixture of complex lipids (see Chapter 2) whereas in contrast the organic phase comprises a single, relatively simple molecule, and as yet no single organic solvent has been identified which exactly mimics the properties of the oral epithelium. Nevertheless the partitioning behavior of a drug between water and organic solvents is an important property that must be taken into account during the feasibility assessment of a drug for oral mucosal drug delivery. This is because it will provide an indication of the relative affinity of the drug for both the saliva and the epithelial layer and many studies have shown the importance of partition coefficients with respect to the loss of drug from aqueous solutions swirled in the oral cavity [28-40]. However, there do not appear to be any reported studies that define the optimal partition coefficient characteristics of a drug for oral mucosal penetration. A number of authors have reported correlations between partition coefficients with extents of absorption from solution from the oral cavity [31-33, 35]. Such studies have shown that within a series of related acidic or basic compounds the ability of a member to pass into human oral mucosa was a function of lipid solubility as measured by its organic phase/water partition coefficient. Workers using a perfusion cell have observed these trends across the buccal mucosa with a small series of alkyl substituted para hydroxybenzoic acid derivatives [41]. Quantitative interpretation of drug loss from the oral cavity during a buccal absorption test have also shown the importance of drug partition coefficient in this process [42, 43].

4. *Ionization*

An inherent assumption of the partition coefficient is that the same drug species exist in both the aqueous and organic phases. In other words the drug must exist in the nonionized form in both phases. The degree of ionization of a drug is a function of both its pKa and the pH of the aqueous phase. Changes in pH can significantly alter the apparent partition coefficient of the drug and its rate of absorption. It has been shown using the buccal absorption test technique that for most of the weak acids and bases studied to date, only the nonionized form of the compound is absorbed across human oral cavity mucosa [28-30, 36, 38-40, 44-62]. Absorption is observed to be highest when pH values dictate that the drug is present predominantly in the nonionized form, and as the degree of ionization increases with a change in solution pH, the absorption decreases in a characteristic sigmoidal fashion. These observations are explained by considering that the nonionized form of the drug possesses a high degree of lipid solubility and therefore an affinity for the oral cavity membrane. In contrast the ionized drug species are poorly lipid soluble and remain confined to the aqueous environment of the saliva in the oral cavity [28-30, 36, 38-40, 44-62]. Similar findings were observed by Barsuhn et al [63] and Rathbone [41] using a human buccal perfusion cell. Quantitative interpretation of drug loss from the oral cavity during a buccal absorption test have also shown the importance of pKa in this process [42, 43, 64, 65].

In general studies performed using the buccal absorption test or buccal perfusion cell have shown that the ability of a compound to partition into the superficial layers of the epithelium is highly dependent upon both the degree of ionization and the lipid solubility of its nonionized form of the drug. In general higher fluxes will be obtained by maintaining the pH so that the drug is in the nonionized form. This can be achieved by the inclusion of pH modifiers to the formulation, however, it should be noted that the presence of a nonphysiological pH at the epithelial surface may also change the properties of the oral mucosa or affect drug solubility, partitioning, or binding, resulting in changes in oral mucosal penetration.

5. Diffusion Across the Epithelial Layer

Once the drug has partitioned into the outer epithelial layer lipids it will set up a concentration gradient and diffuse along that gradient according to Fick's laws of diffusion. Due to the barrier properties of the epithelium we assume that passage across the epithelium is the slowest, and therefore rate-controlling, step in the process of drug absorption across oral mucosa [66-73]. In this case, the rate of transport from the saliva into and across the oral mucosa can be described by the following approximation of Fick's first law of diffusion:

$$J = \frac{DK_P}{h} \Delta C_e \qquad (3)$$

where J is the flux of drug across the epithelium (typically in units of g/cm^2/second, D is the diffusivity of drug in the epithelial layer (cm^2/second), ΔC_e is the difference in drug concentration between one side of the epithelium and the other (g/cm^3), K_p is the membrane:saliva partition coefficient and h is the effective diffusional pathlength of the epithelium (cm). Equation 3 in this simple form is valid only (i) for homogenous materials, (ii) where the concentration difference is constant with time and (iii) where the diffusivity is not dependent on concentration; frequently, none of these are the case in transport across the epithelium. The epithelium is generally recognized as a nonhomogeneous structure, in which the properties of the epithelium near the surface are very different from those of the epithelium near the basal lamina. In addition the drug moves through a tortuous path through the intercellular spaces of the epithelium rather than the more direct route through the cells. For these reasons one often refers to an effective diffusivity and an effective epithelium thickness in order to simplify calculations.

In Equation 3, both the diffusivity and the concentration difference are closely tied to properties of the drug and components of the epithelium as we have seen in this and other chapters. It is apparent from Equation 3 that the flux is constant if the diffusivity and concentration difference (ΔC_e) are constant. Methods by which a formulation scientist can control the concentration difference and ensure maximum flux have been discussed previously in this chapter. In order to increase the flux of drugs across the epithelium two approaches appear feasible. The first is to decrease the diffusional resistance in the structured lipids by making them more fluid. This can be achieved by the use of penetration enhancers such as oleic acid which are known to impart disorder into structured bilayers. This has been discussed in chapter 4 of this book. It should be noted that the overall change in rate and/or extent of absorption should only be gauged by a total assessment which takes account of the physicochemical properties of the drug. For example, very lipophilic drug penetration will not be controlled solely by diffusion through the epithelium and therefore speeding up this process will not necessarily improve absorption into the systemic circulation. Thus such an approach may not be worthwhile. A second approach may involve the formation of supersaturated drug reservoirs which therefore increase the solubility of the drug in the saliva immediately adjacent to the epithelial membrane. Such an approach is still in its infancy and a well optimized oral mucosal drug delivery system may conceivably involve the co-formulation of penetration enhancers in combination with a stabilized supersaturated solution of the drug. Currently, however, through simple formulation changes it is possible to alter D, K_p, and ΔC_e. In any formulation exercise designed to optimize delivery, it is these parameters that should be varied. The composition of the formulation should maximize the thermodynamic activity of the drug in the preparation. This is not always an easy task, because by increasing C we may decrease K_P. A balance has to be achieved between these two parameters.

6. *Molecular Size and Weight*

Molecular size and weight influence the diffusivity of the drug through the epithelial layer. Diffusivity can be viewed as a rough measure of the ease with which a molecule can move about within a medium (in this case, the epithelial layer). As a general rule, the larger the molecule, the more difficult it is to move about, and the lower the diffusivity. For large molecules (and especially for large, nonspherical molecules) in nonhomogeneous media (such as the epithelium), the dependence of diffusivity on molecular weight would be evident because of physical hindrance of movement as the molecular size of the drug approaches the dimensions of the pathways available for diffusion. It is likely that for hydrophilic drugs the rate of absorption would be related to its molecular size. Indeed, small molecules (<75-100 Da) appear to cross oral mucosa rapidly [74-76], however, permeability falls off rapidly as molecular size increases and has been observed to decrease sharply as molar volume is increased beyond 80 mL/mol [75]. For lipophilic drugs the relationship between size and permeability has not been demonstrated across oral mucosa, however, investigators have suggested that such a relationship is likely to exist [6]. In the case of oral mucosal drug absorption it is likely that the effect of molecular size on penetration is much less significant than partitioning and solubility.

7. Partitioning Into and Out of the Basal Lamina

The previous discussion on partitioning focused on the phase boundary between the saliva and epithelium. While this is probably the most important phase boundary, it should be realized that once the drug has crossed the epithelium, it must partition into the underlying layers comprising basal lamina, lamina propria and circulatory system. These tissues are more hydrophilic than the epithelium and can be a potential barrier to oral mucosal transport of extremely lipophilic drugs [77-83]. When the drug reaches the basal lamina it will encounter a phase change; it has to transfer from the predominantly lipophilic intercellular regions of the epithelium into the more aqueous environment of the basal lamina. For lipophilic drugs, transfer into this viable layer may be a slow process and one that will be influenced by a number of factors including the magnitude of the epithelium:basal lamina partition coefficient, the intrinsic solubility of the drug in the aqueous environment of the basal lamina and/or a significant energy barrier to resolvation at the interface at the epithelium:basal lamina boundary.

8. Partitioning Into and Transport Away by the Blood

The partitioning into and transport away by the blood is considered to be rapid and does not contribute any barrier to the whole permeation process.

B. Biopharmaceutical Properties

Thus far we have considered the physicochemical properties of the drug that affect its selection as a drug candidate based on its ability to penetrate the oral mucosa. Although this is important, other factors, not related to the absorptive properties of the drug need to be considered preformulation. These include organoleptic properties of the drug and excipients, texture of the delivery system, irritation or allergenic properties, other adverse effects such as discoloration or erosion of teeth, or the potential to alter the natural microflora. Any of these properties may limit the drug candidate list for this route.

1. Organoleptic Properties

The organoleptic properties of a drug or the delivery system may result in poor patient compliance or acceptance of the product. The detection of a bad taste when the drug or delivery system excipients reach the taste buds would be detrimental to the success of the delivery system. This could be overcome through the formulation of a unidirectional delivery system which prevented release of the drug into the oral cavity. The texture of the delivery system may also affect patient compliance or acceptability. A rough textured delivery system such as slowly eroding buccal tablet or stiff films would inevitably be continually explored by the tongue which may result in erratic release profiles and/or dislodgment.

2. Daily Dose Size

The barrier properties of the epithelium results in the oral mucosa being an efficient barrier to drug penetration allowing only small quantities of drug to penetrate, even over a period of a day. This means that an upper limit on daily delivery exists. For example, realistically a unidirectional buccal drug delivery system would not cover an area of buccal mucosa larger than 2 cm^2 and would be unlikely to be retained on the buccal mucosa for longer than 24 hours. The total amount of drug that could be systematically delivered across buccal mucosa from a 2-cm^2 system in one day has been estimated to be 10–20 mg [84]. Therefore, buccal drug delivery is suitable only for drugs whose daily dose is on the order of a few mg. Clearly the resultant plasma concentration of the drug will depend upon the clearance. However, even if one assumes a small volume of distribution and a relatively long half-life, plasma levels in excess of a few microgram per mL would seem very unlikely via buccal mucosa. Indeed more realistic drug plasma levels might be in terms of nanograms or picograms per mL. The sublingual region is more permeable than buccal mucosa but at this present time it is not technologically feasible to retain a delivery system in this region for periods of much longer than a few minutes. It should be also noted that the physical size of the delivery system itself will also define the amount of drug that can be incorporated into such a system. However, it would seem feasible to formulate a total dose of an amount up to 100 mg into a systemic oral mucosal drug delivery system depending upon the composition and dimensions of the system.

3. Drug Biological Half-life

To assess the effect of half-life on a drugs suitability for oral mucosal delivery, it is necessary to model the time course of plasma concentration. We have done this (Figure 1) with an extension to the kinetic model described in Chapter 7, resulting in three additional equations:

$$\frac{dA_b}{dt} = k_{23}A_m - \frac{CLA_b}{V_b} \tag{4}$$

$$A_b = 0; \;\; t = 0 \tag{5}$$

$$C_b = \frac{A_b}{V_b} \tag{6}$$

Symbols are defined in Figure 1. Solutions giving C_b as a function of time were obtained with the computer program MINIM by numerical integration of the differential equations. We have used experimentally determined transfer rate constants for pethidine ($k_{12} = 5.6 \times 10^{-5}$ second^{-1}; $k_{21} = 2.0 \times 10^{-4}$ second^{-1}; $k_{23} = 2.4 \times 10^{-4}$ second^{-1}) which were determined from transfer data resulting from the continual perfusion of 3.14 cm^2 of human buccal membrane for 2 hours with an aqueous solution (12 mL) containing 0.33 mg pethidine/mL and buffered to pH 10.5. Pethidine was chosen because of its lipophilic nature and pKa, which allowed essentially only the un-ionized form to exist in the perfusing aqueous solution at pH 10.6. We had previously screened a number of opioid analgesics using a buccal perfusion cell, and pethidine exhibited the fastest disappearance profile. Pethidine was therefore used as the model drug in our calculations. We assumed a volume of distribution V_b = 280 L and clearance (CL) = 16.3 mL/second in a 70 kg subject. We initially used this approach to assess the feasibility of pethidine for buccal delivery and then produced hypothetical profiles to assess the effect of half-life on drug candidate feasibility. Predicted plasma concentration profiles for a range of dose sizes are shown in Figure 2. It is evident from this profile and the preceding section on daily dose size that pethidine would not be a realistic candidate for buccal drug delivery as the dose required for therapeutic effect would be too large for incorporation into a delivery system. In addition issues regarding the safety of such a system if it became dislodged and swallowed would have to be considered. It can also be seen that the time of onset for this drug is in the range of hours. This may be acceptable if prolonged delivery was the aim and rapidity of onset unimportant, however, a drug exhibiting such characteristics would not be useful via this route if it were required to be used for rapid relief of symptoms. Figure 3 shows the effect of varying biological half-life on the

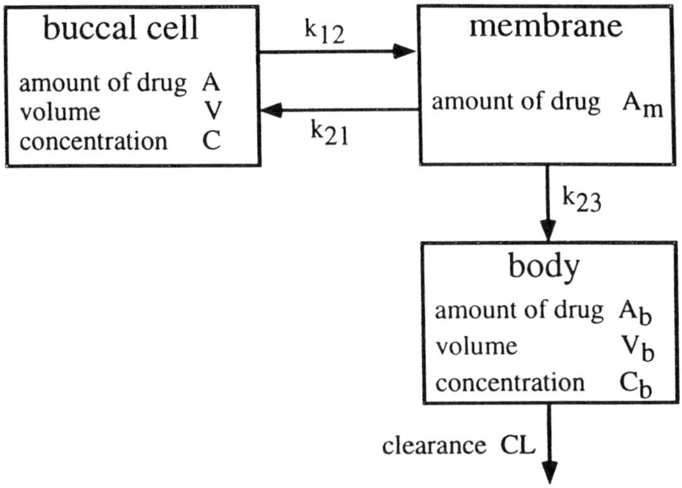

Figure 1. Model for prediction of plasma concentration profiles during absorption via buccal mucosa. The body is represented by a one-compartment pharmacokinetic model.

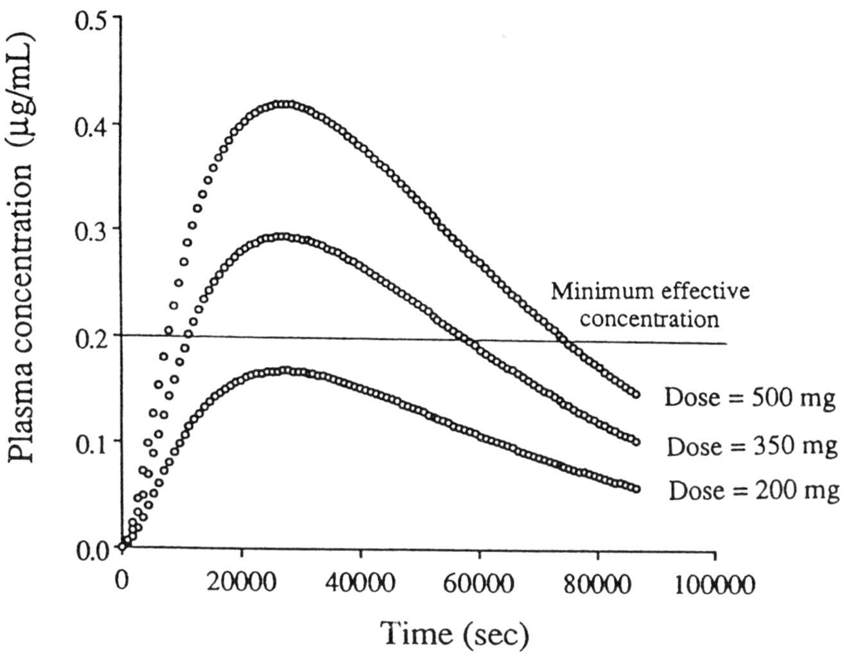

Figure 2. The effect of dose size on the predicted plasma profile of a hypothetical drug administered via the buccal mucosa.

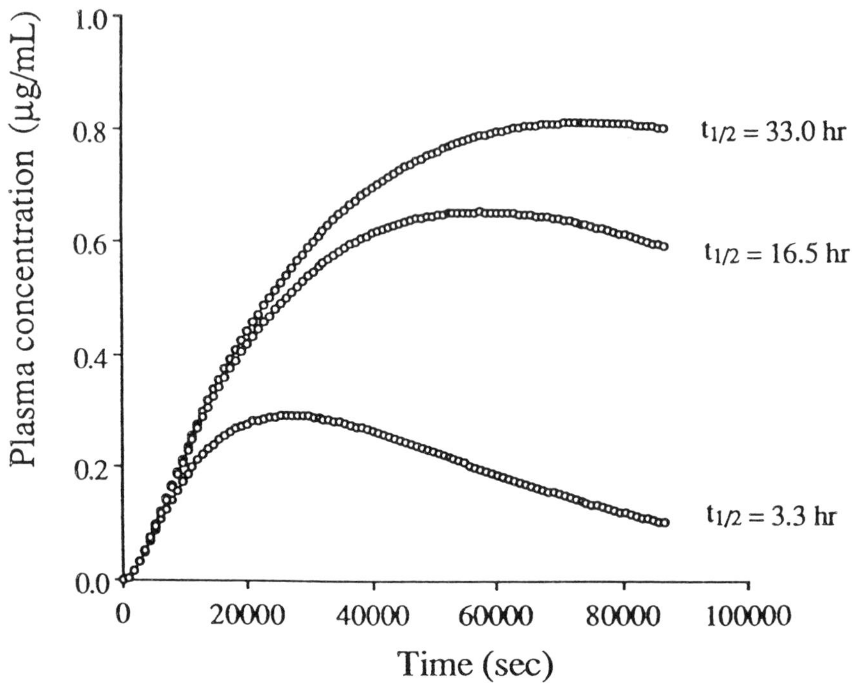

Figure 3. The effect of biological half-life ($t_{½}$) on the predicted plasma profile of a hypothetical drug administered via the buccal mucosa. Dose size = 350 mg.

predicted plasma profile. These profiles were generated by altering the clearance value of the drug (CL = 16.33 mL/second; $t_{½}$ = 3.3 hours, CL = 3.27 mL/second; $t_{½}$ = 16.5 hours, CL = 1.63 mL/second; $t_{½}$ = 33 hours). Figure 3 shows that there is little difference in the onset time of the drug, however, the time to reach peak concentration and the magnitude of that peak concentration both increase with a decrease in biological half-life. For a drug with a half-life of 3.3 hours peak levels are reached relatively rapidly. We therefore conclude that drugs with short biological half lives may be considered potentially useful candidates for buccal delivery.

4. *Toxicity to Oral Mucosa*

If a pharmacologically active material is to be presented to the oral mucosa under a unidirectional occlusive oral mucosal drug delivery system over an extended period there is the potential for an irritant or allergic response to the drug. Many reviewers have claimed the oral mucosa is a robust tissue capable of fast recovery following local stress [3-5] and discussed the possibility of changing the application site of a delivery system over the total surface available. In addition because of the small size of an oral mucosal drug delivery system the damaged areas will be correspondingly small. However, limits have to be determined and set for the acceptability of any undesirable effects that may arise due to the drug. It should be noted that the irritancy/sensitization debate should not only be limited to the drug but also to the components of the delivery system which are also in intimate contact with the oral mucosa. Again the toxic effects of excipients, e.g., penetration enhancers, would be enhanced by the occlusive nature of the system and by extended contact times of the system in contact with the mucosa.

V. ORAL MUCOSAL DRUG DELIVERY SYSTEM DESIGN: THEORETICAL CONSIDERATIONS

The function of any systemic oral mucosal drug delivery system is to provide desired blood levels that are therapeutically efficacious. As discussed earlier many factors affect the bioavailability of a drug administered via the oral mucosa, however, once a suitable drug candidate has been identified the delivery can be optimized through rational delivery system design.

When formulating an oral mucosal drug delivery system several factors must be considered (Table 2). A delivery system that handicaps speaking, eating or drinking could lead to involuntary dislodgment of the dosage form. The tongue is a highly innervated area and any delivery system administered to the oral cavity is likely to be explored by this organ which may affect release rates or retention times.

As discussed previously the mucosa presents a significant barrier to drug absorption which essentially restricts systemic oral mucosal delivery of most drugs to prolonged delivery. To date this has not been an easy task, however, with recent technological advances in system design the concept of the delivery system controlling the amount of drug reaching the systemic circulation via oral mucosa is becoming a reality. The appropriate release profile from an oral mucosal drug delivery system can be engineered using any number of different approaches (Figure 4). Physical and chemical properties of the system components must be matched to the properties of the incorporated drug and can be optimized to achieve the desired release profile. Polymer and excipient selection is therefore critical to a successful formulation.

The design of oral mucosal delivery systems has been reviewed by several authors [1, 27, 85, 86]. Delivery systems can be of two types; bidirectional release or unidirectional release. With the bidirectional release design the drug is simultaneously released into both the saliva immediately adjacent to the

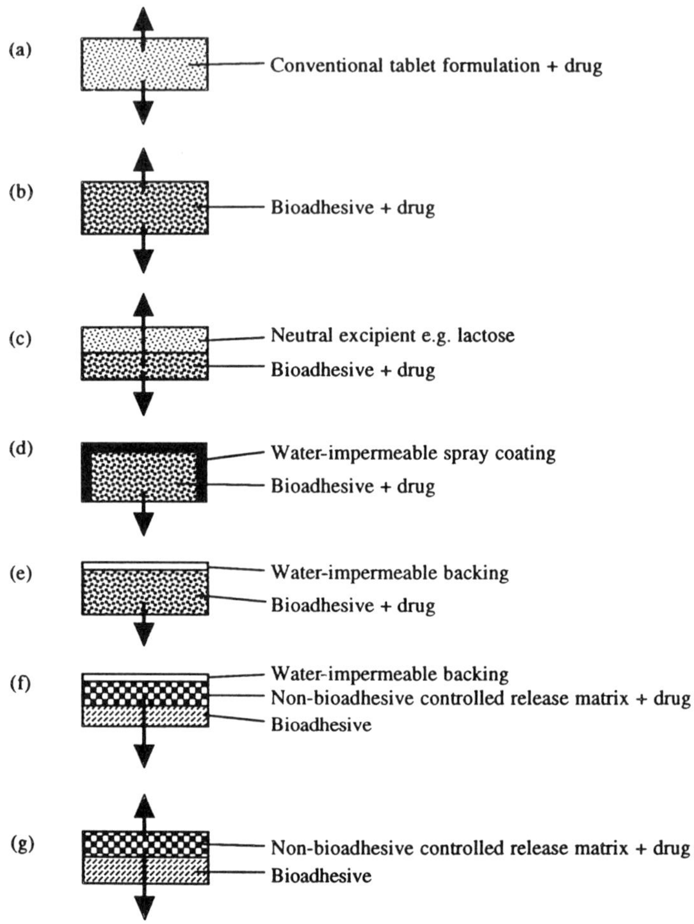

Figure 4. Schematic representation of possible designs of oral mucosal drug delivery systems for systemic delivery.

absorbing membrane and the bulk fluids of the oral cavity. This can lead to a large proportion of the dose being removed from the oral cavity by involuntary swallowing. The formulation of such a system may or may not include a mucoadhesive (Figure 4a, b, c and g). If no mucoadhesive is included, the tablet must be retained in position by a conscious effort by the patient. Such an approach does not allow the patient to eat or drink and handicaps speaking and the administration period of such a formulation is restricted to limited periods. Prolonged release is beyond the scope of such formulations [85]. This limitation can be overcome by the inclusion of a mucoadhesive to the bidirectional release formulation. This will extend the retention time of the delivery system to several hours and introduces the concept of prolonged release from bidirectional release systems. A tablet containing a mucoadhesive has the tendency to stick to the patients finger when locating the delivery system. To overcome this problem a layer which has no adhesive properties can be added to the tablet design e.g., lactose (Figure 4c). Upon administration the lactose layer rapidly dissolves leading to bidirectional release.

With the unidirectional approach the drug is protected from the environment of the oral cavity either by the application of a coating of water-impermeable polymer (Figure 4d), or through laminating the delivery system using a water-impermeable backing material (Figures 4e and 4f). The advantages of the latter approach are (i) retention of the delivery system can be extended to 12 hours or more, (ii) drug can be delivered across a specific, localized region of the oral cavity, (iii) the local environment at the selected site of administration can be controlled by modifying pH and ionic composition, and (iv) permits co-administration of permeability enhancers which will modify absorption in a well-defined area. Using such systems a local micro environment can thus be created between the dosage form and the mucosa to enhance absorption [86]. An advantage of this approach is that irritation or damage to the mucosa by the drug or its excipients will be restricted to the limited area.

VI. CLASSIFICATION OF ORAL MUCOSAL DRUG DELIVERY SYSTEMS

Since the middle of last century, numerous delivery systems have been proposed for the systemic administration of drugs via the oral mucosa. Numerous systems differing in their design and in their applications have been developed. Different types of classifications have been proposed in the literature, based either on physiological or pharmaceutical considerations. Each of them present some advantages but also some limitations because they generally enlighten upon only one property of the delivery systems under consideration. The advantages and the limitations of the three commonly encountered classification are discussed below.

A. Classification Based on Physiological Considerations

Because it has many physiological functions, the structure of the oral cavity is complex. Different membranes line the oral cavity which exhibit different characteristics. Regional variations exist, and both keratinized and nonkeratinized tissues of varying thickness and composition are found which result in regional differences in permeability [87] e.g., the floor of the mouth and the ventral surface of the tongue are more permeable than the buccal membrane.

Based on such characteristics, oral mucosal drug delivery has been conveniently subdivided in: (i) sublingual delivery, which is the administration through the membrane of the ventral surface of the tongue and the floor of the mouth, (ii) buccal delivery, which is the administration through the buccal mucosa, mainly composed of the lining of the cheeks, and (iii) gingival delivery, which is restricted to the administration through the mucosa of the gingivae.

B. Classification Based on the Mobility of the Oral Mucosal Drug Delivery System

Recently it has been proposed that classification of oral mucosal drug delivery systems can be based on the mobility of the drug delivery system in the oral cavity [88]. Typically, two types of systems can be described: (i) a non-attached or mobile drug delivery system that would be physically maintained within the oral cavity in contact with the mucosal surface by a conscious effort of the patient and (ii) an attached or immobilized drug delivery system that can be retained on the mucosal surface by the adhesive properties of the system itself. The classification system is based on the potential of the dosage form to be accepted for use by the patient and also on the clinical reliability of the dosage form, which is related to the extent and the duration of the contact with the mucosa.

In the first category, numerous mobile dosage forms for oral mucosal drug delivery, including solutions, fast dissolving tablets and chewing gum formulations have been shown to be clinically effective for the administration of drugs which are easily absorbed through the mucosa. Following their administration, such formulations must be kept in contact with the concerned mucosal area by a conscious effort of the patient, because such formulations have no inherent retentive characteristics. Therefore, several factors are expected to decrease their effectiveness: (i) the short residence time because of their removal from the oral cavity following swallowing, (ii) high inter- and intra-individual variability in bioavailability due to modification of delivery rates by physiological factors, e.g., tongue and cheek movements or variable salivary secretion and (iii) released drug is not protected from the environment of the oral cavity.

Obviously, the lack of duration of contact between the mobile system and the mucosal absorption surface is a major concern. It is interesting to point out that the physical nature of the delivery system influences the capacity of the patient to retain the system in the oral cavity. For instance, keeping a solution or a fast-dissolving tablet in the mouth induces an intense saliva secretion and makes it difficult to avoid rapid dilution and swallowing of the solution. Alternatively, maintaining a solid dosage form within the oral cavity is much easier. For example, although not intended for a therapeutic use, the traditional betel nut in use in different Pacific and Asian countries can be kept in the mouth for long periods. Similarly, the ease with which chewing gum is retained in the mouth can be partly attributed to its semi-solid nature, which discourages the patient to swallow it. Other factors include the fact that chewing movements are generally semiconscious, pleasant and fit into well established social habits; as can be seen from their intensive use in many countries. Such characteristics are highly favorable to the use of chewing gum as an oral mucosal drug delivery system.

The second category contains attached or immobilized drug delivery systems that can be retained on the oral mucosal surface for a prolonged period of time by the adhesive properties of the system itself. Such systems offer advantages over non-attached systems. These include: (i) the immobilization allows an intimate contact to be developed between the dosage form and the mucosa, (ii) a high drug concentration can be maintained at the absorptive surface for a prolonged period of time, (iii) the dosage form can be immobilized specifically at any part of the oral mucosa: buccal, labial, sublingual or gingival mucosa and (iv) the system itself can be designed to protect the drug from prevailing environmental conditions.

The design of immobilized systems is rather sophisticated because it is necessary to impart two specific properties to the system, immobilization and controlled release behavior. Such a combination of different properties within a single system can be achieved by the use of polymers. Immobilization can be achieved by bioadhesion or mucoadhesion. Development of mucoadhesive drug delivery systems intended for oral administration have been the subject of intensive research recently. This concept has been applied to different devices including sustained release tablets, semi-solid dosage forms, films, patches, powders [89] and microspheres [90].

C. Classification Based on Structural Characteristics of the Oral Mucosal Drug Delivery System

Oral mucosal drug delivery systems can also be classified according to the structural characteristics of the pharmaceutical dosage form. Since the pioneering work of Sobrero on the absorption of nitroglycerin from solutions [5] numerous types of dosage forms have been designed including solutions in the form of mouthwashes or sprays, tablets, lyophilized tablets, bioadhesive tablets, microspheres, chewing gums, gels, pastes, films and patches. The merit of such a classification is to address the design of the oral mucosal drug delivery system and the underlying manufacturing techniques. However, this classification is not very informative on the performance of the oral mucosal drug delivery system.

VII. HISTORICAL OVERVIEW

In 1847 Sobrero reported that nitroglycerin was absorbed from the oral cavity from solutions [91]. Since that time various drug delivery systems for buccal delivery have been proposed for clinical applications (Table 3). Historically, the sublingual and the buccal routes of administration were mainly used for the administration of nitroglycerin and steroids, since they avoided first-pass hepatic metabolism which limited the efficacy of these drugs when administered by the gastrointestinal route. Most of the commercially available products for the sublingual or buccal delivery of drugs are fast-dissolving dosage forms including fast-dissolving tablets and lyophilized systems (e.g., Expidet®, Lyocs®; Table 3). In addition solutions or sprays have also been formulated and used in clinical practice for the administration of nitroglycerin and its derivatives and prochlorperazine.

When examining delivery systems from a chronological point of view, it is possible to distinguish between two main periods in the development of oral delivery systems (Table 4). The first period, which began at the end of the 19th century, was concerned with the development of oral mucosal drug delivery systems based on conventional dosage forms which were developed for other routes of administration. Solutions and tablets were the main types of delivery system developed during this period. Nowadays such delivery systems/vehicles have been refined for oral mucosal delivery by using alternative methods of administration (e.g., sprays for the administration of solutions), the inclusion of excipients such as mucoadhesives (e.g., Buccastem®) or by their production using more advanced manufacturing processes (e.g., lyophilized tablets, Lyocs®). Their advantages and limitations will be discussed later in this chapter.

The second period began in the last decade. This corresponded to a renewal of interest in oral mucosal delivery of drugs. This is probably due to several reasons. Firstly, new drugs have been developed which are associated with formulation problems and which cannot be administered via the gastrointestinal route. Numerous biologically active peptides belong to this category and are generally characterized by short biological half-lives, are sensitive to the gastrointestinal environment and are subject to extensive first-pass metabolism. To overcome these problems, it has been suggested that the buccal route of administration may be an alternative to the parenteral administration of such drugs and much attention has been paid to the different features of the oral cavity as a route of administration [5]. Attempts have been

Table 3. Some Commercially Available Drug Delivery Systems for Systemic Delivery Via the Oral Mucosal Route.

Mucosa	Drug	Proprietary name (manufacturer)	Dosage form
Sublingual	Nitroglycerin	Nitrostat (Parke Davis)	Tablet
	Nitroglycerin	Lenitral Spray (Besins Iscovesco)	Spray
	Nitroglycerin	Susadrin (Forest)	Bioadhesive tablet
	Isorbide dinitrate	Risordan (Rhone-Poulenc Rorer)	Tablet
	Isorbide dinitrate	Sorbitrate (ICI)	Chewable tablet
	Isorbide dinitrate	Isocard Spray (Dexo)	Spray
	Erythrithyle trinitrate	Cardiwell (Wellcome)	Tablet
	Nifedipine	Adalat (Bayer)	Tablet
	Buprenorphine	Temgesic (Reckitt and Colman)	Tablet
	Apomorphine, HCl	Apomorphine (Chabre)	Tablet
Buccal	Prochlorperazine	Buccastem (Reckitt and Colman)	Bioadhesive tablet
	Prochlorperazine	Tementil (Rhone-Poulenc Rorer)	Solution
	Phloroglucinol	Spasfon-Lyoc (Lafon)	Lyocs
	Oxazepam	Seresta Expidet (Wyeth)	Lyophilized tablet
	Lorazepam	Temesta Expidet (Wyeth)	Lyophilized tablet
	Methyltestosterone	Metandren (Ciba-Geigy)	Tablet
	Nicotine	Nicorette (Leo)	Chewing gum
Gingival	Buprenophine[a] Melatonin[a]	Cydot (3M)	Patch

[a]Example compounds incorporated into the delivery system to demonstrate the delivery system's viability.

Table 4. Chronological Appearance of Dosage Forms for Oral Mucosal Drug Delivery Reported in the Literature.

Dosage forms	Year	Reference
Solution	1847	[91]
Tablet	1877	[139]
Lyophilized tablet	1978	-
Chewing gum	1978	[140]
Bioadhesive tablet	1983	[122]
Solution-spray	1984	-
Laminated systems and patches	1987	[135]
Hydrogel	1988	[125]
Adhesive film	1988	[132]
Hollow fiber	1989	[105]
Microspheres	1992	[90]

made to elucidate the more important determinants for the successful systemic oral administration of drugs, including: (i) the limitations of the oral cavity as a site for systemic delivery, (ii) the mechanisms, pathways and barriers to drug permeation and (iii) the design of dosage forms able to improve patient compliance, improve drug bioavailability, control drug delivery and appearance in the systemic circulation, decrease side effects and/or decrease ineffectiveness associated to other administration routes. The reader is referred to Volume 12, Issues 1 and 2 of *Advanced Drug Delivery Reviews* (1993) and Volume 13, Issues 1 and 2 of *Advanced Drug Delivery Reviews* (1994) for a comprehensive compilation of material on this subject.

Second, technological advances in oral mucosal drug delivery system design have led to the formulator being able to overcome the major problems associated with the oral cavity as a site for systemic drug delivery i.e., the secretion of saliva and retention of the delivery system. In addition technological advances have also resulted in the formulation of more rationally designed oral mucosal drug delivery systems. Nowadays a number of different controlled release technologies are available that can be used for the development of oral mucosal drug delivery systems. It is notable that most of the systems which appeared in the 1980's were controlled release products (Table 4), which included bioadhesive systems in the form of tablets, films, patches and hydrogels. However, it should be noted that when such systems were commercialized they mostly incorporated drugs which were already administered via the buccal route. This is because the newer formulations afforded a means for improving the drug delivery characteristics and/or patient compliance of such drugs. This highlights the fact that the list of suitable drug candidates for oral mucosal drug delivery is small.

VIII. CONVENTIONAL DOSAGE FORMS

Traditionally, the use of the oral mucosal route for systemic administration has been restricted to a very limited number of drugs. Consequently, oral mucosal drug delivery systems have been derived from those used from other routes of administration and more or less adapted to some of the specific features of the oral cavity. Falling into this category are the solutions and different types of tablets. They are rather unsophisticated dosage forms and were generally easy to manufacture because they could be produced by standard manufacturing techniques. However, several factors tend to decrease their performance as an oral mucosal drug delivery system including: (i) the residence time of such formulations is very short because such dosage forms are non-attached systems which can be readily removed from the oral cavity by swallowing, (ii) high inter- and intra-individual variability in bioavailability can be expected with these formulations due to modification of delivery rates by physiological factors, e.g., variable salivary secretion or tongue movements and (iii) the released drug is not protected from the environment of the oral cavity and therefore subject to its influences. Such factors decrease the efficiency of such dosage forms for oral mucosal drug delivery.

The main aim of a conventional oral mucosal delivery system is to rapidly create a high concentration of drug in contact with a relatively large mucosal surface. The target mucosal surface is generally the sublingual area or the tongue. Such delivery systems are well suited when the mucosa is highly permeable to the drug and for such systems, systemic absorption is mainly influenced by the rate and extent of drug release. Obviously, in the case of solutions the drug is immediately available in its most absorbable form and is available at its maximal concentration at the beginning of the administration period. However, following administration, the drug concentration declines very rapidly due to extensive dilution by saliva and resultant swallowing by the patient.

Conventional tablet formulations or molded tablets have been for systemic oral mucosal delivery and generally have been administered to the sublingual route. For example, fentanyl has been incorporated in such a system and has been shown to produce reliable sedation and anxiolysis when administered prior to a surgical operation in children [92]. The rate of disintegration of such tablets is the primary consideration in their formulation. In the case of nitroglycerin, in vivo availability from fast-disintegrating tablets composed of soluble excipients (lactose, mannitol, sucrose) has been shown to be strongly dependent upon disintegration rate [93, 94].

In order to obtain a high drug concentration very rapidly in the oral cavity, different formulation methods have been developed to accelerate the disintegration rate or dissolution rate of tablets. Fast-dissolving molded tablets consisting of drug and polyethylene glycol blends with a melting point around the body temperature have been investigated for the delivery of nitroglycerin [93, 94] and progesterone [95]. More recently, dosage forms comprising a freeze-dried mixture of oxazepam and lorazepam, fast-dissolving excipients and micronized radiolabeled ion exchange resin (Expidet®) have been investigated. Wilson et al [96] followed the clearance, residence time and the distribution pattern of this dosage form in humans using gamma-scintigraphy following its application on the surface of the tongue. The formulation was observed to completely dissolve within 15 seconds. The authors reported that the clearance of 50% of the formulation from the oral cavity was 190 seconds and 50 seconds depending upon the amount of ion exchange resin incorporated into the dosage form (2.5 mg and 10 mg, respectively). The extent of absorption of oxazepam and lorazepam from the oral cavity was estimated by measuring the amount remaining in the mouth by performing washings. At each of the time points investigated (30, 60, 90 and 120 seconds), about 90% of drug was recovered, suggesting that negligible absorption of the drug took place during the time that the formulation was in contact with the tongue. Therefore, such a system may only prove useful if the incorporated drug is rapidly absorbed. However, the above example highlights that for such oral mucosal drug delivery systems it is necessary to carefully balance the rate of drug release with the rate of drug absorption.

IX. MODERN APPROACHES

The development and the use of fast-dissolving dosage forms in therapeutic practice have shown that buccal administration of drugs is feasible. However, the clinical success of oral mucosal drug delivery depends on the ability of the delivery system to achieve, and to maintain for a defined period of time, sufficient plasma drug concentration levels that are likely to elicit a therapeutic response. An oral mucosal drug delivery system must be able to deliver an adequate amount of drug according to a desired absorption profile (rate and duration). This amount of drug depends mainly on the formulation features of the delivery system. Therefore, the drug release pattern from the delivery system is crucial and must be carefully considered. Obviously, the conventional dosage forms described above have difficulty in meeting this requirement.

Because of the aforementioned limitations of conventional dosage forms, research in the oral mucosal drug delivery area has focused on the development of rationally designed drug delivery systems which achieve the therapeutic aims of delivery and, at the same time, overcome the unfavorable environmental conditions found in the oral cavity. In the last decade, several alternative oral mucosal drug delivery systems have been designed. The different strategies have been based on: (i) prolonging the duration of the absorption process, (ii) developing bi- or unidirectional release systems and

(iii) preparing user-friendly, patient acceptable, oral mucosal delivery systems. The dosage forms described below are generally a combination of those different strategies.

A. Chewing Gum

Chewing gums are mobile drug delivery systems. The main target mucosa for drug absorption is the sublingual mucosa. However, drug is released into saliva and its subsequent spreading may cause the drug to be absorbed across other mucosae of the oral cavity. Chewing gum formulations consist generally of a gum base of cellulosic or acrylic polymer. The polymer is blended with sugars and drug added. Drug release from chewable formulation is generally rapid but not as immediate as in the case for the fast-dissolving tablets. A study by Christrup et al [97] showed that about 57% of ascorbic acid incorporated in a chewable preparation was released after 5 minutes. This percentage was not significantly increased after 30 minutes of chewing. Similar trends were observed with noscapine derivatives [98]. However, in this case, the percentage released depended on the solubility of the compound. The percentages released were about 80%, 25% and 20% for the water soluble noscapine hydrochloride, the embonate salt and the poorly soluble noscapine base, respectively. The release period can be extended by associating the drug to an ion-exchange resin. This principle has been used for the formulation of a nicotine containing chewing gum (Nicorette®). Release was controlled by the rate and vigor of chewing and reached about 90% after 30 minutes chewing [99, 100]. Thus, the patient can control the drug intake to match his needs.

The bioavailability of different drugs incorporated into chewing gum formulations has been investigated. These drugs have included ascorbic acid [97], salicylamide [101], verapamil [102], noscapine [98], methadone [103] and nicotine [99, 100, 104]. In the case of methadone [18], it has been shown that there were no significant differences in the AUC of the plasmatic profiles obtained after administration of chewing gum or sublingual tablets. A nicotine containing chewing gum (Nicorette®, Leo) has been marketed as an aid to give up smoking.

Despite some interesting, indeed promising, results, chewable formulations, have some drawbacks that are inherent within the design of the dosage form itself. These include (i) the drug is released into the saliva and disappears rapidly from the oral cavity because of involuntary swallowing, (ii) the concentration of drug in the oral cavity is always decreasing as a result of salivary dilution, (iii) the drug is not protected from the environment found in the oral cavity, (iv) drug release from chewable formulations has been shown to be strongly influenced by the way the patient chews the formulation [99, 106, 107] and (v) administration of such dosage forms is restricted to short periods of time because the presence of the delivery system in the oral cavity is a handicap for drinking, eating and speaking. As a result of these limitations, controlled release of drugs over long periods of time are difficult to achieve with such formulations. However, such formulations do afford extended delivery periods compared to solutions and fast dissolving tablets.

B. Hollow Fibers

As an alternative to chewable formulations, Burnside et al [105] reported the design of a microporous hollow fiber of polysulfone (molecular weight cutoff = 500 000 Da) intended for the delivery of histrelin, an LHRH agonist. This fiber is intended to be placed in the buccal cavity for oral mucosal drug delivery. Preliminary experiments showed that peptide delivery rates could be adjusted and prolonged for up to 6 hours. However, the lack of intimate contact of the delivery system with the mucosa may be detrimental to peptide absorption and the delivery system does not afford protection of the drug from the environment of the oral cavity and thus the peptide may be subject to enzymatic degradation in the saliva.

C. Bioadhesive Tablets

Bioadhesive tablets are immobilized drug delivery systems. They can be formulated into monolithic, partially coated or multilayered matrices [108]. Monolithic tablets are easy to manufacture by conventional techniques and provide the possibility of holding large amounts of drug. Drugs can be co-formulated with an absorption enhancer if required. A method for partial coating of a monolithic tablet has been proposed. The technique affords protection of every face of the tablet which is not in contact with the mucosa [109]. Such systems allow unidirectional drug release and avoid drug release into the salivary fluids.

Multilayered tablets allow a variety of geometrical arrangements. In the case of bilayered tablets, drug release can be rendered unidirectional. The drug can be incorporated in the adhesive layer which comes in contact with the mucosal surface. This drug containing mucoadhesive layer is then protected from the oral cavity environment by a second upper inert layer which faces into the oral cavity. Alternatively, the drug can be incorporated into the upper non-adhesive layer. In this case, drug release would occur into the oral cavity.

Retention of an oral mucosal drug delivery system is a requirement for the use of the oral mucosa as a platform for prolonged drug delivery. As such much attention has been paid to the adhesive characteristics of oral mucosal tablets [109-120]. The use of cellulosic or acrylic polymers generally offers almost immediate, high adhesion performances for prolonged periods of time, even when drug content is high. Factors influencing the drug release from bioadhesive tablets are the same as those encountered in hydrophilic matrices, and include the nature of the polymer, the drug/polymer ratio and the swelling kinetics of the system. Various drugs intended for systemic delivery have been incorporated in bioadhesive oral mucosal tablets including propranolol [117, 118], timolol [119], metronidazole [113], metoclopramide [120], insulin [121], nitroglycerin [122], codeine [110] and morphine sulfate [123].

There are limitations associated with oral mucosal adhesive tablets and include: (i) the small surface of contact with the mucosa, (ii) their lack of physical flexibility, (iii) the high drug release rates, which can be required for some drugs, are difficult to obtain and (iv) the extent and the frequency of contact might cause irritation following chronic application on the buccal or sublingual mucosa.

D. Laminated Systems and Patches

In response to some of the drawbacks of tablets, different flexible, adhesive films and laminated adhesive patches have been developed.

Different polymers can be used for the development of mucosal patches including cellulose derivatives (e.g., methylcellulose, sodium carboxymethyl-cellullose, hydroxyethylcellulose), natural gums (guar gum, Karaya gum, agarose), polyacrylates including poly(acrylic acid), poly(methacrylic acid), poly(vinylpyrrolidone), poly(ethylene glycol) and gelatin. These polymers exhibit mucoadhesive properties in the presence of water. Polyacrylic based hydrogels have been extensively studied. Kellaway et al [124-126] have prepared hydrogels by reacting polyacrylic acid (MW 450 000) with sucrose, glycerol or a non-ionic surfactant for the delivery of oxytocin. De Vries et al investigated the physicochemical determinants of the bioadhesive properties of copolymer hydrogels made of acrylic acid and butyl acrylate in various molar ratios [127, 128]. Yang et al [129] prepared polyetherurethane hydrogels which had high loading capacity and release profiles over periods of 12 hours for heparin. Cassidy et al [130] investigated the buccal delivery of diclofenac sodium by means of a hydroxyethyl methacrylate based copolymer hydrogel. They obtained a steady-state flux through the human buccal mucosa of 2.1 $mg/cm^2/hour$. Generally, such hydrogels are intended to be incorporated into laminated patches.

Drug loaded adhesive films can be prepared quite easily by using adhesive polymers. Kurosaki et al [131] reported the use of a simple film of hydroxypropyl cellulose for the delivery of propranolol. Rodu et al [132] prepared a simple film by complexing hydroxypropylcellulose with tannic and boric acid (Zilactin®).

Adhesive patches can be designed either for unidirectional release into the oral mucosa or for bidirectional release into the oral cavity as well as into the oral mucosa [133]. The adhesive part of the system can be used as a drug carrier or as an adhesive for the retention of a drug loaded non-adhesive layer. In this respect, a peripheral adhesive ring is feasible. The use of an impermeable backing layer will maximize the drug concentration gradient and prolong adhesion because the system is protected from saliva. Typically the size of such systems would be 1-3 cm^2 but may have dimensions as large as 10-15 cm^2 depending on the site of administration. Poly(acrylic acid) based patches have been used successfully for the delivery of opioid analgesics. Bioavailability ranged from 35% to 50% in dog, compared to the oral bioavailability which was less than 5% [134]. Veillard et al [135] developed a patch in conjunction with 3M-Riker consisting of a rate-limiting membrane, a polycarbophil adhesive layer and an impermeable backing. Merkle et al [133, 136, 137] experimented with a number of polymers and different geometry's for the design of patches for the delivery of different peptides, such as protirelin and octreotide. Studies on octreotide illustrated some of the drawbacks of such systems. The relative bioavailabilities of octreotide in rats from different patches ranged between 17% and 24% when compared to buccal administration of an aqueous solution. Such a result suggests that retardation in the drug release occurred because of insufficient diffusion of the drug through the adhesive layer. Such a phenomenon is not likely to favor drug absorption from such products. Therefore, a recent tendency consists of the association of a fast-dissolving unit and a bioadhesive part in the same controlled release delivery system [138].

X. ACKNOWLEDGMENTS

We are grateful to Dr Robert Purves, Department of Pharmacology, University of Otago, New Zealand for assistance in the preparation of this manuscript and to Professor Christopher Squier for developing Table 1.

REFERENCES

1. M. E. de Vries, H. E. Boddé, J. C. Verhoef, and H. E. Junginger, Developments in buccal drug delivery, *Crit. Rev. Ther. Drug Carr. Sys. 8*:271 (1991).
2. M. J. Rathbone, and J. Hadgraft, Absorption of drugs from the human oral cavity, *Int. J. Pharm. 74*:9 (1991).
3. C. A. Squier, The permeability of oral mucosa, *Crit. Rev. Oral Biol. Med. 2*:13 (1991).

4. H. P. Merkle, and G. J. M. Wolnay, Muco-adhesive patches for buccal peptide administration, *Minutes, European Symposium, Buccal and nasal administration as an alternative to parenteral administration* (D. Duchéne ed.) Editions de Santé, Paris, 1992 p. 110.
5. M. J. Rathbone, B. K. Drummond, and I. G. Tucker, The oral cavity as a site for systemic drug delivery, *Adv. Drug Del. Rev. 13*:1 (1994).
6. D. Harris, and J. R. Robinson, Drug delivery via the mucous membranes of the oral cavity, *J. Pharm. Sci. 81*:1 (1992).
7. C. A. Squier, N. W. Johnson, and R. M. Hopps, The organization of oral mucosa, *Human Oral Mucosa: Development, Structure and Function*, Blackwell Scientific Publications, Oxford, 1976, p. 7.
8. P. W. Wertz, P. S. Cox, C. A. Squier, and D. T. Downing, Lipids of epidermis and keratinized and nonkeratinized oral epithelia, *Comp. Biochem. Physiol. 83B*:529 (1986).
9. P. W. Wertz, and C. A. Squier, Cellular and molecular basis of barrier function in oral epithelium, *Crit. Rev. Ther. Drug Carr. Sys. 8*:237 (1991).
10. L. M. C. Collins, and C. Dawes, The surface area of the adult human mouth and thickness of the salivary film covering the teeth and oral mucosa, *J. Dent. Res. 66*: 1300 (1987).
11. C. A. Squier, N. W. Johnson, and R. M. Hopps, Regional differences of the oral mucosa. *Human Oral Mucosa: Development, Structure and Function*, Blackwell Scientific Publications, Oxford, 1976, p. 73.
12. J. Meyer, and S. J. Gerson, A comparison of human palatal and buccal mucosa, *Periodontics 2*:284 (1964).
13. C. A. Squier, and D. Nanny, Measurement of blood flow in the oral mucosa and skin of the Rhesus monkey using radiolabeled microspheres, *Arch. Oral Biol. 30*:313 (1985).
14. W. M. Edgar, Saliva: its secretion, composition and functions, *Br. Dent. J. 172*:305 (1992).
15. L. A. Tabak, M. J. Levine, I. D. Mandel, and S. A. Ellison, Role of salivary mucins in the protection of the oral cavity *J. Oral Pathol. 11*:1 (1982).
16. I. D. Mandel, and S. Wotman, The salivary secretions in health and disease, *Oral Sci. Rev. 8*:25 (1976)
17. J. O. Tenovuo, *Human Saliva: Clinical Chemistry and Microbiology* (J. O. Tenovuo ed.) CRC Press, Boca Raton, Florida, 1989, Volumes I and II.
18. C. Arglebe, Biochemistry of human saliva, *Adv. Oto-Rhino-Laryngol. 26*:97 (1981)
19. J. M. Goodson, Dental applications, *Medical Applications of Controlled Release. Volume II: Applications and Evaluation* (R. S. Langer, and D. L. Wise, eds.) CRC Press Boca Raton, Florida, 1984, p. 115.

20. H. H. Chauncey, F. Lionetti, R. A. Winer, and V. F. Lisanti, Enzymes in human saliva. I. The determination, distribution and origin of whole saliva enzymes, *J. Dent. Res. 33*:321 (1954).
21. H. H. Chauncey, F. Lionetti, and V. F. Lisanti, Enzymes in human saliva. II. Parotid saliva total esterases, *J. Dent. Res. 36*:713 (1957).
22. M. S. Burstone, Esterases of the salivary glands, *J. Histochem. Cytochem. 4*:130 (1956).
23. H. H. Chauncey, Salivary enzymes *J. Am. Dent. Assoc. 63*:360 (1961).
24. I. Lindquist, and K. B. Augustinsson Esterases in human saliva, *Enzyme 20*:277 (1975).
25. S. C. Tan, Human saliva esterases. Genetic studies, *Hum. Hered. 26*:207 (1976).
26. I. Lindquist, C. E. Noed, and P. O. Soder, Origin of esterases in human whole saliva, *Enzyme 22*:166 (1977).
27. H. P. Merkle, and G. J. M. Wolnay, Intraoral peptide absorption, Biological Barriers to Protein Delivery, K. L. Audus, and T. J. Raub, eds. Plenum Press, New York, 1993, p. 131.
28. A. H. Beckett, and A. C. Moffat, The influence of alkyl substitution in acids on their performance in the buccal absorption test, *J. Pharm. Pharmacol. 20*:239S (1968)
29. A. H. Beckett, and E. J. Triggs, Buccal absorption of basic drugs and its application as an in vivo model of passive drug transfer through lipid membranes, *J. Pharm. Pharmacol. 19*:31S (1967).
30. A. H. Beckett, and A. C. Moffat, The influence of substitution in phenylacetic acids on their performance in the buccal absorption test, *J. Pharm. Pharmacol. 21*:139S (1969).
31. A. H. Beckett, and A. C. Moffat, Correlation of partition coefficients in n-heptane-aqueous systems with buccal absorption data for a series of amines and acids, *J. Pharm. Pharmacol. 21*:144S (1969).
32. A. H. Beckett, and A. C. Moffat, Kinetics of buccal absorption of some carboxylic acids and the correlation of the rate constants and n-heptane:aqueous phase partition coefficients, *J. Pharm. Pharmacol. 22*:15 (1970).
33. A. H. Beckett, and M. E. Pickup, A model for steroid transport across biological membranes, *J. Pharm. Pharmacol. 27*:226 (1975).
34. A. H. Beckett, O. Grech, and D. Mihailova, The influence of nitrogen, chain and ring substitution on some physico-organic properties and on buccal absorption of amphetamines, *J. Pharm. Pharmacol. 27*:67P (1975).
35. J. C. Dearden, and E. Tomlinson, Buccal absorption as a parameter of analgesic activity of some p-substituted acetanilides, *J. Pharm. Pharmacol. 23*:73S (1971).

36. M. H. Bickel, and H. J. Weder, Buccal absorption and other properties of pharmacokinetic importance of imipramine and its metabolites, *J. Pharm. Pharmacol. 21*:160 (1969).
37. I. W. Mathison, P. H. Morgan, N. J. Wojciechowski, J. P. Bandura, and J. R. Wennemark, Physiocochemical and pharmacological studies of some 8-substituted decahydroisoquinolines, *J. Med. Chem. 19*:385 (1976).
38. D. C. Hicks, The buccal absorption of some β-adrenoceptor blocking drugs, *Br. J. Pharmacol. 47*:680P (1973).
39. K. Chan, The effect of physicochemical properties of pethidine and its basic metabolites on their buccal absorption and renal elimination, *J. Pharm. Pharmacol. 31*:672 (1979).
40. R. Achari, and A. H. Beckett, Buccal uptake, urinary excretion and physicochemical properties of zipeprol and its n-dealkylated products, *Biopharm. Drug Disp. 3*:203 (1982).
41. M. J. Rathbone, Human buccal absorption. II. A comparative study of the buccal absorption of some parahydroxybenzoic acid derivatives using the buccal absorption test and a buccal perfusion cell, *Int. J. Pharm. 74*:189 (1991).
42. E. Lien, R. T. Koda, and G. L. Tong, Buccal and percutaneous absorption, *Drug Intell. Clin. Pharm. 5*: 38 (1971).
43. J. G. Wagner, and A. J. Sedman, Quantitation of rate of gastrointestinal and buccal absorption of acidic and basic drugs based on extraction theory, *J. Pharmacokin. Biopharm. 1*:23 (1973).
44. J. C. Garnham, T. Kaspi, C. M. Kaye, V. M. S. Oh, The different effects of sodium bicarbonate and aluminium hydroxide on the absorption of indomethacin in man, *Postgrad. Med. J. 53*:126 (1977).
45. C. M. Kaye, and A. D. Long, The influence of pH on the buccal absorption and plasma and renal elimination of acebutolol, *Br. J. Clin. Pharmacol. 3*:196 (1976).
46. C. M. Kaye, M. A. Kiddie, and P. Turner, Variable pharmacokinetics of mexiletine, *Postgrad. Med. J. 53*:56 (1977).
47. W. Schürmann, and P. Turner, The buccal absorption of atenolol and propranolol, and their physicochemical characteristics, *Br. J. Clin. Pharmacol. 4*:655P (1977).
48. W. Schürmann, and P. Turner, A membrane model of the human oral mucosa as derived from buccal absorption performance and physicochemical properties of the β-blocking drugs atenolol and propranolol, *J. Pharm. Pharmacol. 30*:137 (1978).
49. J. A. Henry, and K. Ohashi, Recovery of propranolol after buccal absorption, *Br. J. Clin. Pharmacol. 8*:406P (1979).

50. J. A. Henry, K. Ohashi, J. Wadsworth, and P. Turner, Drug recovery following buccal absorption of propranolol, *Br. J. Clin. Pharmacol. 10*:61 (1980).
51. K. Ohashi, and P. Turner, Buccal absorption characteristics of some selective and non-selective β-adrenoceptor agonists and antagonists, *Br. J. Clin. Pharmacol. 9*:120P (1980).
52. B. J. Davis, and A. Johnston, Buccal absorption of verapamil - evidence for membrane storage, *Br. J. Clin. Pharmacol. 7*:434P (1979).
53. B. J. Davis, and P. Turner, The spectrofluorimetric estimation and buccal absorption of SL 75212, a novel β-adrenoceptor antagonist, *Br. J. Clin. Pharmacol. 8*:405P (1979).
54. D. J. Temple, and K. R. Schesmer, The buccal absorption characteristics of fomocaine, *Arch. Pharm. (Weinheim). 311*:485 (1978).
55. W. Meyer, C. M. Kaye, and P. Turner, A study of the influence of pH on the buccal absorption and renal excretion of procainamide, *Eur. J. Clin. Pharmacol. 7*:287 (1974).
56. J. M. Sutherland, W. D. Hooper, M. J. Eadie, and J. H. Tyrer, Buccal absorption of ergotamine, *J. Neurol. Neurosurg. Psych. 37*:1116 (1974).
57. T. Kaspi, A. Blackett, and P. Turner, Spectrofluorometric assay and buccal absorption of LM 5008, a new potential antidepressive drug, *Br. J. Clin. Pharmacol. 8*:412P (1979).
58. A. Blackett, N. Brion, and P. Turner, Recovery of acetylsalicylic acid and indalpine (LM 5008) after buccal partitioning, *Int. J. Clin. Pharm. Res. 3*:5 (1983).
59. G. Edwards, A. M. Breckenridge, K. K. Adjepon-Yamoah, M. L 'E. Orme, and S. A. Ward, The effect of variations in urinary pH on the pharmacokinetics of diethylcarbamazine, *Br. J. Clin. Pharmacol. 12*:807 (1981).
60. A. G. Arbab, and P. Turner, Influence of pH on absorption of thymoxamine through buccal mucosa in man, *Br. J. Clin. Pharmacol. 43*:479P (1971).
61. O. Al-Sayed-Omar, A. Johnston, and P. Turner, Influence of pH on the buccal absorption of morphine sulphate and its major metabolite, morphine-3-glucuronide, *J. Pharm. Pharmacol. 39*:934 (1987).
62. S. A. Sprake, and D. F. Evered, Transport of cycloserine across the mucosa of rat colon and the human mouth, *J. Pharm. Pharmacol. 31*:113 (1979).
63. C. L. Barsuhn, L. S. Olanoff, D. D. Gleason, E. L. Adkins, and N. F. H. Ho, Human buccal absorption of flurbiprofen, *Clin. Pharmacol. Ther. 44*:225 (1988).
64. K. R. M. Vora, W. I. Higuchi, and N. F. H. Ho, Analysis of human buccal absorption of drugs by physical model approach, *J. Pharm. Sci. 61*:1785 (1972).

65. N. F. H. Ho, and W. I. Higuchi, Quantitative interpretation of in vivo buccal absorption of n-alkanoic acids by the physical model approach, *J. Pharm. Sci. 60*:537 (1971).
66. C. A. Squier, The permeability of keratinized and nonkeratinized oral epithelium to horseradish peroxidase, *J. Ultrastruct. Res. 43*:160 (1973).
67. C. A. Squier, and L. Rooney, The permeability of keratinized and nonkeratinized oral epithelium to lanthanum in vivo, *J. Ultrastruct. Res. 54*:286 (1976).
68. C. A. Squier, and B. K. Hall, The permeability of mammalian nonkeratinized oral epithelia to horseradish peroxidase applied in vivo and in vitro, *Arch. Oral Biol. 29*:45 (1984).
69. C. A. Squier, and B. K. Hall, The permeability of skin and oral mucosa to water and horseradish peroxidase as related to the thickness of the permeability barrier, *J. Invest. Dermatol. 84*:176 (1985).
70. C. A. Squier, and B. K. Hall, In vitro permeability of porcine oral mucosa after epithelial separation, stripping and hydration, *Arch. Oral Biol. 30*:485 (1985).
71. M. W. Hill, and C. A. Squier, The permeability of rat palatal mucosa maintained in organ culture, *J. Anat. 128*:169 (1979).
72. M. J. Rathbone, and I. G. Tucker, Mechanisms, barriers and pathways of oral mucosal drug permeation, *Adv. Drug Del. Rev. 12*:41 (1993).
73. I. A. Siegel, K. T. Izutsu, and E. Watson, Mechanisms of nonelectrolyte penetration across dog and rabbit oral mucosa in vitro, *Arch. Oral Biol. 26*:357 (1981).
74. I. A. Siegel, and H. P. Gordon, Penetration of oral mucosa by organic compounds, *J. Dent. Res. 58*:109 (1979).
75. I. A. Siegel, Permeability of the rat oral mucosa to organic solutes measured in vivo, *Arch. Oral Biol. 29*:13 (1984).
76. M. C Alfano, J. F. Drummond, and S. A. Miller, Localization of rate-limiting barrier to penetration of endotoxin through nonkeratinized oral mucosa in vitro, *J. Dent. Res. 54*:1143 (1975).
77. Tolo, K, A study of permeability of gingival pocket epithelium to albumin in guinea pigs and Norwegian pigs, *Arch. Oral Biol. 16*:881 (1971).
78. Tolo, K, Transport across stratified nonkeratinized epithelium, *Periodont. Res. 6*:237 (1971).
79. Tolo, K, Penetration of human albumin through the oral mucosa of guinea pigs immunized to this protein, *Arch. Oral Biol. 19*:259 (1974).
80. M. E. de Vries, H. E. Boddé, J. C. Verhoef, M. Ponec, W. I. H. M. Craane, and H. E. Junginger, Localization of the permeability barrier inside porcine buccal mucosa: a combined in vitro study of drug permeability, electrical resistance and tissue morphology, *Int. J. Pharm. 76*:25 (1991).

81. M. C. Alfano, A. I. Chasens, and C. W. Masi, Autoradiographic study of the penetration of radiolabeled dextrans and inulin through nonkeratinized oral mucosa, *J. Periodont. Res. 12*:368 (1977).
82. W. A. McDougall, The effect of topical antigen on the gingiva of sensitized rabbits, *J. Periodont. Res. 9*:153 (1974).
83. P. Brandtzag, and K. Tolo, Mucosal penetrability enhanced by serum-derived antibodies, *Nature 266*:262 (1977).
84. J. R. Robinson, M. A. Longer, and M. Veillard, Bioadhesive polymers for controlled drug delivery, *Biological Approaches to the Controlled Delivery of Drugs* (R. L. Juliano, ed.) Annals of the New York Academy of Sciences, Volume 507, New York, 1987, p. 307.
85. H. E. Junginger, M. E. de Vries, and H. E. Boddé, Moderne arzneiformen zur lokalen aund systemischen wirkung in mund- und rachenraum, *Deutsche Apotheker Zeitung 131*:1337 (1991).
86. H. P. Merkle, R. Anders, and A. Wermerskirchen, Mucoadhesive buccal patches for peptide delivery *Bioadhesive Drug Delivery Systems* (V. Lenaerts, and R. Gurney, eds.) CRC Press, Boca Raton, Florida, 1990, p.105.
87. A. Siegel, Permeability of the oral mucosa, *The Structure and the Function of Oral Mucosa* (J. Meyer, C. A. Squier, and S. J. Gerson (eds.), Pergamon Press, Oxford, 1984, p. 95.
88. G. Ponchel, Formulation of oral mucosal drug delivery systems for the systemic delivery of bioactive materials, *Adv. Drug Del. Rev. 13*:75 (1994).
89. M. Yamamoto, K. Okabe, J. Kubo, T. Naruchi, H. Ikura, Y. Suzuki. and T. Nagai, The bioadhesive and residence properties and drug penetration effect of powders preparations for the oral cavity containing hydroxypropyl cellulose, *S. T. P. Pharma 5*:878 (1989).
90. S. P. Vyas, and C. P. Jain, Bioadhesive polymer-grafted starch microspheres bearing isorbide dinitrate for buccal administration, *J. Microencapsul. 9*:457 (1992).
91. A. Sobrero, Sur plusieurs composés détonnants produits avec l'acide nitrique et le sucre, la dextrine, la lactine, la mannite et la glycérine, *Comptes Rendus Hebdomadaires des Séances de l'Académie des Sciences, 24*:247 (1847).
92. T. H. Stanley, and M. A. Ashburn, Novel delivery systems: oral transmucosal and intranasal transmucosal, *J. Pain Sympt. Management 7*:163 (1992).
93. M. Lagas, and A. M. J. A. Duchateau, Sublingual nitroglycerin. I. Comparative evaluation of the physical stability of commercially available tablets, *Pharmaceutisch Weekblad Scientif. Ed. 10*:246 (1988).

94. M. Lagas, and A. M. J. A. Duchateau, Sublingual nitroglycerin. II. In vitro and in vivo availability of Nitrostat and Nitrobaat tablets, *Pharmaceutisch Weekblad Scientif. Ed. 10*:254 (1988)

95. D. H. Maddox, B. A. Burnside, and A. D. Keith, Buccal Delivery of progesterone, *Proceed. Intern. Symp. Control. Rel. Bioact. Mater. 17*:291 (1990).

96. C. G. Wilson, N. Washington, J. Peach, G. R. Murray, and J. Kennerley, The behavior of a fast-dissolving dosage form (Expidet) followed by γ-scintigraphy, *Int. J. Pharm. 40*:119 (1987).

97. L. L. Christrup, S. N. Rasmussen, and M. R. Rassing, Chewing gum as a drug delivery system. IV. Excretion of ascorbic acid in urine after administration of chewing gum and chewing tablets, *Farmaci Sci. Ed. 16*:44 (1988).

98. L. N. Jensen, L. L. Christrup, N. Menger, and H. Bundgaard, Chewing gum and lozenges as delivery systems for noscapine, *Acta Pharm. Nord. 3*:219 (1991).

99. M. A. H. Russel, M. Raw, and M. J. Jarvis, Clinical use of nicotine chewing gum, *Brit. Med. J. 280*:1599 (1980).

100. C. Graffner, Some clinical results with respect to buccal administration, *Minutes European Symposium on Buccal and Nasal Administration as an Alternative to Parenteral Administration*, Paris, 10-11 Dec. 1991, Editions de Santé, Paris, 1992 p. 191.

101. L. L. Christrup, J. Bonde, H. Eriksen, S. N. Rasmussen, M. R. Rassing, and K. Simonsen Chewing gum as a drug delivery system. III. Bioavailability of salicylamide administered in tablets and chewing gum, *Farmaci Sci. Ed. 16*:6 (1988).

102. L. L. Christrup, J. Bonde, S. N. Rasmussen, and M. R. Rassing, Relative bioavailability of(+/-)-verapamil hydrochloride administered in tablets and chewing gum, *Acta Pharm. Nord. 2*:371 (1990).

103. L. L. Christrup, H. R. Angelo, J. Bonde, F. Kristensen, and S. N. Rasmussen, Relative bioavailability of methadone hydrochloride administered in chewing gum and tablets, *Acta Pharm. Nord. 2*:83 (1990).

104. N. L. Benowitz, P. Jacob, and C. Savanapridi, Determinants of nicotine intake while chewing nicotine polacrilex gum, *Clin. Pharmacol. Ther. 41*:467 (1987).

105. B. A. Burnside, A. D. Keith, and W. Snipes, Microporous hollow fibers as a peptide delivery system via the buccal cavity, *Proceed Int. Symp. Control. Rel. Bioact. Mater. 16*:93 (1989).

106. C. G. Wilson, and N. Washington, Scintigraphic studies of nasal and buccal administration, *Minutes European Symposium on Buccal and Nasal Administration as an Alternative to Parenteral Administration,* Paris, 10-11 Dec. 1991, Editions de Santé, Paris, 1992, p. 174.

107. C. G. Wilson, and N. Washington, Drug delivery to the oral cavity, *Physiological Pharmaceutics. Biological Barriers to Drug Absorption*, Ellis Horwood, Chichester, 1989, p. 21.
108. G. Ponchel, and D. Duchéne, Development of a bioadhesive tablet. *High Performances Biomaterials. A Comprehensive Guide to Medical and Pharmaceutical Applications* (M. Szycher, ed.), Technomic, Lancaster, 1992, p. 231.
109. Y. Jacques, D. Chulia, A. Verain, and P. Ozil, A propos d'un comprimé mucoadhésif destiné ˆ la cavité buccale, *Pharm. Acta Helv. 64*:163 (1989).
110. K. V. Ranga Rao, A. Ben-Amor, and P. Buri, Studies on buccoadhesive tablet formulation of codeine phosphate, *S. T. P. Pharma 5*:899 (1989).
111. G. Ponchel, F. Touchard, D. Duchéne, and N. A. Peppas, Bioadhesive analysis of controlled release systems. I. Fracture and interpenetration analysis in poly(acrylic acid)-containing systems, *J. Control. Rel. 5*:129 (1987).
112. N. A. Peppas, G. Ponchel, and D. Duchéne, Bioadhesive analysis of controlled release systems. II. Time-dependent bioadhesive stress in poly(acrylic acid)-containing systems *J. Control. Rel. 5*:143 (1987).
113. G. Ponchel, F. Touchard, D. Wouessidjewe, D. Duchéne, and N. A. Peppas, Bioadhesive analysis of controlled release systems. III. Bioadhesive and release behavior of metronidazole-containing poly(acrylic acid)-hydroxypropyl methylcellulose systems, *Int. J. Pharm. 38*:65 (1987).
114. F. Lejoyeux, G. Ponchel, and D. Duchéne, Influence of some technological parameters on the bioadhesive characteristics of poly(acrylic acid) matrices, *S. T. P. Pharma 5*:893 (1989).
115. J. D. Smart, An evaluation of some mucosa-adhesive dosage forms for drug delivery to the oral cavity, *J. Pharm. Pharmacol. 42*:141P (1990).
116. P. Forget, P. Gazzeri, F. Moreau, M. Sabatier, C. Durandeau, J. P. Merlet, and P. Aumonier Comprimés mucoadhésifs. Mesure de l'adhésivité in vitro. *S. T. P. Pharma 4*:176 (1988).
117. W. -G. Chen, and G. C. -C. Hwang, Adhesive and in vitro characteristics of propranolol bioadhesive disc system, *Int. J. Pharm. 82*:61 (1992).
118. O. Kislal, and N. Celebi, Studies on bioadhesive tablet formulation of propranolol HCl, *Proceed. Int. Symp. Control. Rel. Bioact. Mater. 19*:397 (1992).
119. P. B. Deasy, and C. T. O' Neill, Bioadhesive dosage form for peroral administration of timolol base, *Pharm. Acta Helv. 64*:231 (1989).
120. N. Garcia-Gonzalez, H. Blanco-Fuente, S. Anguiano-Igea, B. Delgado-Charro, F. J. Otero-Espinar, and J. Blanco-Méndez, In vitro characterization of bioadhesive metoclopramide tablets for buccal

application prepared with polyacrylic acid and hydroxypropyl methylcellulose, *S. T. P. Pharma Sci. 2*:494 (1992).

121. T. Nagai, and R. Konishi, Buccal / gingival drug delivery systems, *J. Control. Rel. 6*:353 (1987).

122. J. M. Schor, S. S. Davis, A. Nigalaye, and S. Bolton, Susadrin transmucosal tablets, *Drug Dev. Ind. Pharm. 9*:1359 (1983).

123. S. Anlar, Y. Capan, and A. A. Hincal, Studies on buccoadhesive tablet formulation of morphine sulfate, *6th Int. Conf. Technol. Pharm. 2*:30 (1992).

124. I. W. Kellaway, and S. J. Warren, Mucoadhesive hydrogels, *Proceed Int. Symp. Control. Rel. Bioact. Mater. 18*:73 (1991).

125. S. J. Warren, I. W. Kellaway and P. Timmins, Mucoadhesive hydrogels for buccal delivery of peptides, *Proceed Int. Symp. Control. Rel. Bioact. Mater. 16*:402 (1989).

126. I. W. Kellaway, and S. J. Warren, and P. Timmins, Hydrogels for buccal administration, *Minutes European Symposium on Buccal and Nasal Administration as an Alternative to Parenteral Administration*, Paris, 10-11 Dec. 1991, Editions de Santé, Paris, 1992, p.101.

127. M. E. de Vries, H. E. Boddé, H. J. Busscher, and H. E. Junginger, Hydrogels for buccal drug delivery: properties relevant for muco-adhesion, *J. Biomed. Mater. Res. 22*:1023 (1988).

128. M. E. de Vries, H. E. Boddé, A. Nascimento, H. J. Busscher, and H. E. Junginger, Mucoadhesive polyacrylic hydrogels for buccal drug delivery. Copolymers compared with polymer mixtures, *S. T. P. Pharma 5*:847 (1989).

129. B. Yang, and K. Knutson, Buccal Delivery system for polar solutes, *Proceed Int. Symp. Control. Rel. Bioact. Mater. 19*:409 (1992).

130. J. Cassidy, B. Berner, K. Chan, V. John, S. Toon, B. Holt, and M. Rowland, Buccal delivery of diclofenac sodium in man using a prototype hydrogel delivery device, *Proceed Int. Symp. Control. Rel. Bioact. Mater. 16*:91 (1989).

131. Y. Kurosaki, T. Takatori, M. Kitayama, T. Nakayama, and T. Kimura, Application of propranolol to the keratinized oral mucosa: avoidance of first-pass elimination and the use of 1-dodecylazacycloheptan-2-one (Azone) as an absorption enhancer of bioadhesive film-dosage form, *J. Pharmacobio-Dyn. 11*:824 (1988).

132. B. Rodu, C. M. Russell, and A. J. Desmarais, Clinical and chemical properties of a novel mucosal bioadhesive agent, *J. Oral Pathol. 17*:564 (1988).

133. H. P. Merkle, and G. J. M. Wolany, Muco-adhesive patches for buccal peptide administration, *Minutes European Symposium on Buccal and Nasal Administration as an Alternative to Parenteral Administration*, Paris, 10-11 Dec. 1991, Editions de Santé, Paris, 1992, p. 116.

134. M. A. Hussain, B. J. Aungst, C. A. Koval, and E. Shefter, Improved buccal delivery of opioids analgesics and antagonists with bitterless prodrugs, *Pharm. Res. 5*:615 (1988).
135. M. M. Veillard, M. A. Longer, T. W. Martens, and J. R. Robinson, Preliminary studies of oral mucosal delivery of peptide drugs, *J. Control. Rel. 6*:123 (1987).
136. R. Anders, and H. P. Merkle, Evaluation of laminated mucoadhesive patches for buccal drug delivery, *Int. J. Pharm. 49*:231 (1989).
137. H. P. Merkle, and G. J. M. Wolany, Buccal delivery of peptide drugs, *J. Control. Rel. 21*:155 (1992).
138. Y. Nozaki, M. Kakumoto, M. Ohta, K. Yukimatsu, and Y. Chien, A new transmucosal therapeutic system: overview of formulation development and in vitro / in vivo clinical performance, *Drug Dev. Ind. Pharm. 19*:221 (1993).
139. W. J. Conine, and M. J. Pikal, Special tablets. Sublingual and buccal tablets, *Pharmaceutical Dosage Forms. I. Tablets. Volume 1* (H. A. Lieberman, and L. Lachman eds.), Marcel Dekker, New York, 1980, p. 259.
140. M. R. Rassing, Chewing gum as a drug delivery system, *Adv. Drug Del. Rev., 13*:89 (1994).

12

Specialized Oral Mucosal Drug Delivery Systems: Patches

Gary DeGrande, Luce Benes, Françoise Horrière, Herve Karsenty, Claire Lacoste
3M Santé, France

Roy McQuinn, Jian-Hwa Guo, Robert Scherrer
3M Pharmaceuticals, USA

I. INTRODUCTION

It is our view that the best illustration of what is involved in the design of oral mucosal (buccal) patches for the systemic delivery of drugs is our own experience. Our work covers the full range from developing new test methods and assessing structure-property relations through studies of drug delivery in animals, tests of patch positioning and comfort in human subjects, and clinical studies of delivery efficacy. Recent publications on the subject have been incorporated into this review, but much of what is reported here has not been published before. Our discussion is prefaced by a summary of the principles of transmucosal drug delivery and the problems that must be overcome to design a successful product. Many of these issues are reviewed in greater detail in earlier chapters of this book.

The oral cavity has a number of features that make it desirable for drug delivery: a rich blood supply that drains directly into the jugular vein, thus bypassing the liver and sparing the drug from first-pass metabolism [1, 2]; ease of drug delivery even in unconscious patients and those who are permitted nothing by mouth [3]; ready termination of delivery by the healthcare practitioner or the patient; and an abundance of usable sites capable of recovering rapidly from any insult [3]. Therefore, despite its potential drawbacks - the physical and metabolic barriers to drug uptake and the numerous ways a drug or its delivery system can be lost [3] - many efforts have been made to utilize the oral surface clinically. The buccal mucosa was first investigated as a potential site for drug delivery several decades ago [4, 5], as it is an ideal surface for the placement of retentive delivery systems [2].

A. Pertinent Features of the Oral Mucosa

The mucosa of the mouth may be thought of as a multilayer laminate [6]. The outer layer is the saliva, which may take the form of an unstirred fluid layer [7]. Several components of the saliva may affect transmucosal delivery (TMD) systems. For example, the high molecular weight mucin known as MG1 [7] may be important in bioadhesion. Saliva also contains several proteins, including some enzymes, that may bind or inactivate a drug, reducing the concentration available to drive absorption [3, 8]. The pH of saliva is between 6.5 and 7.5 [3].

The next layer, the epithelium, may be either partly keratinized or entirely nonkeratinized, the former type being less permeable to hydrophilic drugs [8]. In the buccal region, the epithelium is nonkeratinized and approximately 500 to 600 μm in thickness [9]. Chronic inflammation and physical damage to the epithelium may reduce its barrier function (increase the permeability) [7]. Underlying the epithelium are a basement membrane (basal lamina) and the lamina propria. The latter is readily permeable to many drugs, whereas the former may limit the rate at which some drugs (e.g., β blockers) are absorbed [6]. The blood flowing through the vessels in the lamina propria acts as a sink for drugs delivered transmucosally [9].

B. Pertinent Features of Drug Uptake from the Oral Mucosa

Drugs applied to the oral mucosa gain access to the circulation principally by passive diffusion according to Fick's law[1] [1, 3]. For the most part, drugs move

---

[1] Specialized transport systems such as carrier-mediated transport or facilitated diffusion are operative for a small number of drugs; cefadroxil being one example [6].

extracellularly and follow, not the shortest path, but the path of least resistance [6], which for most agents is through the neutral lipids and glycolipids that separate the cells. The lipid solubility of a candidate drug therefore is one important measure of its suitability for a TMD system [6]. Also, because passive diffusion involves nonionized species, the pKa of a candidate drug is important [6, 7].

C. Pertinent Considerations in the Design of a TMD System

Successful transmucosal drug delivery requires at least three things: (i) a bioadhesive to maximize the intimacy of contact with the mucosa for a time sufficient for optimal drug delivery and to retain the delivery system in the oral cavity; (ii) a vehicle to release the drug at an appropriate rate under the conditions prevailing in the mouth; and (iii) strategies to overcome the low permeability of the oral mucosa (increase bioavailability).

The drug selected for a TMD system must have physicochemical properties, including size and pKa, that will allow it to move through the mucosa at a rate sufficient to produce a sustained therapeutic concentration in the blood [1, 6, 10]. It must either resist or be protected from the various metabolic barriers in the form of salivary and tissue enzymes [8]. The drug and the other materials must not damage the teeth or oral tissues (e.g., by keratinolysis, discoloration, irritation, allergenicity, or alterations in the microflora) and they must not produce an objectionable flavor [3, 11].

A TMD system may be unidirectional (i.e., release the drug only into the mucosa) or bidirectional (i.e., release drug into the mouth as well). The system must be of a surface area and thickness acceptable to the patient while holding and releasing sufficient drug for therapeutic needs. We find that flexible patches having a surface area of 0.5 to 1 cm^2 are comfortable, although larger patches may be tolerated. The shape and conspicuousness of the system are other considerations. Lastly, the TMD system must remain in the desired position.

The principal mechanism for bioadhesion of oral TMD patches appears to be physical entanglement of the adhesive polymer of the patch in the mucus glycoprotein chains overlying the mucosa [11]. Primary (covalent) and secondary (electrostatic, hydrogen, hydrophobic) chemical bonding appear to be less important mechanisms. The binding properties of a given polymer are affected by its molecular weight, configuration, cross linking density, charge and degree of ionization, concentration, and extent of hydration [11]; and the duration of adhesion is affected by the type and amount of the adhesive polymer, its viscosity, and the method of patch manufacture [12].

D. Comparison of Transmucosal with Other Drug Delivery Systems

Although direct comparative data in humans are limited, animal models demonstrate that transmucosal drug delivery has unique characteristics not easily obtained with other methods, including rapid onset of drug delivery, sustained release of the drug, and rapid decline in the serum concentration of the drug when the TMD patch is removed. Preliminary data [13, 14] show that TMD systems can provide a significantly faster initiation and decline of delivery than do transdermal patches. Transmucosal delivery appears to have low intersubject variability, particularly in comparison with oral controlled release formulations. Transmucosal delivery of larger molecules such as low molecular weight (LMW) heparin has been demonstrated. Thus, TMD systems hold particular promise as an alternative for some drugs now deliverable only by injection.

II. DEVELOPMENT OF A PATCH FOR TRANSMUCOSAL DELIVERY

The TMD patch developed by 3M Pharmaceuticals has been given the name Cydot™. It is either a unidirectional or a bidirectional bioadhesive dosage form able to deliver an active drug for either systemic or local action while suffering little or no erosion. The thin flexible patch can be a simple matrix in which the drug is dispersed, a multilayer matrix with each layer having a different concentration of the same drug or different drugs, or a reservoir. A patch shape (circular, elliptical, square, or rectangular) can be chosen according to its intended site of placement, the surface area of the site being the predominant consideration. A protective backing shields the patch from saliva, reducing erosion and drug loss via the oral route (see Figure 1).

The matrix patch is a mixture of elastomeric compound(s) and polymeric resin(s) in which the active drug is dispersed. The reservoir patch has a similar bioadhesive matrix containing a cavity in which various pharmaceutical formulations can be placed (Figure 1). Investigation of such patches has shown that it is possible to deliver many kinds of drugs (small and large [200 to 10,000 Da], lipophilic and hydrophilic) at various doses (0.25 - >30 mg) to obtain plasma drug concentrations in the range of picograms to micrograms per milliliter [15]. If necessary, additives (e.g., solubilizers and penetration enhancers) can be incorporated. The easiest molecules to deliver are the small ones that are active at low plasma concentrations and have an appropriate partition coefficient.

Two primary types of manufacturing processes have been developed to produce the TMD system: solvent cast and direct milling (with or without

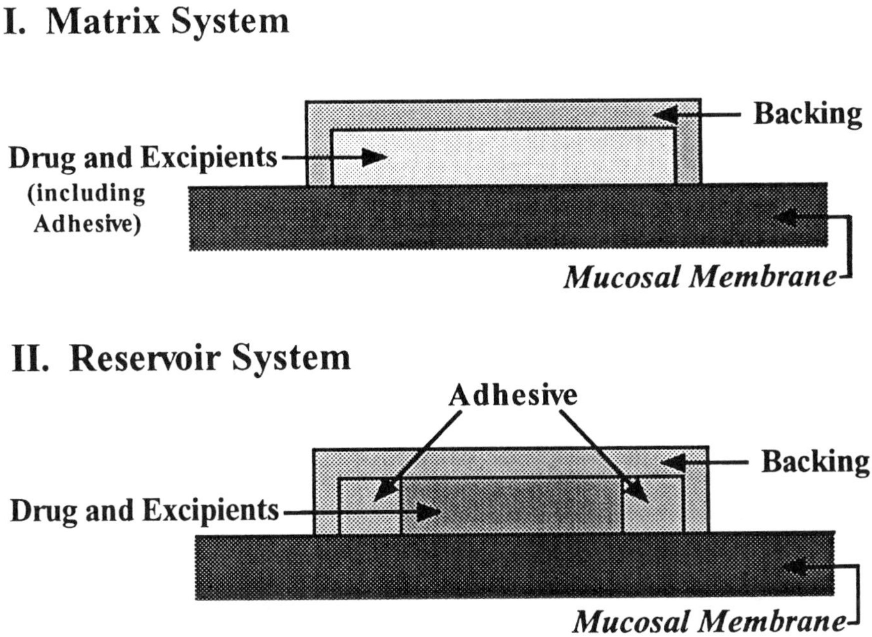

Figure 1. Alternative matrix and reservoir patch designs. These extend formulation options and the list of potentially deliverable therapeutic agents.

solvent). The intermediate product is a sheet from which patches are punched. A backing is then applied to each patch to control the direction of drug delivery and to minimize deformation and disintegration during residence in the mouth.

Figure 2 shows three of the possible patch designs. The design in Panel A has a barrier on the top and edge, making drug diffusion unidirectional. Panel B shows a patch with a semipermeable barrier that allows drug delivery. Such a design would be useful for delivery of drug to treat intraoral disease. The design in Panel C has a drug retentive barrier on the top only; as a function of the drug, this patch will deliver drug transmucosally and/or orally.

III. IN VITRO TESTING

It has been our experience that one can easily be misled by in vitro testing results and that the value of a particular formulation/patch design must be verified by in vivo testing. In vitro studies are still useful, however, in that they

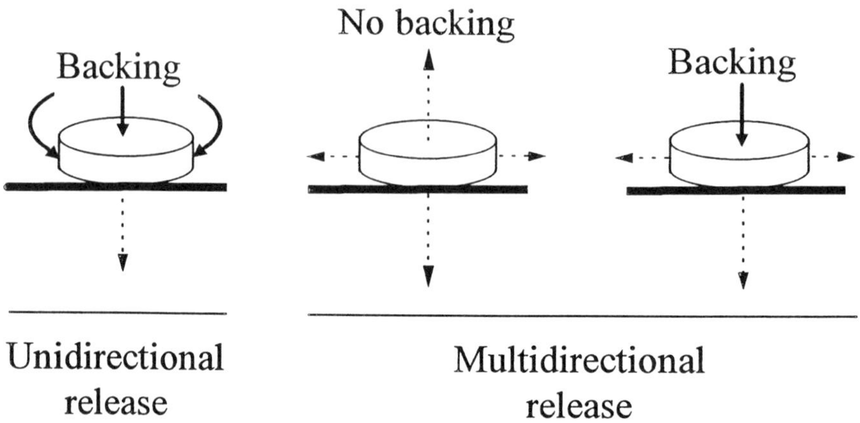

Figure 2. By varying the extent and permeability of a backing, a patch can be designed to provide delivery ranging from primarily systemic to predominantly local (oral cavity).

yield a general qualitative evaluation of basic properties such as adhesion and drug release and provide a valuable aid for formulation optimization. Recent developments such as the use of diffusion cells for assessing drug permeation through slices of excised animal buccal tissue may create a more prominent role for in vitro methods of studying drug permeation and the development of delivery devices. The use of cultured buccal epithelium to study drug transport and metabolism likewise may assist in the rapid development of buccal drug delivery products, as discussed in Chapter 6 of this book.

A. Characterization of Bioadhesion

1. Initial adhesion

One advance that was a marked help in patch design was the finding that bioadhesive patches adhere to a hydrogel film comprised of a blend of polyvinylpyrrolidone (PVP) and cellulose acetate [16]. The extent of adhesion to a wet hydrogel film qualitatively parallels the experience of human subjects wearing the patches. The porous film allows hydration through the adhering side of the patch during studies of initial adhesion, duration of adhesion, swelling rate, and drug release. Adhesion is measured using an Instron machine (Model 4201, Instron Co., Canton, MA).

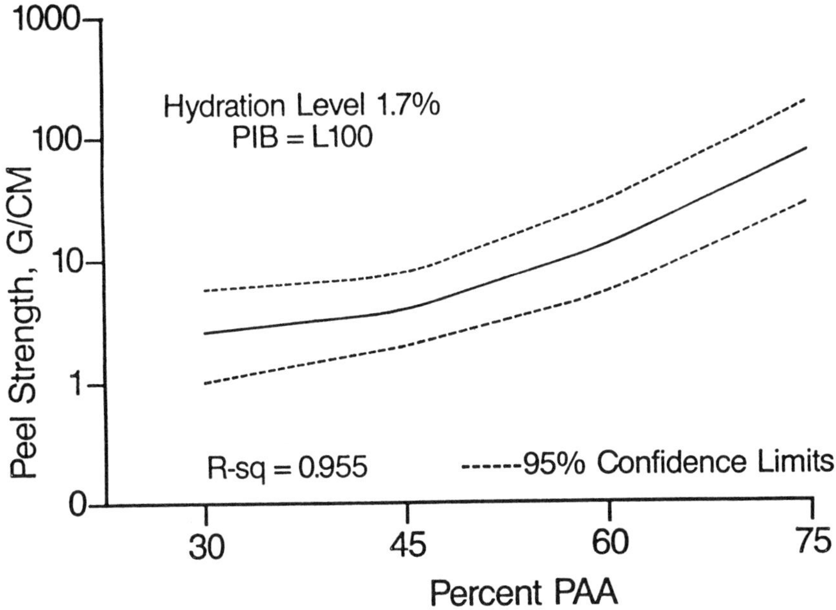

Figure 3. Effect of PAA concentration on force required to remove a PAA/PIB patch from a wet hydrogel film.

As an illustration of the relative value of various bioadhesive polymers in the formulation of a patch, Guo [17] compared polyacrylic acid (PAA), hydroxypropyl methylcellulose, chitosan, and acacia in patches made with a combination of polyisobutylene (PIB) and polyisoprene (PIP). The PAA is Carbopol™ 934P (B. F. Goodrich). The average peeling strength of samples made with this PAA was 0.021 kg/mm, nearly triple the value for hydroxypropyl methylcellulose. This result is in agreement with that of Smart et al [18], who used a surface tension technique similar to the Wilhelmy plate method and found that PAA was the second strongest among 11 adhesive materials tested. These results confirmed the choice of PAA for formulating the patches. A study was conducted to assess the effects of the PAA concentration on adhesion in an experiment using the Instron adhesion test [19]. The maximum force tolerated without detachment (peeling strength) rose with the percentage of polymeric resin (Figure 3). The need for other ingredients to maintain patch integrity limited the upper concentration of PAA that could be used effectively in the formulation.

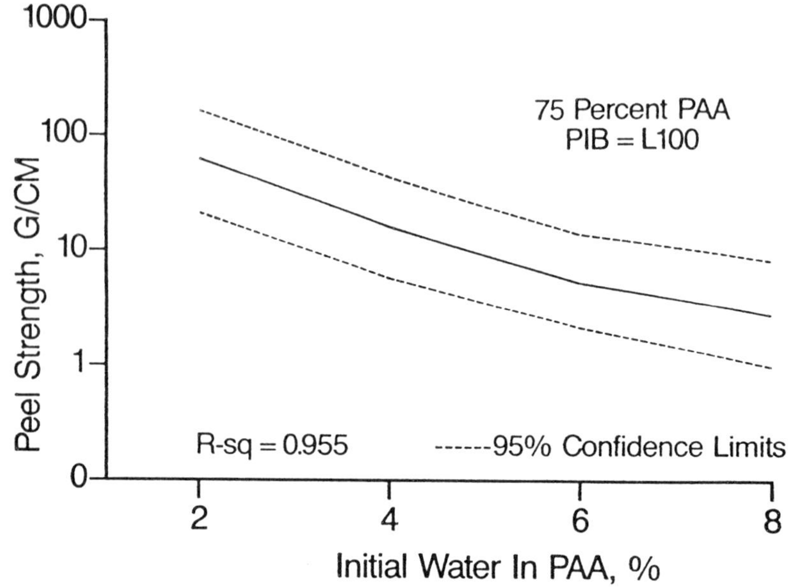

Figure 4. Effect of prehydration of PAA on peel strength of PAA/PIB patches adhering to a wet hydrogel film.

The effect of the initial extent of hydration of the PAA on mucoadhesion was determined. The PAA was prehydrated in a high humidity atmosphere to 1.7%, 4.1%, or 8.9% water. It was then milled with PIB at various concentrations, and the resulting material was tested for bioadhesion as described above. The peeling strength was dramatically affected by hydration, correlating inversely with the water content of the polymer. The results at a fixed PAA content are shown in Figure 4 [19].

2. *Duration of adhesion*

Because bioadhesive materials are affected by water and some may dissolve in the oral cavity, it is important to establish the duration of the adhesive force provided by the chosen polymer [12]. A variety of methods can be employed for these measurements [18, 20, 21]. We used the Instron instrument to assess adherence between polymer patches and the hydrated PVP/cellulose acetate hydrogel after various hydration times. Adhesion was expressed as the average peeling strength (kg/mm) or load (kg) [17]. For tests of the duration of adhesion, in vitro findings were also assessed in animals and human volunteers.

The relation of patch composition to duration of adhesion is a complex one, in part relating to the rate of patch hydration (Section III.B.). An example of an in vitro study is described by Guo [17]. Patches having PAA/PIB/PIP ratios of 60/35/5 and 50/43.75/6.25 behaved similarly in that the initial maximum adhesion was found after 2 to 8 hours of contact with the test medium, with no significant change for 24 hours thereafter. In fact, the patches retained more than 50% of their bioadhesive strength after 72 hours of contact. Later, however, adhesion decreased with contact time. Scanning electron micrographs of milled patches showed a looser structure with increasing swelling and a longer soaking time in the buffer solution [22].

B. Characterization of Patch Hydration

For evaluation of the rate of water uptake, the unprotected patch was covered by an aqueous medium, and its weight was plotted as a function of time. The swelling ratio and initial swelling rate were then calculated. Two degrees of acidity were used. Phosphate buffer, pH 7.0 is near the pH of the saliva, whereas phosphate buffer, pH 2.6 approximates the conditions created around the patch on the gingiva by the ionization of the PAA. There was a striking difference in the extent of hydration as a function of pH (Figure 5). At pH 2.6, the extent of hydration after 10 hours was approximately 200%, whereas

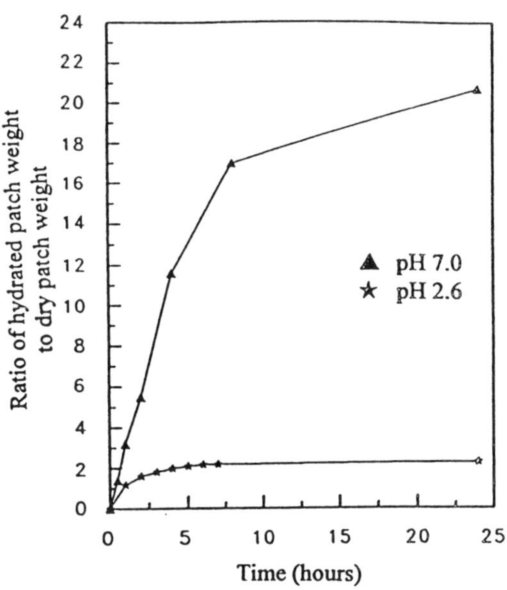

Figure 5. Rate of uptake of water into PAA/PIB/PIP patches at pH 2.6 and 7.0.

at pH 7.0, this value was 1000%. The extent of hydration at pH 7.0 is unlikely to be so high in the in vivo situation.

The extent of patch hydration also correlated with the PAA concentration: the higher the polymer concentration, the greater the hydration. Patch diameter and density likewise increased with increasing hydration. The immersion of a patch covered by an impermeable backing resulted in less swelling than was seen in patches without a backing. In another procedure, patches placed on a hydrogel membrane through which they are hydrated likewise became hydrated and swelled more slowly.

C. Characterization of Drug Release

Two methods have been used to characterize drug release from patches. One is simple dissolution using a modified paddle method. For some formulations, special flasks containing 100 mL of the dissolution medium were used. The medium, rotation speed, time of sampling, and method of analysis were adjusted as a function of the formulation. A second method uses a diffusion cell for determining drug release and is considered an improvement over dissolution in that only one face of the patch is in contact with the medium via a hydrated hydrogel, a situation that more closely mimics the moist surface of the buccal cavity. For this study, the patch was covered by a protective backing and applied to a hydrated hydrogel film (PVP/cellulose acetate). The patch absorbed medium via the hydrogel, then released the drug through the hydrogel into the receptor phase.

In general, there was a correlation between drug release and patch hydration, suggesting that swelling is an important mechanism. As an example, with the dissolution method, buprenorphine was released from the patches in a linear fashion over approximately 10 hours; by 24 hours, nearly 75% of the drug had been released (Figure 6) [17]. However, the microenvironment properties of the patch (e.g., pH) might be affected by the interaction between the active drug and the polymers, implying that the release profile could change from drug to drug.

The effect of patch thickness on drug release was studied with the diffusion method, using a fixed weight of melatonin in patches having identical diameters (0.5 cm^2) but different thicknesses. Melatonin represented 1%, 2%, or 4% of the patch weight. As expected, the release rate of melatonin was proportional to its initial concentration in the patch. This in vitro phenomenon has been confirmed

Figure 7. Comparison of rates of release of melatonin from patches of identical diameter and drug content but different thickness so that the concentration of melatonin is 1%, 2% and 4%.

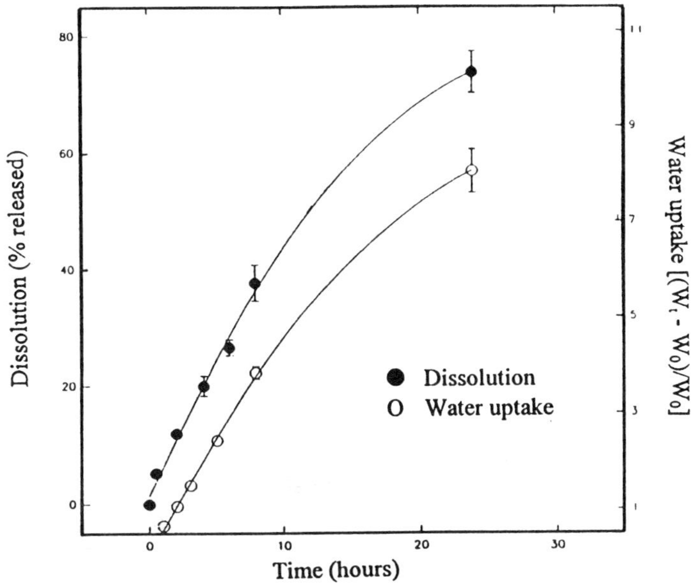

Figure 6. Dissolution (●) and swelling (O) profiles of buccal patches containing buprenorphine.

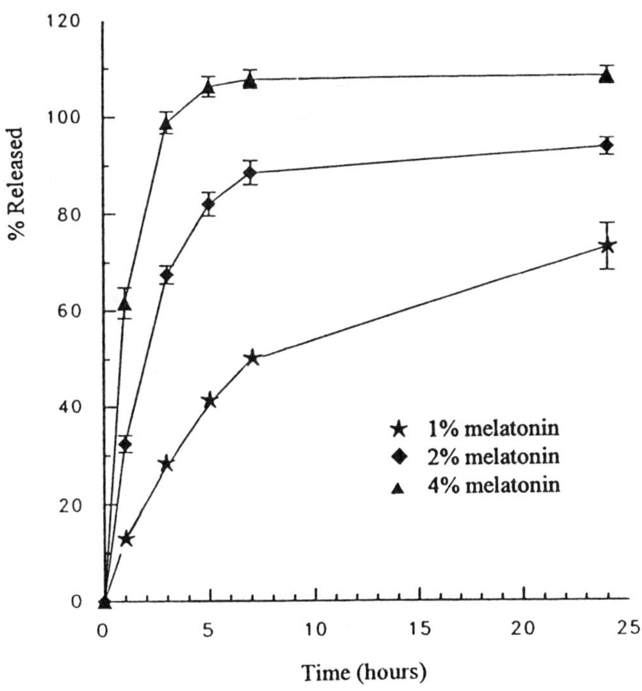

in vivo (Section VI.B.1). The profile and total extent of release suggest the establishment of a concentration gradient within the patch (Figure 7).

D. Additional Studies and Discussion

The effects of the two patch manufacturing processes on the properties of patches containing melatonin were compared. The maximum detachment forces were similar, but the release of melatonin was faster from patches made by the solvent cast process than from milled patches. This effect of the manufacturing process was also reflected in the faster hydration of the former type of patch, probably because of a looser structure.

Patches with a high PAA content and high PIB/PIP ratio have low surface energy and water wetting angles. Initially, therefore, one might expect these patches to be more adhesive. However, we were unable to predict the adhesion of buccal patches on the basis of their surface properties alone. Because the wetting angle and surface energy indicate only the initial ability of a patch to adhere to a substrate, the relation between bioadhesion and the morphologic structure of the patches must be considered [17].

Adhesion increased during the first few hours of contact with the test medium, an observation that may reflect increasing interpenetration of the macromolecular chains at the polymer-polymer interface [23]. Jabbari et al [24], using the technique of attenuated total reflection infrared spectrophotometry, found that chain interpenetration is indeed important in the bioadhesion of PAA at a mucin interface, as the mucin swells the crosslinked PAA matrix. The later decrease in adhesion can then be explained by the relaxation of PAA, as shown by electron microscopy. However, considerable bioadhesive strength was still present in the patches after 24 hours, indicating that the patches would provide sufficient mucosal adhesion to permit once daily administration.

The release profile for buprenorphine from the TMD patch was similar to that reported for lidocaine in buccal patches containing 30 mg of a freeze dried 1:2 mixture of hydroxypropyl cellulose and PAA [25]. The curve obtained with the current patches (see Figure 6) suggests a sustained delivery of buprenorphine over a 24 hour period, with the ultimate release of nearly 75% of the drug. The correlation between drug release and water uptake curves also suggests that patch swelling is the principal determinant of buprenorphine release.

In summary, these studies suggest that the strength and duration of adhesion and the rate of drug release can all be controlled by manipulating the PAA:elastomer ratio and that patches composed of these materials have the physical properties necessary for controlled buccal delivery of a variety of drugs.

IV. IN VIVO AND PRECLINICAL STUDIES

A. Animal Models and Testing Methods

Even small changes in the nature or the ratio of components in a mucoadhesive drug delivery system or in the method of manufacture can have a profound effect on the extent of delivery of drug in vivo as well as in vitro [12]. Therefore, it is necessary to refine patch designs by in vivo testing to select formulations suitable for clinical trials.

Considerable effort has been devoted to the identification of an animal model that reflects the behavior of human buccal epithelium [25, 26]. This topic has been discussed in detail in Chapters 1 and 7. We have relied on two models, the rat with a ligated esophagus and the Beagle dog, as our primary in vivo screening systems. The rat model is useful in the earliest development of drugs such as LMW heparin for which transmucosal delivery is problematic because of molecular weight and other factors. Because the animal is small, even modest amounts of drug absorption can be detected by assay of the plasma. The same feature makes the rat a good screening tool for promoters of drug absorption. This model allows one to answer the question, "can this drug, in any formulation, be observed to cross a mucosal membrane?" If not, there would seem to be little point in putting it into a patch.

The Beagle dog is useful in that it is a relatively large and docile animal that is tolerant of frequent handling and oral manipulation. Moreover, repeated blood samples can be obtained easily. Most important, its oral mucosal tissue is generally nonkeratinized and essentially lipoidal, like that of the human, and the tissues of the two species have nearly equivalent permeabilities for a large number of compounds. Several drugs that have low bioavailability after oral administration to humans or dogs, such as nitroglycerin [27], flurbiprofen [28], insulin and other peptides [29, 30], and opiates [31, 32], have been administered buccally to the dog with encouraging results. Moreover, the duration of adhesion and extent of patch hydration on the dog oral mucosa are good [63].

B. Results of Initial Studies of TMD Patch in Dogs

1. Tolerance

Daily application of a placebo patch for 14 hours on six sites on the upper gum over a 4 week period induced only slight inflammatory reactions detectable by microscopic examination. No macroscopic change in the oral cavity was noted. At the end of the observation period, total reversal of the inflammatory reaction was found. No additional reaction was observed in animals receiving a 1 mg melatonin patch instead of a placebo.

2. *Bioavailability*

A variety of model pharmaceutical compounds were chosen for preliminary testing which represented a large range of molecular weights (180-4000 Da) and water solubilities. The results of these preliminary determinations are shown in Table 1. Typical plasma concentration profiles of some of the drugs that demonstrated good bioavailability from buccal patches are depicted in Figure 8.

3. *Avoidance of oral delivery*

Drug in a buccal patch may diffuse directly into the saliva and be swallowed; if the drug in question is destroyed in the stomach, this portion of the dose will be lost. To investigate this possibility, buccal patches containing fluorescein were prepared with and without a protective backing, and the diffusion of the

Table 1. Compounds Screened for Buccal Patch Delivery in the Beagle Dog.

Compound	MW	Solubility in water	Oral bioavailability	Buccal bioavail-ability
Theophylline	180	1 g/120 mL	High	Moderate
Propranolol	259	High	Variable	Poor
Nitroglycerin	227	Low	Low	High
Digoxin	781	Low	Variable	High
Imiquimod	240	FB[a]: insoluble	Low	None
		HCl: high		Moderate
Estradiol	272	Low	Very low	High
Morphine	285	FB[a]: insoluble	Variable	Moderate
		HCl: 1 g/ 15 mL		
		SO_4: 1 g/17 mL		
Buprenorphine	468	FB[a]: insoluble	Low	High
		HCl: moderate		High
Melatonin	232	Moderate	Low	High
LMW Heparin	~ 4000	Moderate	Low	High

[a]Free base

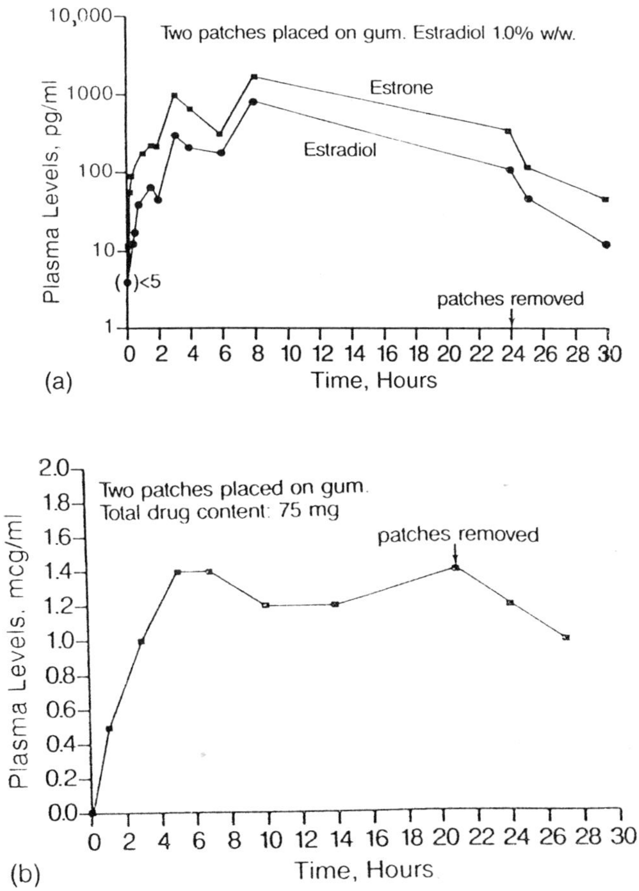

Figure 8. Examples of drug delivery to dogs from TMD patches; (a) estradiol, (b) theophylline.

water soluble dye was monitored under ultraviolet light after patch application to the gingiva or lip of Beagle dogs. In animals receiving patches without the occlusive backing, fluorescein could be detected outside the patch within approximately 30 minutes. The dye spread rapidly throughout the oral cavity, so that after 1 to 2 hours, most of the inside of the animal's mouth on the side of the patch demonstrated fluorescence, and by 5 hours, the patch was showing signs of dye depletion. In contrast, patches with an occlusive backing permitted only a gradual circumferential spread of fluorescein, such that by 8 hours after application, the zone of diffusion was approximately twice the diameter of the patch. These results suggest that swallowing of dye leached by saliva from the occlusive backed patches was not likely to have been a significant contributor to plasma concentration. Conversely, these results demonstrate the potential for local oral delivery from an unoccluded patch.

V. TOLERANCE AND ACCEPTABILITY OF MUCOSAL ADHESIVE PATCH IN MOUTHS OF HUMAN SUBJECTS

Two critical aspects of developing a patch for transmucosal drug delivery in the mouth are that the device be reasonably comfortable, interfering as little as possible with usual daily activities, and that it be tolerated by the tissues with which it is in contact. These features were assessed using a volunteer panel and later in a follow up to a clinical trial.

A. Use of Wear Panel to Evaluate a Patch Formulation and Placement Sites

A volunteer panel comprised of 10 men and 10 women was assembled to evaluate the acceptability of wearing a patch in different sites in the mouth and to assess the duration of adhesion that could be achieved at each site. Five placement sites were chosen: the cheek, the upper and lower lips, and the upper and lower gingiva. The site order was randomized, and a 0.5 cm^2 placebo patch with a protective backing was applied on days 1, 2, 3, 15, and 16 opposite the subject's preferred chewing side. The sites were examined before patch placement and again the following day. If the patch was still in place at 24 hours, it was removed, and the site was examined immediately. There were no dietary restrictions. A diary was kept by each subject.

Local tolerance for the patches at all sites was rated excellent by the clinical examiner. In most subjects, either no visible reaction was present or only mild erythema was noted, although moderate erythema, abrasion, ulceration, or edema were seen in a few subjects. None of the patches had to be removed because of local intolerance, and all of the reactions resolved spontaneously.

On a scale of 1 to 5, subjects rated the patch "comfortable" (1) or "fairly comfortable" (2) in 73 of the 100 experiences (all placement sites for all subjects). The subjects reported little or no interference of the patches with their daily activities (78% of placements). In 28% of the site experiences, the subjects had ceased to be aware of the patch within 15 minutes. The median duration of adhesion by site ranged from 21.5 hours for patches placed on the upper gingiva to 4.6 hours for those placed on the lower lip.

B. Postclinical Evaluation of Subject Acceptance

In one clinical study, subjects wore patches on the upper gingiva for 12 hours a night on three consecutive nights. The combined experience with more than 1600 patches was that 63% of the subjects felt the presence of a patch on their gums for no more than 15 minutes, 73% rated the overall comfort as good or excellent, and 79% thought that wearing a TMD patch created no or only slight interference with normal activities, including eating, drinking and sleeping [64].

VI. SPECIFIC DEVELOPMENT PROJECTS

We chose to explore further the TMD delivery of buprenorphine, melatonin and low-molecular-weight (LMW) heparin. The opiate analgesic buprenorphine has poor bioavailability after oral administration and is frequently used in patients who have poorly functioning or otherwise compromised gastrointestinal tracts, necessitating administration by injection. Similarly, melatonin, a naturally occurring hormone secreted during sleep and having a square wave pulse pharmacokinetic profile, has been cited as a candidate in need of novel delivery systems [33]. Low-molecular-weight heparin, which is used to prevent venous thrombosis, must now be given by subcutaneous injection, so a TMD formulation would be desirable clinically. Also, because LMW heparin has an average molecular weight of approximately 4000, the preliminary studies with this drug allowed assessment of the feasibility of delivering macromolecules with a TMD patch.

A. Development of a Patch for Transmucosal Delivery of Buprenorphine

Buprenorphine, a highly lipid soluble drug that is a more potent analgesic than morphine, is used clinically in the management of acute and chronic pain and is being investigated as a treatment for opiate dependence. It has low and variable oral bioavailability in both dogs and humans, presumably because of extensive first-pass metabolism, as well as a rapid rate of plasma clearance [34, 35]. At present, it is given by intravenous infusion, intramuscular injection, or, in Europe, sublingual tablets. The tablets dissolve rapidly, producing a drug plasma profile similar to that obtained with intramuscular injections.

Cassidy and Quadros and their associates [32, 36, 37] investigated the buccal penetration of buprenorphine from a mucoadhesive non woven reservoir device containing the drug in solution. They found the transmucosal flux of the drug to be similar, at approximately 40 $\mu g/cm^2$ per hour, in dogs and humans. We have tested the feasibility of delivering this drug by a mucoadhesive patch in order to provide a more stable and sustained serum concentration.

1. *Studies in dogs*

Buccal patches (0.5 cm^2) with a protective backing were prepared consisting of 2%, 4%, or 8% (w/w) buprenorphine hydrochloride or 8% buprenorphine free base; the amount of drug in a single patch was 1 to 4 mg. Single patches of each formulation were applied for 8 hours in a crossover study to the inside upper lip or gingiva of four Beagle dogs. Serum buprenorphine was measured by radioimmunoassay, and the residual buprenorphine was determined in the recovered patches for estimating the amount delivered.

Nearly all of the patches adhered well to the mucosal surfaces for the 8 hour wear period with little or no patch erosion. Mucosal irritation was minimal. Measurable serum concentrations of buprenorphine (≥ 25 pg/mL) usually were present within 0.5 hours after patch application, and maximum concentrations usually were observed by 4 hours. The serum concentration profile frequently was characterized by multiple peaks during the wear period, but after removal of the patches, the concentration declined rapidly. There was considerable inter-animal variability in both C_{max} and serum AUC within a treatment group (Table 2). Nevertheless, it was clear that the amount of drug delivered depended on the initial load in the patch (Figure 9a), that the systemic exposure to the drug (as measured by the serum AUC) was related to the drug load (dose) (Figure 9b), that the free base and hydrochloride formulations delivered essentially the same amount of drug, and that more drug was delivered when the patch was applied to the lip rather than the gingiva. Regardless of the treatment regimen, all dogs exhibited opiate related symptoms (miosis, sedation, unsteady gait, and, in some cases, vomiting).

Table 2. Pharmacokinetic Summary of Buprenophine in Beagle Dogs After 8 Hour Application of Buccal Patches (Mean ± SD).

Drug form, (% w/w)	Site	C_{max} (ng/mL)	t_{max} (hour)	AUC (ng/hour/mL)
HCl (2)	Lip	4.47 ± 4.84	5.5 ± 3.0	18.46 ± 18.50
HCl (4)	Lip	7.82 ± 7.58	1.5 ± 1.7	21.15 ± 21.86
HCl (8)	Lip	44.60 ± 60.54	5.3 ± 0.5	155.64 ± 210.14
HCl (8)	Gum	11.79 ± 6.38	3.3 ± 3.2	33.78 ± 11.26
Free base (8)	Lip	49.00 ± 35.43	2.7 ± 1.2	209.09 ± 149.75

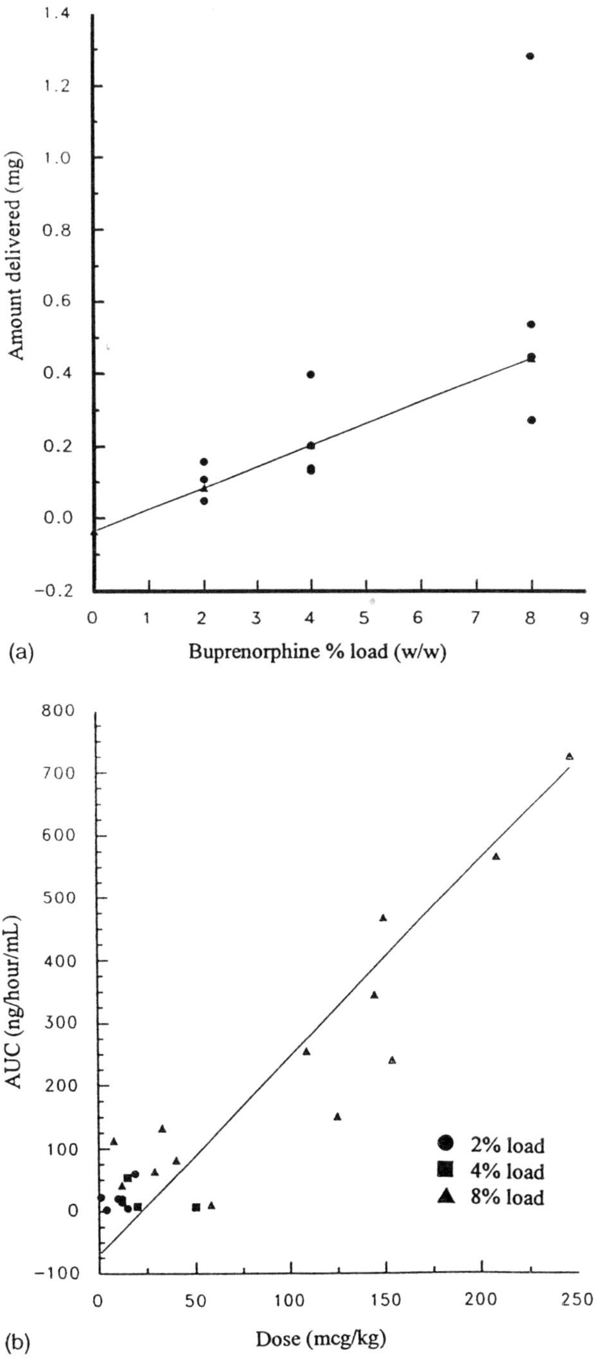

Figure 9. Transmucosal delivery of buprenophine to dogs from buccal patch as a function of drug load; (a) amount delivered, (b) AUC versus dose delivered.

2. *Studies in human volunteers*

A recently completed study of the mucoadhesion, local tolerance, and drug delivery properties of 0.5 cm^2 patches containing 2.9 mg of buprenorphine free base has been described [65]. Each of the seven human volunteers received a single buccal patch on two occasions. In one study period, the patch was placed either on the maxillary alveolar area above and between the lateral incisor and the canine tooth or on the maxillary labial area opposite the lateral incisor. In the second study period, the patch was placed on the other site. Patches remained in place for 12 hours and then were analyzed for residual drug by high performance liquid chromatography. The serum drug concentration was measured by radioimmunoassay at 0, 0.5, 1, 2, 3, 4, 5, 6, 8, 10, 12, 16, and 24 hours after patch application. Because opioids produce a concentration dependent miosis, the diameter of the subjects pupils was measured every hour for the first 6 hours after patch application and at 9, 12, and 24 hours.

Patches applied to the gingiva remained in place for the planned 12 hour period, whereas all of the patches applied to the lips exhibited considerable lift within 2 to 8 hours. The only reaction seen at the application sites was slight erythema, and the subjects found the comfort and taste of the patches acceptable at both locations. The adverse events were attributable to the opiate, not the patch. One subject reported several such events, including irregular breathing, during the first part of the study while a patch was in place on the gingiva. He was replaced for the second part of the study with another subject who likewise had a patch applied to the gingiva.

Pharmacologically relevant drug concentrations, as determined by the percent of miosis, were obtained after 1 to 3 hours and generally were sustained for 12 to 24 hours. Measured serum concentrations of buprenorphine were within the therapeutic range by 2 to 4 hours after patch application. Peak or near peak concentrations usually were attained by 4 to 6 hours and remained relatively unchanged over the remainder of the wear period.

Because of the better mucoadhesion, drug delivery was superior from patches applied to the gingiva (Table 3), with a mean AUC value of 5594 ±1419 pg hr/mL versus 3958 ± 780 pg hr/mL for patches applied to the lip. The mean serum drug concentrations 12 hours after patch removal were 79.0 ± 18.2 pg/mL for the gingival patches and 54.4 ± 17.1 pg/mL for the labial patches. Analysis of the patches after removal showed delivery of approximately 14% and 7% of the drug in the gingival and labial patches, respectively.

Because the serum drug concentrations generally were within the range associated with clinically significant analgesia (200-800 pg/mL) for 8 to 14 hours after application of a single patch, it seems probable that therapeutic amounts of buprenorphine can be delivered rapidly and in sustained fashion in this way.

Table 3. Pharmacokinetic and Pharmacodynamic Results of Application of a Single 0.5 cm^2 Patch Containing 2.9 mg of Buprenorphine to Human Subjects.

Subject	C_{max} pg/mL	t_{max} hour	AUC pg/hour/mL	% M_{max}	tm_{max}	Total delivered (µg)
Gingival application						
1	413	8	4622	53.2	9	520
2[a]	779	10	7377	48.5	9	380
3	428	10	5509	33.9	9	500
4	694	4	7032	38.5	6	560
5	468	12	4769	18.5	24	440
6	266	12	3456	39.3	12	30
7	419	12	6392	61.9	12	510
Mean	495	10	5594	42.0	12	420
SD	178	3	1419	11.6	6	182
Lip application						
1[b]	355	12	4736	36.1	9	70
3[c]	328	8	4144	41.4	12	280
4[d]	410	5	3977	30.6	12	320
5[e]	288	12	2657	12.3	24	190
6[f]	393	12	4257	44.4	12	140
Mean	355	10	3958	33.0	14	200
SD	49	3	780	12.7	6	102

[a]Patch removed 10 hours after application, [b]Patch became attached to gingiva approximately 2 hours after application, [c]Patch became attached to gingiva approximately 4 hours after application, [d]Patch lost adhesion and was removed 6.5 hours after application, [e]Patch became attached to gingiva between 6 and 8 hours after application, [f]Patch became attached to gingiva approximately 8 hours after application.

B. Development of a Patch for Transmucosal Delivery of Melatonin

The compound that has been studied most extensively in the 3M TMD system is melatonin (*N*-acetyl-5-methoxytryptamine), a pineal neurohormone that is secreted with a nocturnal circadian rhythm. Sleep disorders, seasonal depression, mood disorders, jet lag, and a number of other disorders have been ascribed to a disruption of normal melatonin secretion. Administration of exogenous melatonin to resynchronize the circadian rhythm has been proposed as a way to alleviate these symptoms. However, because of the variable but extensive first-pass metabolism of orally administered melatonin, a convenient, reliable nonparenteral method for administering the hormone is needed [33].

1. Effect of patch formulation on melatonin release in dogs

Development of a melatonin patch provided the basis for a simultaneous assessment of the importance of a variety of factors in patch design. Such things as the manufacturing method (solvent cast versus direct milling), the type of PAA, and the PAA content could be correlated with drug release rates, retention time, patch swelling, degree of patch hydration, and serum melatonin concentrations. Some of these experiments were described earlier in this chapter. One conclusion that appears warranted is that the optimum concentration of PAA in a patch depends on the objectives for that patch. For example, a higher PAA content favors initial adhesion strength and faster drug release at the expense of a greater swelling rate and shorter duration of adhesion. Viewed from another perspective, an important function of the hydrophobic components of these TMD systems appears to be control of the rate of hydration and thus of other important patch characteristics.

To study the effect of patch thickness, the same amount of melatonin was mixed throughout the matrix to produce concentrations ranging from 1% to 4% in patches 0.92 to 0.25 mm in thickness. After an 8 hour wear period, residue analysis of the patches demonstrated better drug delivery from thinner patches, even taking into account the difficulty in recovering the entire patch with the thinner designs (see Figure 7).

2. Pharmacokinetic profile of melatonin delivery in dogs and human subjects

An early comparison of melatonin patches in dogs and human subjects established that there is a good correlation in the pharmacokinetic profiles and extent of drug release in the two species.

A buccal patch containing 10 mg of melatonin was applied for 10 hours during the daytime to the gingiva of six Beagle dogs and six healthy male volunteers. In both dogs and humans, there was a rapid increase in the plasma concentration of melatonin (near peak concentrations by 2 to 4 hours post application) followed by a slightly ascending plateau until the maximum concentration was reached. There was a rapid decline as soon as the patches were removed. The C_{max} was 11,900 pg/mL and 2188 pg/mL in dogs and humans, respectively. The drug kinetics were equivalent in the two species when normalized for the difference in body weight.

Daytime application of patches containing melatonin doses ranging from 0.5 to 2 mg in 12 male volunteers led to plasma profiles that were qualitatively similar to those observed with 10 mg patches. The plasma concentration of the hormone appeared to be proportional to the dose, and the C_{max} reached 190, 400, and 825 pg/mL for the 0.5, 1, and 2 mg doses, respectively.

3. Comparative kinetics of melatonin following daytime and nocturnal patch application in human volunteers

The plasma concentration profiles of melatonin after nocturnal patch application (see Figure 10) did not appear to differ significantly from those obtained after daytime application, and the C_{max} values were equivalent with 0.25 to 2 mg doses (150-750 pg/mL). However, further investigation revealed

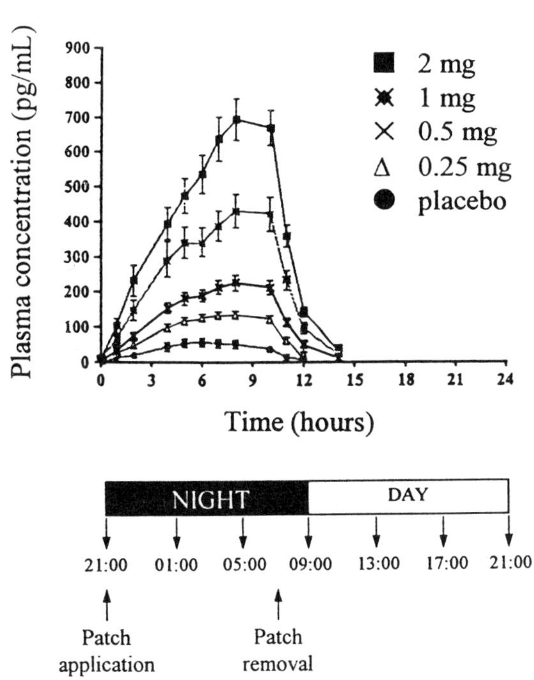

Figure 10. Melatonin kinetics after nocturnal TMD patch application in 20 healthy subjects: dose - response relationship. Points represent mean ± SEM.

some differences that appeared to be related to the time of day the patch was applied. Endogenous melatonin secretion, which is entirely nocturnal, tends to complicate the kinetics of exogenous melatonin from a nocturnally applied patch by adding to the total amount in the plasma. Also, patches applied during the day became more hydrated than those applied nocturnally and were subjected to greater erosion. Thus, the amount of melatonin delivered by daytime patches was higher than that delivered by nocturnal ones (49% versus 26% of the available compound).

It is probable that some of the daytime melatonin was delivered by the oral route. This observation comes from analyses of the plasma concentration of sulfatoxymelatonin, the main hepatic metabolite of melatonin. The metabolite kinetics of exogenous melatonin delivered at night via the TMD patch were much like those of endogenous melatonin, i.e., an approximate 1:1 molar ratio of melatonin to sulfatoxymelatonin (Figures 11 and 12). In contrast, after daytime patch application, the metabolite profiles were

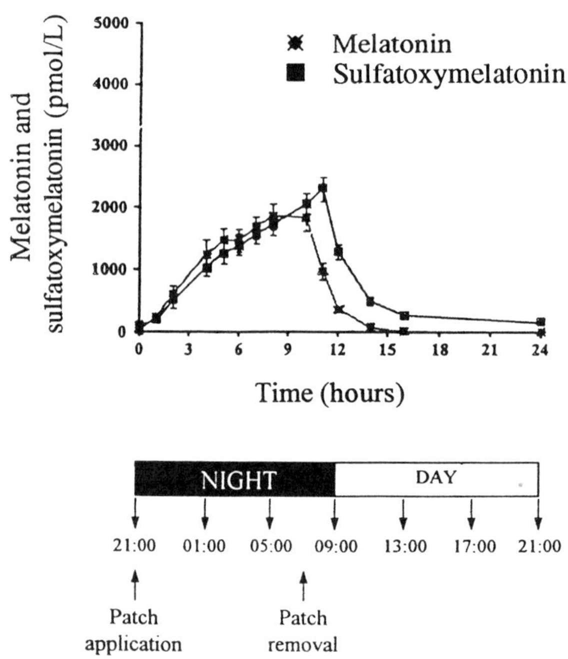

Figure 11. Kinetics of melatonin and its metabolite after nocturnal TMD melatonin patch application in 20 healthy subjects. Points represent mean ± SEM; melatonin dose = 1 mg.

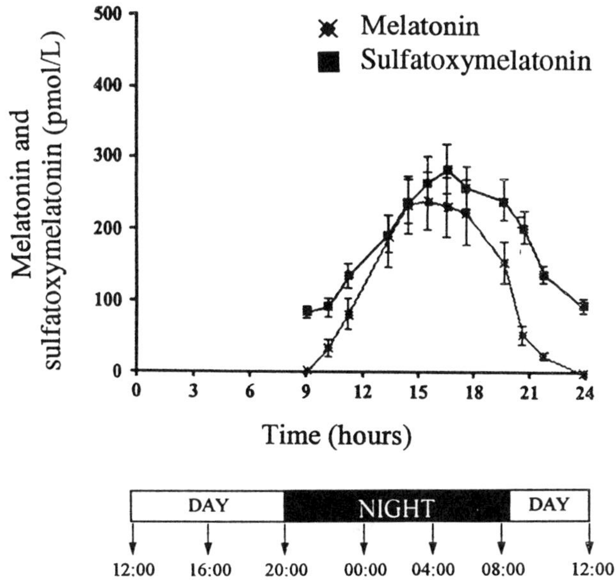

Figure 12. Endogenous melatonin and sulfatoxymelatonin profiles observed in 20 healthy subjects wearing placebo TMD patches. Points represent mean ± SEM.

qualitatively similar, but the metabolite plasma concentrations were higher, indicating greater first-pass metabolism and implying some oral delivery.

C. Development of a Reservoir Patch for Transmucosal Delivery of LMW Heparin

Development of a TMD form of heparin, a sulfated mucopolysaccharide composed of D-glucosamine and D-glucuronic acid residues, presents a considerable challenge, not only because of its molecular weight, but because it is a highly charged molecule. Most of our work with heparin has been with LMW heparin, i.e., the 4000 Da form.

1. Studies in rats

Our attention was directed first to determining if there was a reasonable possibility of success in creating a TMD system for heparin by using a model that involves a more or less direct application of the agent in the buccal cavity. The experimental technique was adapted from Aungst et al [38], who used it to study absorption promoters for buccal insulin delivery. Anesthetized rats underwent surgical ligature placement on the esophagus in order to avoid gastric absorption of a buccally administered gel formulation. This method was useful for rapid evaluation of the feasibility of transmucosal delivery of the drug and for defining the conditions necessary for such delivery: pH range, gel composition, and the effects of promoters. We demonstrated that the ability of heparin to cross the mucosa is poor without the aid of penetration enhancers and that some surfactants can improve drug delivery tenfold.

2. *Studies in dogs*

Three dogs received two reservoir patches placed simultaneously on the right and left cheek mucosa for 8 hours. Each patch contained 13.4 mg (1500 anti-Factor Xa units) of LMW heparin. Anti-Xa activity in the plasma after patch placement proved the ability of this system to deliver LMW heparin through the buccal mucosa (Figure 13): the plasma anti-Xa concentration reached 0.8 units/mL after 6 hours and then decreased slowly until patch removal 2 hours later. Because the plasma concentration required for prophylaxis of thromboembolism is approximately 0.1 to 0.2 anti-Xa U/mL, the prototype buccal patch is a suitable delivery system. However, some mild irritation of the mucosa attributable to the penetration enhancer was observed, making further studies necessary to enhance patient comfort and compliance. These data also suggest that other macromolecules such as peptides could be delivered with this technology, providing an interesting alternative to parenteral administration.

D. Discussion

The 3M mucoadhesive patch can adhere for more than 8 hours to the oral epithelium, and in many cases, adhesion for as long as 24 hours has been observed in humans. There is an inverse relationship between patch hydration and the duration of bioadhesion, but good hydration may improve the drug delivery rate. Tolerance of the patch was good, with minimal and acceptable erythema observed in a few cases. Unless they were specifically formulated to erode, erosion of the patches was minimal, and recovery of intact patches from the mucosal site was good. Controlled and sustained delivery from these patches containing a variety of pharmaceuticals yielding pharmacologically relevant serum concentrations has been demonstrated in laboratory animals and human volunteers.

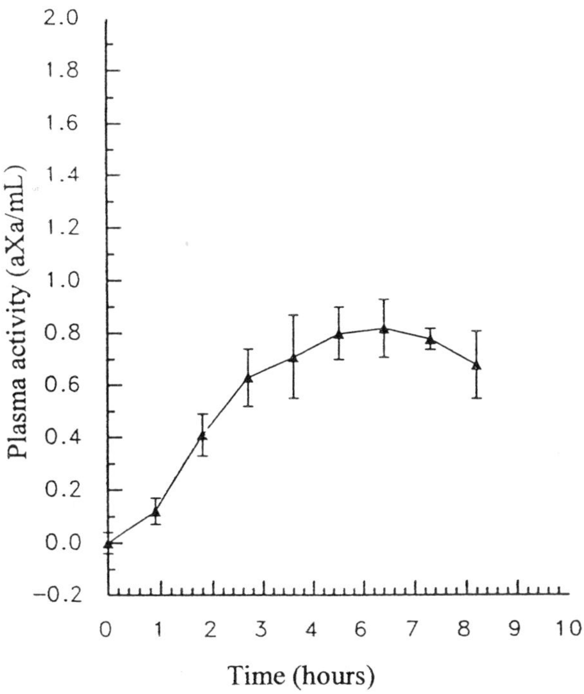

Figure 13. Mean (± SEM) plasma anti-Xa activity in dogs (n = 3) after buccal administration of ~ 3000 anti-Xa units of LMW heparin.

VII. ADDITIONAL MUCOSAL PATCHES REPORTED TO BE USEFUL FOR DRUG DELIVERY

Transmucosal delivery systems were recently reviewed by Ponchel [10]. An interesting feature of the review is a list of commercially available products used for sublingual and buccal delivery. There are no buccal patches on the list, which is an indication of just how new the field is. A recommended treatise, particularly from the standpoint of solutions to practical problems associated with the development of mucoadhesive patches, is that by de Vries [39].

One of the most challenging and potentially rewarding areas is buccal peptide and protein delivery systems, which have been reviewed by Merkle and associates [40-42]. One review [41] includes a chronological listing of patents on unidirectional mucoadhesive delivery systems. Another [42] has a comprehensive listing of drugs for which buccal or sublingual absorption has been studied. A chronological listing of bioadhesive material introductions in the literature is also included. Ho et al [43] emphasize mechanistic insights into buccal delivery in their review and include a good discussion of enhancers. A review by Leung, Nagai, and Machida [44] discusses nasal and ocular transmucosal routes in addition to buccal delivery.

There are several recent studies on peptides. Lee and Chien studied luteinizing hormone releasing hormone (LHRH), looking at its stability in the presence of enzymes [45], the effect of permeation enhancers [46], and delivery from a bilayer system through porcine oral mucosa in vitro [47]. Chen and Hwang [48] looked at bioadhesive patches for the delivery of leuenkephalin with various enhancers and an enzyme inhibitor using canine buccal mucosa. Sodium glycocholate was the most effective enhancer. A third peptide discussed in the recent literature is thyrotropin releasing hormone (TRH), which was studied by Li and coworkers [49]. Those investigators used mucoadhesive patches derived from Dow Corning pressure sensitive adhesive. Testing in anesthetized rats showed an increase in serum thyroid stimulating hormone (TSH) by 30 minutes after patch application and eventual concentrations of TSH that were fourfold to sevenfold greater than baseline. A multilaminated buccal patch has been described that has been modified to deliver propanolol and phenacetin systemically and triamcinolone acetate locally [50].

A recent patent application [51] describes a novel patch system based on PAA in a matrix of polytetrafluoroethylene support (PTFE web). Other excipients, such as permeation enhancers and agents to control the rate of patch swelling, can easily be added. The PTFE web matrix is soft and pliable and biologically inert and undergoes little or no disintegration in the mouth.

VIII. CONCLUSION

Various new drug delivery systems for the oral mucosa have been studied recently, including slowly dissolving tablets, lozenges, patches and chewing gum [10, 52]. Some of these devices are designed for the local delivery of anesthetics, corticosteroids or antimicrobial drugs for the treatment of intraoral diseases [53-56]. Others, such as some TMD patches, are effective for systemic delivery of drugs such as opiates, melatonin, propranolol, or heparin [57, 58] but also have the potential for local delivery. Particular effort has been directed toward the use of systems that deliver peptide or proteinaceous drugs which must presently be given parenterally to avoid degradation by digestive enzymes [30, 40, 43, 59-62]. As the material presented here indicates, defining an appropriate patch formulation is an arduous process, but the transmucosal delivery of drugs by mucoadhesive oral patches holds great clinical promise.

REFERENCES

1. P. W. Wertz, D. C. Swartzendruber, and C. A. Squier, Regional variation in the structure and permeability of oral mucosa and skin, *Adv. Drug Del. Rev. 12*:1 (1993).
2. D. Harris, and J. R. Robinson, Drug delivery via the mucous membrane of the oral cavity, *J. Pharm. Sci. 81*:1 (1992).
3. M. J. Rathbone, B. K. Drummond, and I. G. Tucker, The oral cavity as a site for systemic drug delivery, *Adv. Drug Del. Rev. 13*:1 (1994).
4. R. Gurny, and H. E. Junginger, Bioadhesion: possibilities and future trends, Presented at the First International Joint Workshop of the Association for Pharmaceutical Technology and the Controlled Release Society, Leiden, The Netherlands, 1989.
5. T. Nagai, and R. Konishi, Buccal/gingival drug delivery systems, *J. Control. Rel. 6*:353 (1987).
6. M. J. Rathbone, and I. G. Tucker, Mechanisms, barriers and pathways of oral mucosal drug permeation, *Adv. Drug Del. Rev. 12*:41 (1993).
7. C. A. Squier, and P. W. Wertz, Permeability and the pathophysiology of oral mucosa, *Adv. Drug Del. Rev. 12*:13 (1993).
8. H. Yamahara, and V. H. L. Lee, Drug metabolism in the oral cavity, *Adv. Drug Del. Rev. 12*:25 (1993).
9. N. F. H. Ho, Biophysical kinetic modeling of buccal absorption, *Adv. Drug Del. Rev. 12*:61 (1993).
10. G. Ponchel, Formulation of oral mucosal drug delivery systems for the systemic delivery of bioactive materials, *Adv. Drug Del. Rev. 13*:75 (1994).
11. R. B. Gandhi, and J. R. Robinson, Oral cavity as a site for bioadhesive drug delivery, *Adv. Drug Del. Rev. 13*:43 (1994).
12. R. Anders, and H. P. Merkle, Evaluation of laminated mucoadhesive patches for buccal drug delivery, *Int. J. Pharm. 49*:231 (1989).
13. L. Benes, G. DeGrande, F. Horriere, H. Karsenty, and D. Lagain, A new buccal delivery system for an indole derivative [abstract]. Proceedings of the International Symposium on Controlled Release of Bioactive Materials, 1992, volume 19, p. 419.
14. L. Benes, N. Ducloux, G. DeGrande, F. Horriere, H. Karsenty, and C. Lacoste, Melatonin delivery-comparison of transdermal and buccal routes of administration. Presented at the Third European Symposium on Controlled Drug Delivery, Noordwijk Aan Zee, The Netherlands, April 1994.
15. M. H. Longer, H. S. Ch'ng, and J. R. Robinson, Bioadhesive polymers as platforms for oral controlled drug delivery III: Oral delivery of

chlorthiazide using a bioadhesive polymer, *J. Pharm. Sci. 74*:406 (1985).

16. R. F. Ofstead, Polymer blends with high water absorption. U. S. Patent No. 4,771,089.
17. J. -H. Guo, Bioadhesive polymer buccal patches for buprenorphine controlled delivery: Formulation, in vitro adhesion and release properties, *Drug Dev. Ind. Pharm. 20*:18 (1994).
18. J. D. Smart, I. W. Kellaway, and H. E. C. Worthington, An in vitro investigation of mucosa adhesive materials for use in controlled drug delivery, *J. Pharm. Pharmacol. 36*:295 (1984).
19. R. A. Scherrer, M. T. Scholz, R. L. McQuinn, J. K. Barkhaus, and N. M. Marecki, A transmucosal drug delivery system based on polyisobutylene and polyacrylic acid. Presented at the Annual Meeting of the American Association of Pharmaceutical Scientists, San Antonio, TX, November 15-19, 1992.
20. R. Gurny, J. M. Meyer, and N. A. Peppas, Bioadhesive intraoral release systems: design, testing, and analysis, *Biomaterials 5*:336 (1984).
21. H. Park, and J. R. Robinson, Physicochemical properties of water insoluble polymers important to mucin epithelial adhesion, *J. Control. Rel. 2*:47 (1985).
22. J. -H. Guo, Investigating the surface properties and bioadhesion of buccal patches, *J. Pharm. Pharmacol. 46*:647 (1994).
23. N. A. Peppas, and P. A. Buri, Surface, interfacial and molecular aspects of polymer bioadhesion on soft tissues, *J. Control. Rel. 2*:257 (1985).
24. E. Jabbari, N. Wisniewski, and N. A. Pappas, Evidence of mucoadhesion by chain interpenetration at a poly(acrylic acid)/mucin interface using ATR-FTIR spectoscopy, *J. Control. Rel. 26*:99 (1993).
25. M. E. de Vries, H. E. Boddé, J. C. Verhoef, and H. E. Junginger, Developments in buccal drug delivery, *Crit. Rev. Ther. Drug Carr. Syst. 8*:271 (1991).
26. A. J. Hoogstraate, and H. E. Boddé, Methods for assessing the buccal mucosa as a route of drug delivery, *Adv. Drug Del. Rev. 12*:99 (1993).
27. W. A. Ritschel, A. N. Shaaya, and H. S. I. Jan, Disposition of nitroglycerin in the Beagle dog after intravenous and buccal administration, *Exp. Clin. Pharmacol. 7*:307 (1985).
28. C. L. Barsuhn, L. S. Olanoff, D. D. Gleason, E. L. Adkins, and N. F. H. Ho, Human buccal absorption of flurbiprofen. *Clin. Pharmacol. Ther. 44*:225 (1988).
29. T. Nagai, and Y. Machida, Mucosal adhesive dosage forms, *Pharm. Int. 6*:196 (1986).

30. G. J. M. Wolany, J. Munzer, A. Rummelt, and H. P. Merkle, Buccal absorption of Sandostatin® (octreotide) in conscious Beagle dogs, *Proc. Int. Symp. Control. Rel. Bio. Mat. 17*:224. (1990).
31. M. A. Hussain, B. J. Aungst, C. A. Koval, and E. Shefter, Improved buccal delivery of opioid analgesics and antagonists with bitterless prodrugs, *Pharm. Res. 5*:615 (1988).
32. J. Cassidy, and E. Quadros, Sustained buccal delivery of buprenorphine in the dog in vivo, *Pharm. Res. 8*:S-155 (1991).
33. D. Dawson, Melatonin and sleep in humans, *J. Pineal Res. 15*:1 (1993).
34. L. E. Mather, Opioid pharmacokinetics in relation to their effects, *Anaesth. Intens. Care 15*:15 (1987).
35. E. R. Garrett, and V. R. Chandran, Pharmacokinetics of morphine and its surrogates X: analyses and pharmacokinetics of buprenorphine in dogs, *Biopharm. Drug Dispos. 11*:311 (1990).
36. E. Quadros, J. Cassidy, V. Tipnis, T. Livingston, and S. Langley, Controlled buccal delivery of buprenorphine in man, *Pharm. Res. 8*:S-155 (1991).
37. J. P. Cassidy, N. M. Landzert, and E. Quadros, Controlled buccal delivery of buprenorphine, *J. Control. Rel. 25*:21 (1993).
38. B. J. Aungst and N. J. Rogers, Comparison of the effects of various transmucosal absorption promoters on buccal insulin delivery, *Int. J. Pharm. 53*:227 (1989).
39. M. E. de Vries, Buccal drug absorption and development of mucoadhesive polymer systems [doctoral dissertation] . University of Leiden, The Netherlands, 1991.
40. H. P. Merkle, R. Anders, and A. Wermerskirchen, Mucoadhesive buccal patches for peptide delivery, *Bioadhesive Drug Delivery Systems* (V. Lenaerts and R. Gurny, eds.), CRC Press, Boca Raton, Florida, 1990, p. 105.
41. H. P. Merkle, and G. J. M. Wolany, Mucoadhesive patches for buccal peptide administration, *Buccal and Nasal Administration as an Alternative to Parenteral Administration*, Éditions de Santé, Paris, 1991, p. 110.
42. H. P. Merkle, R. Anders, A. Wermerskirchen, S. Raehs, and G. Wolany, Buccal routes of peptide and protein drug delivery, *Adv. Parent. Sci 4*:545 (1990).
43. N. F. H. Ho, C. L. Barsuhn, P. S. Burton, and H. P. Merkle, Mechanistic insights to buccal delivery of proteinaceous substances, *Adv. Drug Del. Rev. 8*:197 (1992).
44. S. H. S. Leung, T. Nagai, and Y. Machida, Mucoadhesive dosage forms for peptide and protein drug delivery, *Adv. Parent. Sci. 4*:741 (1990).

45. Y. Lee, and Y. W. Chien, Oral mucosal delivery of LHRH I: Physicochemical and enzymatic stability of LHRH in buccal mucosal extracts and stabilization, Proceedings of the American Association of Pharmaceutical Scientists Meeting, San Diego, Nov. 6-10, 1994, p. S-300.
46. Y. Lee, and Y. W. Chien, Oral mucosal delivery of LHRH II: Enhancement of permeation by bile salts and evaluation of mechanism, Proceedings of the American Association of Pharmaceutical Scientists Meeting, San Diego, Nov. 6-10, 1994, p. S-300.
47. Y. Lee and Y. W. Chien, Oral mucosal delivery of LHRH III: Long acting delivery by bi-layer mucoadhesive polymer systems, Proceedings of the American Association of Pharmaceutical Scientists Meeting, San Diego, Nov. 6-10, 1994, p. S-300.
48. W. Chen, and G. C. Hwang, In vitro evaluation of buccal bioadhesive patches II: delivery study of leuenkephalin through dog buccal mucosa, Proceedings of the American Association of Pharmaceutical Scientists Meeting, Orlando, Nov. 14-18, 1993, p. S-201.
49. C. Li, V. A. Raul, P. I. P. Bhatt, P. L. Koch, and T. P Johnson, Transbuccal delivery of a model tripeptide, Proceedings of the American Association of Pharmaceutical Scientists Meeting, Orlando, Nov. 14-18, 1993, p. S-201.
50. W. Chen, and G. C. Hwang, In vitro evaluation of buccal bioadhesive patches I: systemic and local delivery of drugs, Proceedings of the American Association of Pharmaceutical Scientists Meeting, Orlando, Nov. 14-18, p. S-201 (1993).
51. R. L. McQuinn, and J. K. Barkhaus, *Int. Publication WO* 93/23011.
52. M. R. Rassing, Chewing gum as a drug delivery system, *Adv. Drug Del. Rev. 13*:89 (1994).
53. M. Addy, Local delivery of antimicrobial agents to the oral cavity, *Adv. Drug Del. Rev. 13*:123 (1994).
54. D. N. Thorburn, and M. M. Ferguson, Topical corticosteroids and lesions of the oral mucosa, *Adv. Drug Del. Rev. 13*:135 (1994).
55. L. P. Samaranayake, and M. M. Ferguson, Delivery of antifungal agents to the oral cavity, *Adv. Drug Del. Rev. 13*:161 (1994).
56. N. J. Medlicott, M. J. Rathbone, I. G. Tucker, and D. W. Holborow, Delivery systems for the administration of drugs to the periodontal pocket, *Adv. Drug Del. Rev. 13*:181 (1994).
57. C. D. Ebert, S. J. Heiber, S. C. Dave, S. W. Kim, and D. Mix, Mucosal delivery of macromolecules, *J. Control. Rel. 28*:37 (1994).
58. W. Chen, and G. C. Hwang, Adhesive and in vitro release characteristics of propranolol bioadhesive disc system, *Int. J. Pharm. 82*:61 (1992).

59. H. P. Merkle, R. Anders, J. Sandow, and W. Schurr, Self adhesive patches for buccal delivery of peptides, *Proceed. Int. Symp. Control. Rel. Bio. Mat. 12*:85 (1985).
60. H. P. Merkle, R. Anders, J. Sandow, and W. Schurr, Drug delivery of peptides: the buccal route, *Delivery Systems for Peptide Drugs* (S. S. Davis, L. Illum, and E. Tomlinson, eds.), Plenum Press, New York, 1986, p. 159.
61. M. M. Veillard, M. A. Longer, T. W. Martens, and J. R. Robinson, Preliminary studies of oral mucosal delivery of peptide drugs, *J. Control. Rel. 6*:123 (1987).
62. H. P. Merkle and G. J. M. Wolany, Mucoadhesive patches for buccal peptide administration, *Buccal and Nasal Administration as an Alternative to Parenteral Administration*, Editions de Santé, Paris, 1992, p. 110.
63. L. Benes, G. DeGrande, F. Horrière, and M. Land, Effect of carbopol concentration on in vitro and in vivo characteristics of the 3M buccal delivery system (Cydot™). Presented at the American Association of Pharmaceutical Scientists Meeting, Miami Florida, Nov. 6–8, 1995.
64. L. Benes, I Chau, G. DeGrande, F. Horrière, and C. Lacoste, Evaluation of patient comfort and acceptance of the 3M transmucosal drug delivery system Cydot™ after repeated application in humans, 7th International Symposium on Recent Advances in Drug Delivery Systems, Salt Lake City, Utah, February 28, 1995.
65. R. McQuinn, D. Kvam, M. Maser, A. Miller, and S. Oliver, Sustained oral mucosal delivery in human volunteers of buprenorphine from thin non-eroding mucoadhesive polymeric disk, *Journal of Controlled Release 34*:243–250 (1995).

13

Specialized Oral Mucosal Drug Delivery Systems: Chewing Gum

Margrethe Rømer Rassing
Royal Danish School of Pharmacy, Denmark

I. INTRODUCTION

The chewing of gum is a well accepted and frequently undertaken activity in both adults and children. It is a potentially useful means of administering drugs both locally to, or systemically via, the oral cavity. As an oral mucosal drug delivery system it offers several advantages. For the administration of drugs intended to treat or prevent local diseases of the mouth, it offers the possibility of releasing drug in a controlled manner over extended times thereby providing a prolonged therapeutic effect. As a delivery system for the systemic administration of drugs via the oral mucosa it has the potential to overcome the problems of short-lived action and variations in drug release and retention times; disadvantages which are associated with conventional systemic oral mucosal drug delivery systems. It may prove to be particularly suitable for the systemic delivery of drugs which are susceptible to metabolism in the gut wall or liver. Under certain circumstances chewing gum could also be used as a convenient alternative to conventional peroral dosage forms. In addition to the convenience, it also offers the advantage that it makes peroral administration of drugs possible without simultaneous intake of water. Furthermore the treatment can, if required, be terminated at any time by expelling the chewing gum. In addition, drugs that are released from chewing gum and swallowed, will be introduced to the gastrointestinal tract either dissolved or suspended in saliva and will thus be present in a readily bioavailable form.

Chewing gum consists of a gum base co-formulated with several other ingredients whose function is to give the gum the right texture, taste, feel and to prevent adhesion to the teeth. The formulation, manufacture and assessment of chewing gum, together with its therapeutic potential and limitations are discussed in this chapter. In addition the future directions and possible applications of chewing gum are highlighted.

II. HISTORICAL AND CULTURAL ASPECTS

The habit of chewing something besides food dates back many centuries. The first kind of chewing gum, *chewing tree resins*, was chewed by the ancient Egyptians [1]. It is known that in A.D. 50, the Greeks chewed mastiche to sweeten their breath and to clean their teeth [2]. The chewing of frankincense was considered to cure different kinds of illnesses including ulcers and gonorrhea [1]. One thousand years ago the Mayan Indians of Yucutan chewed chicle from the sabodilla trees, and the early American Indians chewed resin from the spruce trees.

In 1848 *"State of Maine Pure Spruce Gum"* became the first commercial chewing gum [1]. In 1869 the first patent for chewing gum was taken out by a dentist, Dr. William F. Semple from Mount Vernon, Ohio. He considered chewing gum was not only a confectionery, but also had a potential role as a dentifrice [3]. In 1879 pepsin powder and chewing gum were blended together to make a medicament to aid digestion. The first fruit flavored chewing gum, *"Kiss-Me"*, was marketed around 1880. William Wrigley launched his first chewing gum products, *"Lotta"* and *"Vassar"*, in 1892 and shortly afterwards introduced a spearmint flavored gum called *"Wrigley's Spearmint"* [2]. *"Dentyne"* was marketed in 1899 with the manufacturers claiming it to be beneficial to the teeth, possessing cleansing and refreshing qualities [2]. Aspirin was manufactured in chewing gum as *"Aspergum"* in 1924 in the USA, and it is still on the market today [4].

No monograph exists for medicated chewing gum in any Pharmacopoeia, but it is listed as a standard term in the guidelines for pharmaceutical dosage forms (1991) issued by the Commission of European Communities (CPMP). In this document chewing gum is defined as a "solid preparation with a basis consisting of gum which should be chewed and not swallowed, providing a slow, steady release of the medicine contained" [5].

Chewing gum has long been regarded as a low class addiction. However, nowadays it is marketed worldwide and in most countries is accepted as a harmless practice. Indeed, the chewing of (sugar free) gum is considered to be beneficial for dental health and it is increasingly being used as a drug delivery system. It should be noted that in some cultural groups the chewing of gum is still considered bad manners and in Singapore chewing gum is even forbidden.

III. COMPONENTS OF CHEWING GUM

Although many different formulations of chewing gum have been reported in the patent literature (e.g., [6, 7]) the characteristic component of all chewing gums is the gum base. Other components added to chewing gum typically include sweetening agents, flavoring agents and aromatics. In medicinal chewing gum an active ingredient is also added. A gum base may comprise a complex mixture of elastomers, natural and synthetic resins, fats, emulsifiers, waxes, antioxidants, fillers and flavoring agents.

The elastomers provide elasticity and cohesion to the chewing gum. Historically the gum base contained natural elastomers, but nowadays the synthetic elastomers such as polyisobutylene and butyl rubber are used. The polymer styrenebutadiene is primarily used in bubble gum.

Natural and synthetic resins have two functions; (i) as mastication substances and (ii) as binding agents between the elastomers and fillers. They contribute to the balance between the properties of elasticity and plasticity. Glycerol esters from pine resins are examples of natural resins and are used in medicated chewing gum because of their lack of taste and good chemical stability. The synthetic resin polyvinyl acetate is a common example of a synthetic resin which is used in medicinal chewing gum. It reduces the tendency of the gum to adhere to the teeth (i.e., it acts as a "detackifier") and to be divided into pieces during chewing (i.e., it prevents "bite through"). It has only a slight taste, its stability is good and it is available in a range of different molecular weights.

Emulsifiers and fats are used to soften the mixture of elastomers, resins and fillers to give the required chewing consistency and mouth feel. Emulsifiers promote the uptake of saliva into the chewing gum during mastication. Monoglycerides, diglycerides and partly hardened vegetable and animal fats are examples. Microcrystalline waxes serve the same purpose as an emulsifier or fat, but it should be noted that the waxes give a different chewing consistency and mouth feel. The advantage of the waxes is that their stability is often better than that of the fats.

Antioxidants may be added to protect the gum base and flavors from oxidation. Ascorbic acid (vitamin C), tocopherol (vitamin E), butylhydroxyanisol (BHA) and butylhydroxytoluene (BHT) have been used in chewing gum for this purpose.

Fillers are important ingredients. Their function is to provide the right texture for the gum base. Talc is used in products containing sour ingredients,

Table 1. Composition of a Commercially Available Medicated Chewing Gum, Fluomin®. (From reference 8).

Ingredients	Weight (%)
Gum base[a]	52.6
Paraffin oil	3.4
Sorbitol	40.8
Mannitol	0.9
Saccharin	0.1
Aroma compounds[a]	2.1
Sodium fluoride	0.1

[a]Details of the composition of the gum base and the aroma compounds were not reported in reference 8.

because of its acid resistance, while calcium carbonate is used in most other types of chewing gum products.

The gum base and typical components included in chewing gum are tasteless. It is important to consider the taste of any incorporated drug when producing medicated chewing gum as this can affect patient compliance. Chemical modification of a drug to one which is only moderately soluble and thereby exhibits a moderate release rate, can sometimes provide the solution to a taste problem. However, experience and know-how about how to match the taste of flavoring agents to mask the taste of a drug is essential in the production of an acceptable chewing gum product. It should be noted that ideally the release rate of any flavor additives and sweeteners should be about the same as the release rate of the drug from the gum base.

A further consideration when manufacturing a medicated chewing gum is the particle size of any solid substance suspended in chewing gum. To avoid an unpleasant gritty feeling during chewing, or the risk of damaging the enamel of the teeth, the particle size should be kept below approximately 100 μm.

An example of the composition of a commercially available medicated chewing gum, Fluomin®, is given in Table 1.

IV. THE MANUFACTURING PROCESS

The manufacturing process begins by softening the gum base at a temperature between 50°C and 70°C in a mixer using slowly turning blades. Corn syrup or glucose syrup is then added together with powdered sugar. The former ingredients keep the gum moist and pleasant to chew and help the sugar combine easily with the gum base. Softeners and flavors are then incorporated.

To successfully manufacture chewing gum the ingredients must be added at the right time and must not be mixed for too long or too short a period.

From the mixers, the warm mass passes onto slow moving cooling belts which are bathed in currents of cool air to reduce the temperature of the mass. The mass then moves to a rolling plant where the gum mass is extruded into a "carpet" of gum. This carpet is rolled out to the right thickness by a series of rollers before it is finally scored into single pieces. The chewing gum is then moved to a conditioning room in which the temperature and humidity are carefully controlled. This gives the product good durability. After a few days of maturing the gum is ready for coating.

In medicated chewing gum the drug is generally incorporated into the gum base, however, it is possible to add the active ingredient during the coating process if the drug is unstable under any of the conditions employed during the manufacturing process.

Some gum manufacturers have developed a granulation and compression method similar to that used in the manufacture of tablets. Gum granulation methods are described in the patent literature (e.g., [9]). This method can be used for the manufacture of medicated chewing gum and is particularly appropriate for drugs that exhibit poor release characteristics.

A unique method of medicated chewing gum manufacture is used for a nicotine containing chewing gum called Nicorette®. The first step in the manufacturing process of this product is the formation of a nicotine cation exchange complex. This is produced by stirring together a mixture of an ion exchanger and nicotine. The loaded ion exchanger is called nicotine polacrilex and is separated from the mixture by filtration. The second step is to place the gum base into a hot kettle which has been fitted with stirrers. After the base has melted, a quantity of powdered sugar and corn syrup are added and the whole mass is mixed. Finally a second quantity of powdered sugar, which had previously been mixed with the nicotine polacrilex, is added to the molten mixture in the kettle and the contents thoroughly mixed. When mixing is complete the chewing gum is extruded and cut into pieces [6].

V. IN VITRO AND IN VIVO ASSESSMENT OF CHEWING GUM

A. Adhesion and Effects of Chewing Gum on Teeth

There is no official method or apparatus to evaluate the adhesion of chewing gum to teeth or to assess adverse effects of chewing gum on the teeth. Chewing gum seems to display minimal adhesion properties to teeth enamel, however, certain additives such as fillers can cause problems to some denture materials.

A mastication device was designed by Kleber et al [10] to evaluate the physical and chemical effects of chewing gum on the teeth. Chewing gum containing different particle sizes of zirconium silicate (0.6-2 μm) were examined to evaluate their polishing effect on ox enamel mounted in the mastication device. The use of zirconium silicate containing chewing gum resulted in highly polished teeth, results which were in contrast to those seen using a commercial chewing gum which contained no polishing agent. The authors also used their mastication device to study the effect of different chewing gums on enamel solubility and dentine abrasion. A large reduction in enamel solubility was observed following the use of fluoride containing chewing gum indicating a reaction between fluoride and enamel had taken place during mastication. Zirconium silicate incorporated in the size of 30 μm in chewing gum was shown to abrade dentine. When tested in vivo the silicate was detectable by the chewer as grit in the gum. In contrast commercially available chewing gum which contained calcium carbonate as a filler did not physically abrade the dentine.

It is evident from these (limited) results that the chewing of gum may have an effect on the teeth. These effects would be dependent on the physical and/or chemical properties of the additives or drug included in the formulation. Such effects should be evaluated during the development of a medicated chewing gum.

B. Release of Drug

1. In Vitro Methodology and Apparatus for Assessing Drug Release From Chewing Gum

There is no official method to evaluate the release of drug from chewing gum, but several different methods have been described in literature.

The first apparatus for studying the release of drug from chewing gum, the *"Masticator M 66"*, was reported in 1973 [11], however, the details of its design were not described.

In a patent from 1989 [12] an apparatus to test the release of drug from chewing gum is described. It consists of a vertical releasable container and a first jaw fixed in the lower end of the container. A second jaw facing the first jaw is vertically movable and rotatable and was designed to subject the sample to both compression and shearing forces. The apparatus includes a means for driving the second jaw and for controlling the temperature of the liquid medium in the container. It has had only limited use.

Christrup and Møller [13] tried to use the device developed by Kleber et al [10] to determine the release of drug from chewing gum but found the device to be inconvenient. Their experiences prompted them to design a new chewing machine which is shown in Figures 1 and 2. The machine consists of a temperature controlled reservoir for the dissolution medium and two pistons. During one chewing cycle, the pistons, one on each side, move towards each

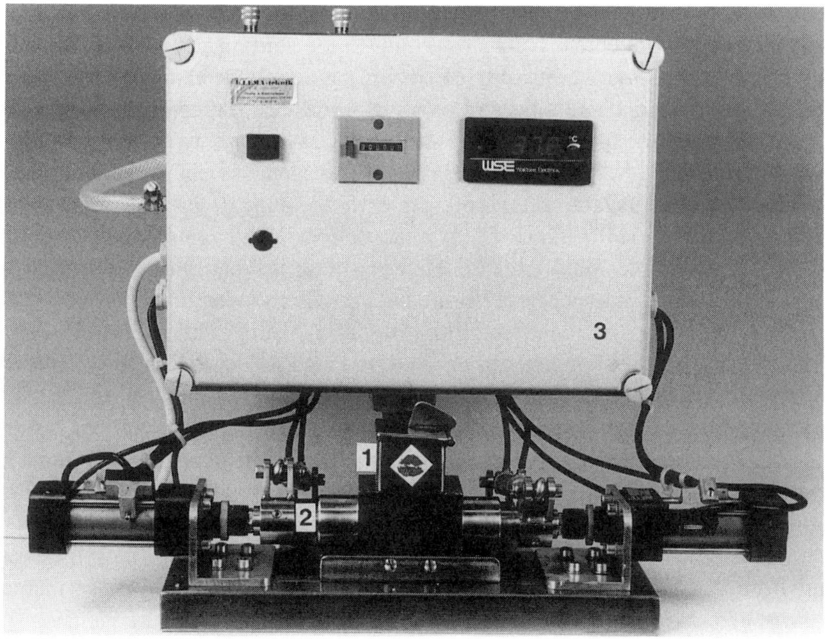

Figure 1. Chewing machine constructed by Christrup and Møller [13] showing dissolution medium reservoir (1), pistons (2) and thermostat and regulator of the rate of chewing cycle (3).

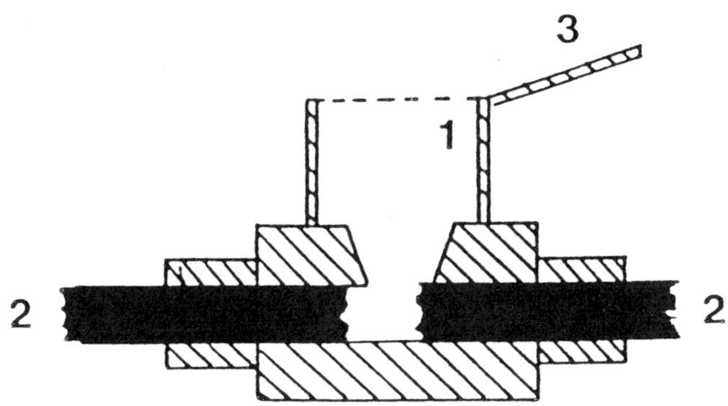

Figure 2. A cross-sectional diagram of the release chamber of the chewing machine constructed by Christrup and Møller [13]. A piece of chewing gum is placed in the reservoir (1), the dissolution medium (10-25 mL) is added and the lid (3) put on. The pistons (2) which move against each other then back to the starting point are driven by compressed air. The normally used frequency is 60 cycles each minute. Samples are taken at specified time intervals from the reservoir and analyzed for drug content.

other. When they meet they press the chewing gum between them and then make a twisting movement before returning to the starting point. To perform a drug release test, a known quantity of chewing gum is placed in the dissolution medium reservoir and pressing and twisting forces are transmitted to the gum via the pistons. At specified time intervals, a sample is removed from the reservoir and the quantity of drug released is determined. The cycle rate (chewing rate) is usually set at 60 per minute, and 20 mL of dissolution medium equilibrated to 37°C are typical volumes and temperatures of the dissolution medium. Many release studies on drugs exhibiting a range of aqueous solubilities have been performed using this chewing machine.

The apparatus designed by Christrup and Møller [13] has now been developed further to allow experiments to be performed which allow 6 pieces of chewing gum to be evaluated at the same time [14]. In addition to the two horizontal pistons, the chewing chambers are supplied with a vertical piston working staggered to the horizontal pistons. This ensures that the gum is always positioned in the right place during the mastication process. No results using the new apparatus have yet been published.

A further apparatus which has been developed to measure the release of drug from chewing gum is shown in Figure 3 [15]. One cycle of the piston consists of one upward and one downward stroke, with cycle frequencies of 7.5-30 every minute. Simultaneously, the plunger constantly rotates during the experiment at 10 to 40 rpm. The ribs allow for circulation of the dissolution medium which is normally 500 mL of purified water equilibrated to 37°C. A rotation speed of 20 rpm and a cycle frequency of 30 cycles/minute were found to give release rates similar to those observed in vivo. The only published data using this machine determines the release of the water soluble agent phenylpropanolamine hydrochloride [15]. Although the authors found a good correlation between the in vitro release rate and the quantity of drug released during an in vivo chewing study, more experiments are needed, particularly those which investigate the release of slightly water soluble drugs, before the machine can be considered fully evaluated.

When comparing the different mastication devices the one developed by Rider et al [15] seems to operate well but more data is needed. The apparatus of Christrup and Møller [13] has been used in many studies with different formulations of chewing gum containing drugs of a wide range of aqueous solubilities. In general the results have shown a high correlation between in vitro and in vivo release data. The latest device that has been developed seems promising, efficient and easy to operate [14]. The fact that 6 pieces of chewing gum can be examined at the same time is advantageous as it provides more results at a faster rate compared to the other devices. In addition, the data obtained with this apparatus would be expected to be more reproducible than the results obtained with the original apparatus developed by Christrup and Møller because of the additional vertical piston that maintains the gum in the correct position.

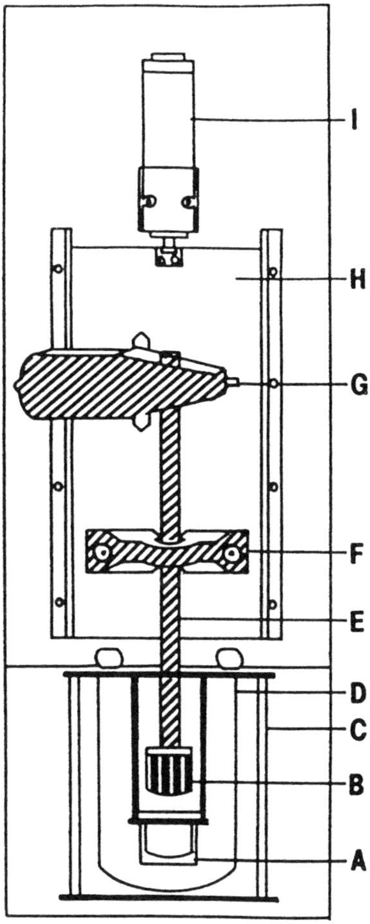

Figure 3. Chewing machine developed by Rider et al [15] to investigate the release of drugs from chewing gum. The machine comprises a Teflon® base (A), Teflon® plunger (B), dissolution vessel support (C), USP dissolution vessel (D), stainless-steel shaft (E), pillow block (F), motor (G), Teflon® plate (H) and piston (I). The plunger rotates constantly (20 rpm) and simultaneously moves up and down usually at 30 cycles each minute.

2. Factors Affecting Release

Several factors have been shown to affect release of drug from chewing gum. The major determinants include the chewing time, chewing rate, aqueous solubility of the drug and the composition of the chewing gum.

a. *Chewing Time and Rate*

Barabolak et al [16] performed a study to identify how people use chewing gum. They employed a self-reporting questionnaire technique to determine the length of chewing time (in minutes) a person chewed a piece of gum. The results were based on 4064 respondents and have a bearing on the design of any release study. The mean chewing time per piece of gum was 36 minutes The authors suggested that when designing a clinical trial a chewing time of 30 minutes should be used if the results were to be extrapolated to ordinary use of chewing gum. However, by selecting a 20 minute chewing time the results would still be applicable to more than 80% of the population of (American) gum chewers.

The rate at which a subject chews gum also affects the amount of drug released. The average chewing rate is about 60 chews every minute. The release of nicotine from Nicorette® chewed at different rates has been investigated. A chewing rate of 1 chew every second, gave a significantly ($p<0.05$) higher release than a chewing rate of 1 chew every 8 seconds [17].

b. *Aqueous Solubility of the Drug*

Table 2 documents the studies which have been performed that examine the effect of aqueous solubility on drug release from chewing gum. Based on the results of these studies, and other chewing gum release studies in general, one can generalize as to the effect of the drugs aqueous solubility on its release from chewing gum. They indicate that the release of water soluble drugs (aqueous solubility greater than 1:10) is, in general, about 75% or more during 5 minutes of chewing, and 90% or more during 15 minutes of chewing at a rate of 60 chews per minute. Drugs with aqueous solubility between 1:10 and 1:300 demonstrate up to 60% release during 10 minutes of chewing and between 50 and 90% when the gum is chewed for 15 minutes. The release of a drug which is only slightly water soluble can only be expected to be small (less than 5%) even if the gum is chewed for 30 minutes.

c. *Percentage of Drug and Mass of Piece*

The release of fluoride from a piece of chewing gum (1 g) containing 0.1 mg and 1.0 mg sodium fluoride (aqueous solubility 1:25) has been compared [20]. Figure 8 shows that the percentage of drug retained in the gum for the two formulations are similar. Indeed the percentage released for the 0.1 mg and 1.0 mg fluoride gum are very similar after 8 minutes at 75% and 80% respectively.

These results are in contrast to those of Christrup and Rassing [24] who showed that an increase in the quantity of salicylamide (slightly soluble in

Table 2. Effect of Aqueous Solubility on Drug Release from Chewing Gum.

Ref.	Drug studied	Aqueous solubility	Percent released (mins of mastication)	Comments
11	Sodium acid phosphate	1:1		For 5 of the drugs the inverse ratio of the release was dependent upon the water solubility of the drug (Figure 4). Calcium gluconate did not follow this general pattern and may have formed a complex with the sweetwner (sucrose).
	L-ascorbic acid	1:3.5		
	Sodium bicarbonate	1:11		
	Amidopyrine	1:18		
	Calcium gluconate	1:30		
	Acetylsalicylic acid	1:300		
18	Noscapine hydrochloride	1:4	78% (5 min)	Release has been studied in vitro (Figure 5) and in vivo (Figure 6). In both cases the fastest release was observed with the drug that was most water soluble.
	Noscapine embonate	1:10000	23% (5 min)	
	Noscapine	sws[a]	8% (5 min)	
19	Hydrocortisone sodium succinate	1:300	95.2% (15 min)	Release of the lipophilic steroids was poor. In contrast the release of the chemically similar, but more water soluble, steroid was rapid and complete (see Figure 7)
	Progesterone	piw[b]	2.2% (15 min)	
	Hydrocortisone	piw[b]	10.2% (15 min)	
	Hydrocortisone hemisuccinate	piw[b]	18.9% (15 min)	
15	Phenylpropanolamine hydrochloride	1:2	75% (5 min) 90% (15 min)	Rapid and complete release was observed
20	Sodium fluoride	1:25	80-90% (10-15 min)	Rapid release was observed by both these investigators.
21	Sodium fluoride	1:25	22% (2 min) 68% (5 min) 94% (10 min)	The slightly higher results of Bruun and Givskov [21] may have been due to differences in the formulations.
22	Chlorhexidine acetate	1:55	40% (5 min) 65% (15 min)	
4	Acetylsalicylic acid	1:300	53.7% (5 min) 66.1% (15 min)	Only a small increase in drug released was observed following a further 15 min of chewing (69.2% after 30 min).
23	Sulfathiazole	1:1060	12-57% (60 min)	

[a]Slightly soluble in water. [b]piw - practically insoluble in water.

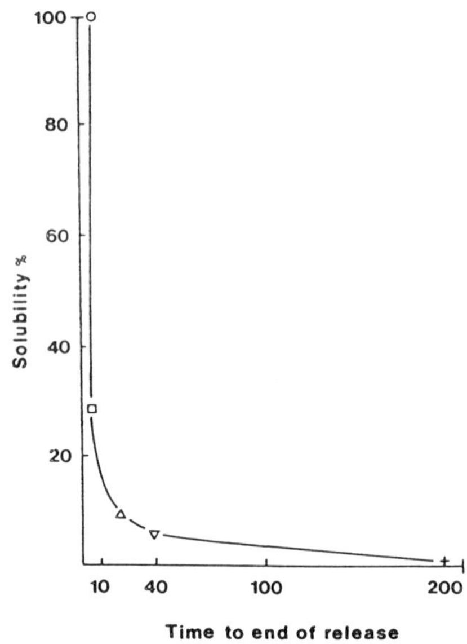

Figure 4. Relationship between aqueous solubility and time to end of release from chewing gum determined in vitro for sodium acid phosphate (O), vitamin C (□), sodium bicarbonate (Δ), amidopyrine (∇) and aspirin (+). Release medium was distilled water maintained at 37°C. (From reference 11).

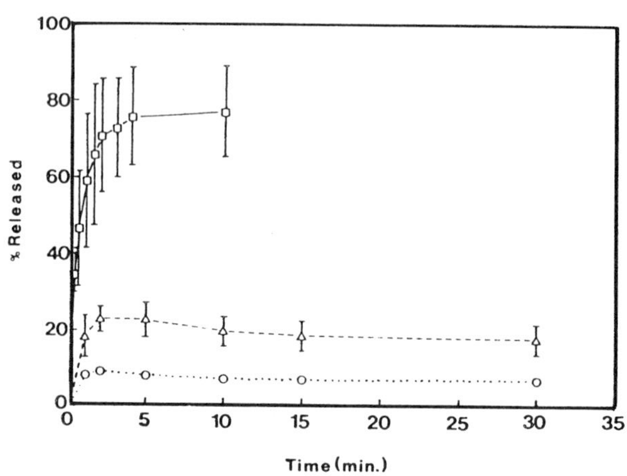

Figure 5. Release of noscapine from chewing gum determined in vitro (60 chewing cycles each minute) using the chewing machine constructed by Christrup and Møller [13]. The release medium was 30 mL phosphate buffer pH 6.9. Samples were removed at specified time intervals and replaced with an equivalent volume of medium. Noscapine hydrochloride (25 mg/1.2 g) at 25°C (n = 5) (□), noscapine embonate (50 mg/1.2 g) at 37°C (n = 5) (Δ) and noscapine base (50 mg/1.2 g) at 37°C (n = 3) (O). Noscapine in the gum residue was extracted and determined by HPLC. Each point shows mean ± SD. (From reference 18).

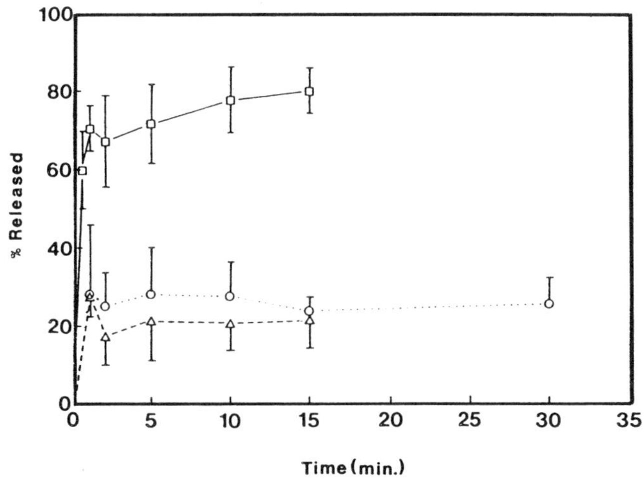

Figure 6. Release of noscapine from chewing gum determined in vivo in healthy volunteers. Noscapine hydrochloride (25 mg/1.2 g, n = 5) (□), noscapine embonate (50 mg/1.2 g, n = 5) (O) and noscapine base (50 mg/1.2 g, n = 3) (Δ). Noscapine in the gum residue was extracted and determined by HPLC. Each point shows mean ± SD. (From reference 18).

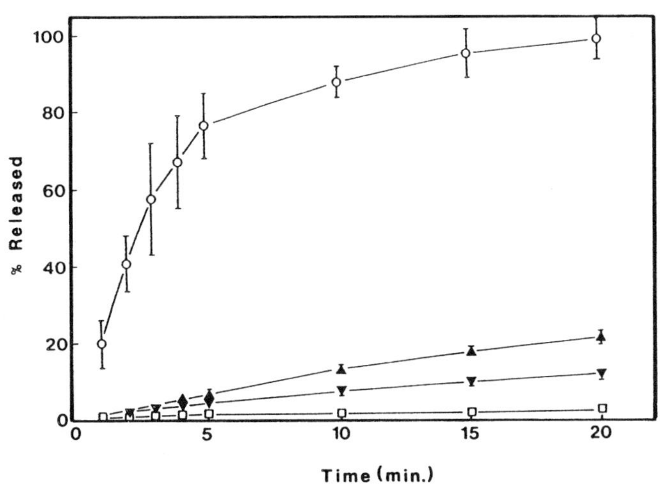

Figure 7. Release of four steroids from chewing gum determined in vitro (60 chewing cycles each minute) using the chewing machine constructed by Christrup and Møller [13]. The release medium was 20 mL distilled water (37°C) from which 3 mL samples were removed at specified time intervals and replaced with an equivalent volume of distilled water. Hydrocortisone sodium succinate (2 pieces of chewing gum 13 mg/800 mg), (O) hydrocortisone (2 pieces of chewing gum 8 mg/800 mg) (▲), hydrocortisone hemisuccinate (2 pieces of chewing gum 10 mg/800 mg) (▼), and progesterone (2 pieces of chewing gum, 5 mg/800 mg) (□). (From reference 19).

Table 3. Composition of Chewing Gum Formulations Investigated by Christrup and Rassing. (From Reference 24).

Formular number[a]	Mass per piece (mg)	Salicyclamide content (mg)	Content of gum base A (%)	Percent released after 15 minutes
1	900	100	30	19.1
14	900	200	30	
6	3000	100	30	23.4
7	3000	200	30	15.2
8	900	100	24	22.2
13	900	200	24	15.9
4	900	100	45	24.8
9	900	100	20	26.6

[a]Refers to the formular number allocated in original reference [24].

water) in a piece of chewing gum of the same composition and weight decreased the percentage released (compare formular numbers 6 and 7, and 8 and 13; Table 3).

The release of nystatin (slightly soluble in water) incorporated in increasing amounts (2.8%-11.1%) was studied in vitro using the chewing machine of Christrup and Møller [13]. Results showed a decrease in the percentage released with increasing amounts of drug (Figure 9) [25]. The released nystatin existed partly dissolved and partly suspended in the release medium.

Benowitz et al [26] reported a release of 53% for the 2 mg nicotine polacrilex chewing gum and 72% for the 4 mg nicotine polacrilex chewing gum. Although the subjects were instructed to chew slowly and steadily for 2 minutes the interindividual variation in percent released was large. In another study investigating nicotine polacrilex chewing gum, pieces containing 2 mg, 4 mg and 8 mg nicotine complex were chewed at a rate of one chew every 3 seconds for 20 minutes with the subjects limiting swallowing to once every minute or so to allow more time for nicotine absorption via the buccal mucosa. The release of nicotine from the chewing gums containing 2 mg, 4 mg and 8 mg nicotine complex was 51%, 59% and 65%, respectively. Such results have implications for patients using this chewing gum since a reduced quantity of swallowed nicotine diminishes the uncomfortable gastrointestinal effects of hiccups and nausea associated with this drug [27]. The slight difference between the two studies investigating nicotine polacrilex chewing gums may reflect different chewing conditions employed in the studies.

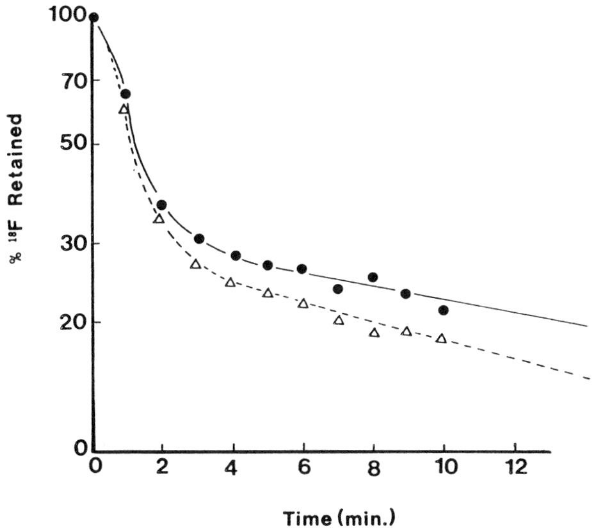

Figure 8. Retained ^{18}F in chewing gum when sodium fluoride chewing gum was chewed by trained volunteers at a constant rate. Key: 0.1 mg F (●) and 1 mg F (Δ). (From reference 20).

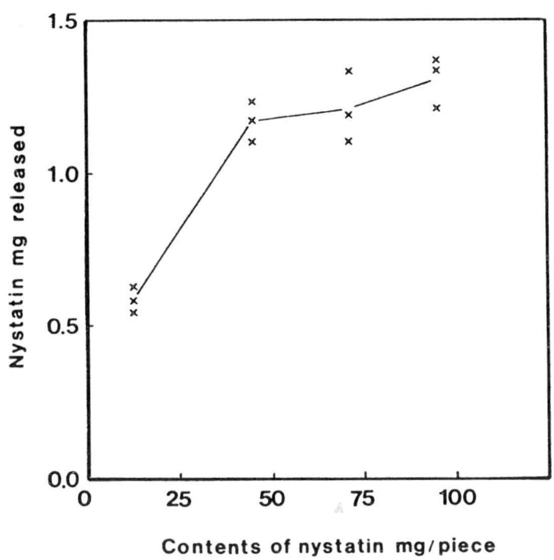

Figure 9. Release of nystatin in vitro using the chewing machine (60 chewing cycles each minute) constructed by Christrup and Møller [13] from different chewing gums as a function of the content of drug in each piece (900 mg). The release medium (phosphate buffer: 10 mL, pH 7.4, 37°C) was removed and replaced with fresh buffer every 2 minutes for 30 minutes. The content of nystatin was determined spectrophotometrically at 323 nm. (From reference 25).

The physical and chemical characteristics of the four drugs (sodium fluoride, salicylamide, nystatin and nicotine bound to an ion exchange resin) which were investigated in these studies are very different. A tentative conclusion that may be drawn from these studies is that an increase in the percentage of a moderate to slightly water soluble drug in chewing gum might reduce the rate of release, while an increase in the percentage of a drug which is freely soluble in water has little or no effect on the rate of release.

The effect of gum mass per piece of chewing gum on the release of incorporated drug has not been studied extensively. However, Table 3 shows that when one compares the release of salicylamide (100 mg) from a piece of gum weighing 3 g with a piece weighing 900 mg (formular number 6 and 8 or formular number 7 and 13; Table 3) the increase in the mass of gum per piece has little or no effect on the percentage of drug released. It should be noted however, that the mastication force required to work a large piece of gum is less than that required to work a small piece.

d. Composition of Chewing Gum

The influence of gum base mass on drug release has been investigated using salicylamide as a model substance [24] (see Table 3). When salicylamide was incorporated into a chewing gum which contained a relatively large percentage of gum base (formular number 4; Table 3) the release after 30 minutes of chewing was significantly lower (25.6%) compared to a gum in which less gum base was present (52.0% - formular number 9; Table 3).

The release of nicotine from two different chewing gum formulations has also been studied. The solid complex of nicotine bound to a cation exchanger, nicotine polacrilex, was incorporated into different chewing gum compositions, two of which are shown in Tables 4 and 5.

Two subjects were instructed to periodically chew gently leaving the gum against the inside of the cheek between chews. The average quantity of nicotine released from the two formulations is shown in Table 6.

The release of nicotine from the two very different formulations was almost identical. For both formulae, a very pronounced feeling of smoking was reported [6]. Note that the physicochemical properties of the two bases were not reported in the original publication.

VI. INCREASED RELEASE

Many of the drugs used today are lipophilic in nature. Lipophilic drugs are partially soluble in the gum bases. Consequently they exhibit a slow release rate from chewing gum and only a small percentage of the total amount of drug incorporated is released even following prolonged chewing times. For such

Table 4. Formular 1, a Sugar Containing Formular Containing 20 mg Amberlite IRP 64M Resin Complexed With Nicotine Base (20% by Weight Nicotine) and 1 g Chewing Gum Mass.

Ingredients	Weight (%)
Natural gum base	22.0
Powdered sugar	64.0
Corn syrup 45 grader Baume	14.0

Table 5. Formular 2, a Sugar Free Formular Containing 20 mg Amberlite IRP 64M Resin Complexed With Nicotine Base (20% by Weight Nicotine) and 3 g Chewing Gum Mass.

Ingredients	Weight (%)
Synthetic gum base	73.7
Powdered sorbitol	19.8
70% Sorbitol solution	3.8
Glycerin	0.7
Flavoring oil	2.0

Table 6. Average Quantity of Nicotine Released From the Two Formulations.

Time (minute)	Formular 1 (% released)	Formular 2 (% released)
2	18	18
5	36	39
10	61	65
20	91	92

drugs it may be necessary to develop methods which increase the release rate and extent of release from chewing gum. Methods for increasing the rate and extent of drugs from chewing gum are discussed in this section.

A. Addition of Buffering Agents

Pack et al [28, 29] proposed that local application of folic acid might be beneficial to patients suffering from gingivitis and suggested chewing gum as a delivery system for folic acid. Three different chewing gum formulations of the slightly water soluble B-vitamin, folic acid (5 mg/piece) were formulated in an attempt to increase the release of folic acid by modifying its solubility in saliva. Formulation A contained sodium bicarbonate (11 mg/piece), formulation B contained both sodium bicarbonate and sodium carbonate (5.5 mg and 6.9 mg/piece, respectively) and formulation C was formulated without the addition of any buffering agents. Both the in vitro (Figure 10) and in vivo release of folic acid from formulations A and B were significantly higher than its release from formulation C. The release profile of folic acid from both formulation A and B was considered satisfactory for its intended purpose [30].

The principle of using acidic/basic substances to enhance the release of incorporated drug from chewing gum was also investigated by Emslie et al [20] who measured the amount of fluoride retained in chewing gum in which two different acids and a basic substance were added. In contrast to the work of Pack et al these authors found that following the addition of 2% citric acid the release of fluoride decreased (Figure 11). This may have been due to the citric acid interacting with the polymers in the chewing gum. Following the addition of 0.5% phosphoric acid to the chewing gum formulation a similar release rate to that of when no acidic substances were added to the formulation was observed (Figure 11). In contrast the addition of 5% calcium carbonate to the formulation was shown to enhance the release of fluoride from the gum (Figure 11). This effect was the opposite to the decrease in release that was expected to be observed following the formation of the less soluble CaF_2.

B. Coating with Hydrophilic Gum

To enhance the release of the slightly water soluble drug nystatin Witzel et al coated particles of finely divided drug with Arabic gum [31]. When uncoated drug was incorporated into chewing gum a release of only 4% was observed in vivo in a panel of 5 subjects. This amount increased to 24% when coated drug was incorporated into the gum.

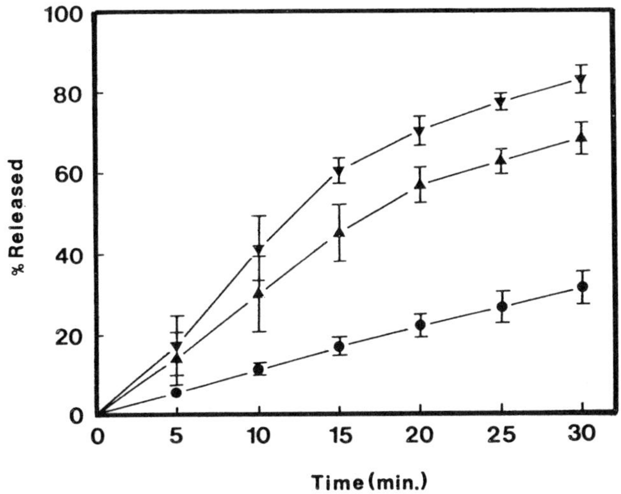

Figure 10. Release of folic acid from chewing gum (5 mg/piece) determined in vitro (60 chewing cycles each minute) using the chewing machine constructed by Christrup and Møller [13]. The release medium (phosphate buffer: pH 7.4, 37°C) was changed every 5th minute. Folic acid chewing gum (●), with 11 mg/piece sodium bicarbonate (▼), and with 5.5 mg/piece sodium bicarbonate (▲). The quantity of folic acid in the medium was analyzed by HPLC. Each point represents the mean ± SD (n = 3). (From reference 30).

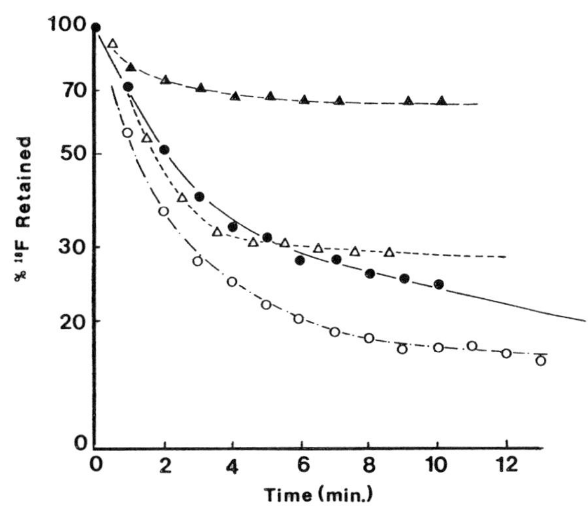

Figure 11. Retained ^{18}F in chewing gum when sodium fluoride chewing gum with different buffering substances was chewed by trained volunteers at a constant chewing rate. Key: 0.1 mg F (▲), 0.1 mg F + 2% citric acid (Δ), 0.1 mg F + 0.5% phosphoric acid (●), 0.1 mg F + 5% calcium phosphate (O). (From reference 20).

C. Solubilizing Agents

The effect of the addition of various solubilizing agents to a chewing gum formulation on release rate has been studied for a number of drugs including nystatin, miconazole, metronidazole and propranolol hydrochloride [25, 32-33].

1. Nystatin

Anderson et al [25] studied the effect of adding various nonionic surfactants on the release of nystatin (slightly water soluble) from chewing gum. The solubilizing agents investigated were the nonionic surfactants Cremophor® RH 40, Tween®60 and Panodan®AB 90. Nystatin and the surfactant were mixed together in a ratio of 1:1 prior to incorporation into the chewing gum base. The in vitro release rate of nystatin in the presence of each of the surfactants increased dramatically compared to a piece of gum in which nystatin was formulated on its own. The quantity of released drug was observed to increase by a factor of 50-70 with up to 95% of the incorporated drug being released (Figure 12).

The addition of a surfactant to the chewing gum formulation [25] promoted a far higher release of nystatin than the coating process described by Witzel et al (see above) [31].

2. Miconazole

The antifungal drug, miconazole (slightly water soluble) is used for the treatment of oral candidiasis. Miconazole chewing gum co-formulated with the different anionic surfactants Panodan® (diacetyl tartaric acid esters of mono- and diglycerides of vegetable fats), and Acidan® (a citric acid ester of monoglyceride of vegetable oil) has been investigated [32]. A detackifying agent, polyethylene glycol (PEG) 6000, was also included in the formulation. The in vitro release of miconazole from chewing gum containing 5% Panodan and 5% PEG 6000 was several times higher than from chewing gum containing pure miconazole. During mastication in vivo for 30 minutes approximately 7% of the incorporated miconazole was released from this formulation. When the gum was chewed for 120 minutes by two persons the release was 15.8% and 14.3%. The miconazole chewing gum formulation was later further tested in healthy volunteers and salivary concentration of miconazole were determined. It was found that the salivary concentrations achieved during chewing of the gum formulation were comparable with the salivary concentrations obtained when 5 mL of a 2% miconazole preparation (Daktarin®, Janssen) was ingested by healthy subjects [34]. Furthermore it was reported that miconazole was

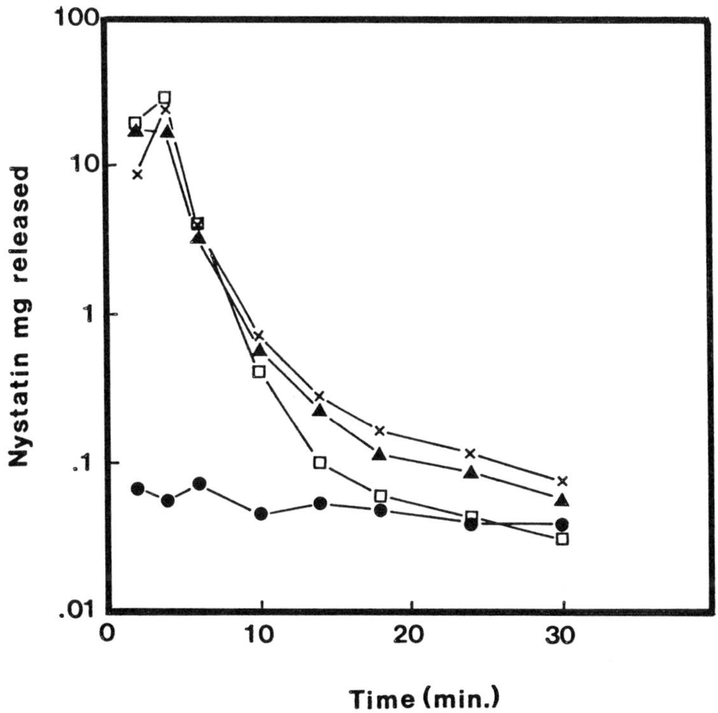

Figure 12. Release of nystatin from chewing gum determined in vitro (60 chewing cycles each minute) using the chewing machine constructed by Christrup and Møller [13]. The release medium (phosphate buffer: 10 mL, pH 7.4, 37°C) was replaced by a fresh 10 mL of buffer every 2 minutes. Nystatin 61.3 mg (●), nystatin 58.2 mg + Cremophor® RH 40 (▲), nystatin 58.7 mg + Tween® 60 (×) and nystatin 58.8 mg + Panodan® AB 90 (□). The ratio of nystatin to solubilizing agents was 1:1. The concentration of nystatin was determined spectrophotometrically at 323 nm [25].

detectable in saliva 450 minutes after the subjects had stopped chewing and expelled the gum [32].

3. Metronidazole and Propranolol Hydrochloride

The hydrophilic agents glycerol and Span® 20 were added to metronidazole (slightly water soluble) and propranolol hydrochloride (aqueous solubility 1:20) chewing gum in order to determine their effect on release [33]. The release was determined in vitro using the apparatus of Christrup and Møller [13]. However, the addition of these additives gave the opposite effect than what was expected; the release of these drugs was retarded in the presence of the additives. An explanation of the results could be that the additives increased the affinity of the drug for the chewing gum base, changed the gum base/water partition coefficient and, consequently, the release rate decreased.

It can be concluded that by testing the addition of different solubilizing agents to chewing gum, it will often be possible to find an agent that substantially increases the release.

D. Solid Dispersion

Pedersen et al [35] investigated several solid dispersions of miconazole in chewing gum. The tested carriers included polyethyleneglycol 6000 (PEG), polyvinylpyrrolidone (PVP), xylitol and carbamide. Different solid dispersions of the drug and carriers were formulated to contain different proportions of drug. The preparations were made either by pounding a mixture of miconazole and the carrier or by a molten, or precipitation, method. The solid dispersion of miconazole in PEG 6000 increased the release rate to a large extent over the first few minutes of mastication. To further modify the release profile of miconazole lecithin was added to the formulation. This resulted in an extended release profile (Figure 13). The solid dispersion principle might be a useful approach for other slightly water soluble drugs.

VII. SUSTAINED RELEASE OF DRUGS

Drugs with a high aqueous solubility are released rapidly from conventional chewing gum. Very few methods have been documented in the literature which reduce the release rate of drugs from medicated chewing gum. One example, however, is the principle of binding a drug to an ion exchange resin to decrease the release of nicotine. In contrast, many different principles have been used in the confectionery industry to reduce the release rate of flavors and sweeteners from chewing gum. Some of the principles are reported in this article to provide ideas which might be useful in the formulation of medicated chewing gum.

A. The Formulation of Chewing Gum

1. Particle Size of the Drug

A reduction of the particle size of an incorporated ingredient might be a valuable approach to retard the release of that substance from chewing gum.

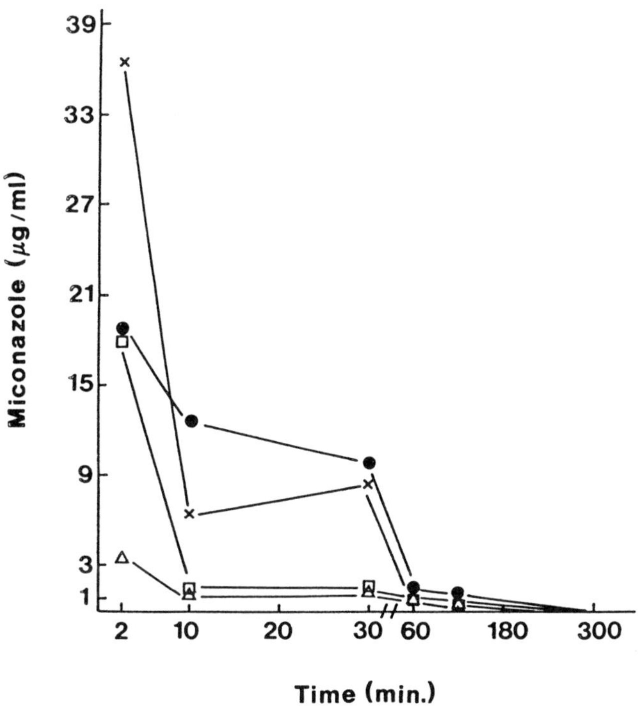

Figure 13. Release of miconazole from chewing gum determined in vivo (results expressed as average saliva miconazole concentrations from six volunteers). Chewing time was 30 minutes with the rate of chewing individualized. Each piece of gum contained 50 mg miconazole; pure miconazole (Δ), 20:80 solid dispersion miconazole:PEG 6000 ( ), 20:80 solid dispersion miconazole:PEG 6000 + lecithin 50 mg (⊞) and pure miconazole + lecithin 50 mg (●). The saliva concentrations of miconazole were determined by HPLC [35].

Reduction of the particle size of the sweetener saccharin acid prior to its incorporation in chewing gum resulted in decreased release rate [36]. As a result the bitter taste associated with saccharin was reduced, and the sweet taste of the chewing gum was reported to last for between 30-60 minutes. The reason forwarded for the prolonged release profile was that the sweetener was protected from contact with saliva by the gum base, and the effect of this protection was greater than the potential increase in dissolution rate due to the increased surface area of the saccharin acid. Consequently the particle size giving the optimal release has to be determined during the development of a medicated chewing gum.

2. *Drug-Ion Exchange Complex*

Nicotine is a liquid with a boiling point of 247°C, basic in nature with a pKa of 3.12 and 8.02 and is freely soluble in water. At pH 7.5, less than 30% of nicotine exists in the absorbable unionized form. When nicotine is incorporated into ordinary gum compositions, its release occurs rapidly [37]. Such a release profile is, however, undesirable for its clinical use which requires that release from a nicotine chewing gum formulated as a smoking substitute should be uniform and last for at least 20 minutes. In addition the released nicotine should produce a "feeling of smoking" not only following absorption but also in the mouth. Several attempts have been made to fulfill these requirements. Nicotine has been incorporated into chewing gum as a base, in the form of different salts, and adsorbed or absorbed, onto or into, different materials such as silicic acid, amorphous silica and bentonite, all without success. However, in July 1970 a patent was taken out by Lichtneckert [6] describing tobacco alkaloids bound to a cation exchanger containing functional carboxylic or sulfonic groups. The cation exchanger used in the marketed Nicorette® chewing gum is Amberlite IRP 64M, a weak acidic methacrylic acid polymer and the nicotine complex product is referred to as nicotine polacrilex. The method of manufacture of nicotine polacrilex and Nicorette® has been described in a previous section (Section IV).

3. *Coating and Embedding*

Different coating principles and different coating agents such as polyvinylpyrrolidone and cellulose compounds have been used in order to obtain a prolonged release of flavors and sweeteners from chewing gum (amongst others [38, 39, 40]). Embedding a drug in a hydrophobic matrix consisting of lecithin, synthetic waxes or mixtures thereof reduced the release rate of a sweetener from chewing gum [41].

A process in which an agent was embedded in gradual release fibers, made by an extrusion technique of a polymer such as polyvinylacetate was used to prolong the release of aspartamine from chewing gum [42].

Broderick et al [43] combined embedding of a sweetener in water-insoluble porous beads of a copolymer of divinylbenzene and styrene with coating of the beads with a water soluble agent such as hydroxypropyl methylcellulose, or water insoluble agents such as shellac and waxes.

The methods described above could, in principle, also be appropriate to decrease the release rate of a drug from medicated chewing gum. However some of these methods are rather complicated and no experience with such methods has yet been published as far as medicated chewing is concerned. For a more detailed review of this subject the reader is referred to reference [44].

4. *Adsorption*

The last principle to be mentioned here is the adsorption principle combined with an embedding technique. A flavor was adsorbed onto an adsorbing material such as silica which was then dispersed throughout a thermoplastic material such as cellulose-2-hydroxypropyl-ether. The release rate of the flavor was reduced to 20% during 20 minutes of mastication compared to 35% for the conventional chewing gum formulation [45].

More experience would be needed to be able to recommend one of the above mentioned principles over another to obtain a well controlled sustained release rate of a drug from medicated chewing gum and to simultaneously avoid stability and formulation problems.

B. The Manufacturing Process

The manufacturing process can also affect the release rate of a drug from a chewing gum formulation and may be a viable method with which to prolong the release profile of a drug.

Salicylamide has been incorporated into chewing gum by mixing it with the hydrophilic components of the base, and by mixing it with the hydrophobic components of the base. It was shown that the release of salicylamide from the latter formular was slower than from the former [24].

It is also known that the use of a more hydrophobic gum base as opposed to a hydrophilic gum base often results in a decreased release rate of any incorporated drug, and for lipophilic drugs an increase in the total amount of drug released as well, which is due to a higher base/water partition coefficient.

VIII. CLINICAL EVALUATION

A. Non-medicated Effects

Before discussing the effect of medicated chewing gum (particularly that used for dental health) it is pertinent to draw attention to the physiological effects of masticating non-medicated chewing gum. The chewing of gum will stimulate the flow of saliva which will lead to an increase in the pH and buffering capacity, and supersaturation of the oral fluids which in turn beneficially affects the balance between enamel demineralization and remineralization in early caries [46]. Several studies have provided evidence for the beneficial effect of chewing gum on dental health. Fröhlich et al [47] found the stimulating effect of sucrose or sorbitol sweetened gum and paraffin chewed for 20 minutes to result in a total saliva volume of 32.2 mL for sugar sweetened gum, 29.5 mL for sorbitol sweetened gum and 27.4 mL for paraffin compared to a resting volume of 7.4 mL (n = 4; 2 replications). The chewing of sugar free gum for 20 minutes after meals and snacks increased the remineralization in experimental caries-like lesions in human enamel particles carried in an intra-oral device. Subjects chewing sugared gum for as long as 30 minutes after meals and snacks also showed a significant enhancement in the remineralization potential of their saliva. However, this effect was not seen in subjects chewing sugared gum for only 20 minutes Subjects in the experimental groups used fluoride-containing toothpaste twice a day [48]. It seems obvious taking the average chewing time into consideration that the use of sugar free chewing gum after meals and snacks should be recommended. It is claimed that sugar free chewing gum containing xylitol has caries reducing properties. This has, however, never been proved.

B. Local Delivery

1. *Chlorhexidine*

The anti-plaque effect of chlorhexidine is well known. Chlorhexidine has, however, two disadvantages, a bitter taste and the fact that it in some individuals it stains the teeth, tongue and tooth colored fillings [49]. The anti-plaque effect of chlorhexidine chewing gum has been studied [50]. With chlorhexidine chewing gum the bitter taste is not so apparent and the possibility of counteracting the staining by the addition of oxidizing agents in the same chewing gum product exists. This was shown in a study where the anti-plaque effect of chlorhexidine acetate chewing gum (5 mg/800 mg piece), with and without urea hydrogen peroxide, was compared to a piece of gum base containing flavoring agents, but no active agent [51]. The results showed that both the chlorhexidine containing chewing gums completely inhibited the growth of plaque, while the placebo gum had no inhibitory effect.

A chlorhexidine chewing gum (5 mg/piece) is marketed. Its use is usually limited to high risk caries groups, e.g., xerostomia patients and only as a supplement to normal oral hygiene.

2. *Carbamide and Sodium Bicarbonate*

Carbamide is an active ingredient of saliva which is degraded in plaque to ammonia by urease produced by plaque bacteria. In a double blind cross-over study Birkhed [52] compared three commercial sugar free chewing gums on the recovery of plaque pH following a sucrose rinse. The gum contained either sorbitol, carbamide/sorbitol or sorbitol/xylitol. Following chewing for 10 minutes after expulsion of the rinse, all three of the gums equally increased plaque pH to between 6.5 and 6.7. The carbamide chewing gum demonstrated the highest pH value over the chewing gum period.

Another neutralizing agent, sodium bicarbonate, also a natural ingredient of saliva, is available on the market as a chewing gum. Because of the beneficial effects of carbamide or bicarbonate containing chewing gum on oral health their use after meals is recommended not only for healthy individuals but also for patients suffering from dry mouth.

3. *Sulfonamides*

Sulfonamides in chewing gum have been shown to provide a bacteriostatic salivary concentration for between 1-1½ hours [23, 53]. Chewing gum may have a potential as a delivery system for sulfonamides in the local treatment of infections in the oral cavity and as a supplement to systemic treatment of tonsillitis or pharyngitis.

4. *Fluoride*

In vitro and in vivo studies have documented a complex cariostatic action of fluoride; it reduces enamel solubility, acts directly on the remineralization process of enamel and influences the metabolic activity of dental plaque bacteria thereby causing a reduced acid production. Chewing gum as a vehicle for fluoride was investigated by Emslie et al in 1961 [20]. The authors observed a partial uptake of the released ^{18}F by dental enamel in caries free teeth of children. The uptake of fluoride in carious teeth and in teeth with gingival recession exposing their roots was much higher.

Ekstrand et al [54] investigated the effect of chewing fluoride containing gum (0.25 mg and 0.5 mg) on the pH change of dental plaque after using a mouth rinse containing 10% sucrose. Plaque pH increased without any change in the microbiological composition in the plaque which suggested that the change in pH was due to a change in the carbohydrate metabolic activity of the dental plaque bacteria. The concept of remineralization of enamel lesions has been supported by clinical studies (amongst others [55, 56]).

Bruun and Givskov [8] have demonstrated that saliva fluoride level has remained above baseline values for over 1 hour following the chewing of one or two sticks of fluoride (0.21 mg and 0.4 mg respectively) chewing gum for 10 minutes.

Chewing gum appears to be an ideal vehicle for the delivery of fluoride. It is convenient to administer, the dose is controllable and there is little likelihood

Chewing gum appears to be an ideal vehicle for the delivery of fluoride. It is convenient to administer, the dose is controllable and there is little likelihood of overdosage since the number of pieces of gum a person will chew is self limiting.

5. *Miconazole*

Miconazole containing chewing gum was investigated by Pedersen and Rassing [32] in a clinical trial using HIV-positive and HIV-negative patients with oral candidiasis. The therapeutic effect of the chewing gum was compared to a commercially available miconazole gel (Brentan® oral gel, Janssen) and shown to be identical. The patients who used chewing gum reported that the mode of administration was convenient and acceptable [34]. A stability problem concerning the surfactant that was included in the formulation has become apparent, however formulation studies which aim to optimize the gum composition are currently being undertaken.

IX. SYSTEMIC DELIVERY

There are several possible reasons for developing chewing gum as a dosage form for the delivery of drugs to the systemic circulation. The first is to improve bioavailability by delivering drugs via the oral mucosa. Since drugs absorbed via the oral mucosa directly enter the systemic circulation it may prove useful for drugs which undergo extensive first pass metabolism in the liver. The second is the formulation of a delivery system that is a convenient alternative to tablets and capsules. In this respect, although the delivery system is administered to and retained in the oral cavity, the drug is intended to be swallowed either dissolved or suspended in saliva and absorbed via the gastrointestinal tract.

A. Drugs Extensively Metabolized in the Liver

Several studies have shown that drugs which are subject to high first pass metabolism and which are well absorbed through the oral mucosa will, when administered in chewing gum, partly avoid metabolism in the gastrointestinal tract and in the liver. Several studies have shown that when drugs of this type are administered in chewing gum they will display greater bioavailability and this results in the possibility of administering a reduced dose. These studies are discussed below but it should not be assumed that the improved bioavailability is due exclusively to absorption through the oral mucosa, since the amount of drug entering the systemic circulation via this route cannot be accurately determined from the protocols used in the studies.

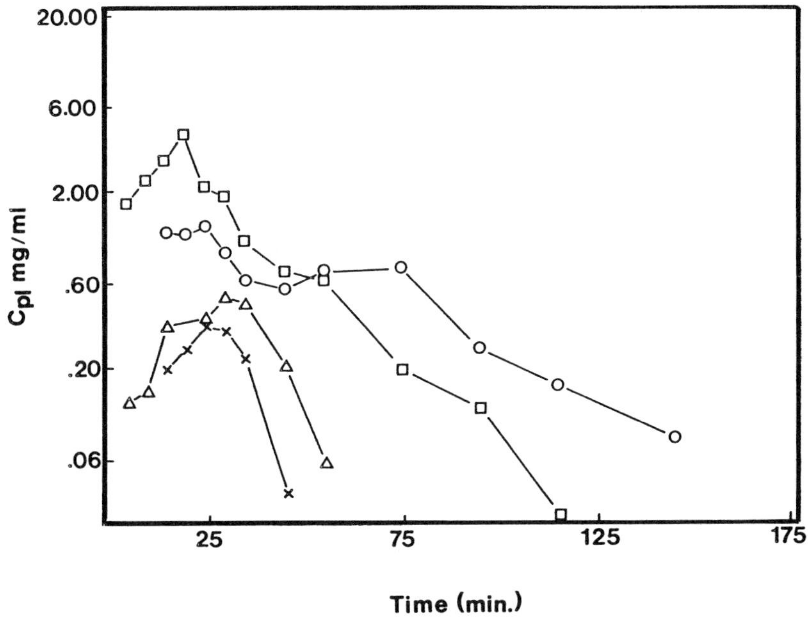

Figure 14. Plasma salicylamide concentration versus time curves obtained following administration of 400 mg salicylamide as an intravenous injection (□), 2000 mg salicylamide as a tablet (O), and 63 mg salicylamide as a chewing gum (X and Δ) to one subject on separate occasions [57].

1. Salicylamide

Christrup et al [57] used salicylamide as a model substance to determine whether a reduced first pass metabolism was observed following administration in chewing gum compared to a tablet. When salicylamide was given perorally, a dose greater than 500 mg needed to be administered to obtain a detectable salicylamide plasma concentration [58, 59]. When a piece of chewing gum (1000 mg salicyclamide) was chewed for 30 minutes between 50-300 mg salicylamide was released and after about 10 minutes a salicylamide plasma concentration of about 0.10 μg/mL was observed (Figure 14). The bioavailability of salicylamide given in tablets (dose = 2000 mg) was much higher than when given in chewing gum (dose = 63 mg). This was probably due to saturation of the metabolizing enzymes in the liver. The relative bioavailability of salicylamide (chewing gum to tablet) is probably not relevant due to the large difference between the dose and the aforementioned saturation phenomenon. However, the absolute bioavailability of salicylamide from chewing gum was estimated to be 30.0% (± 11.1% SD). It is interesting to note

Table 7. Pharmacokinetic Data Reported in the Study of Bouquet et al. (From Reference 61).

Formulation	T_{max} (hours)	$AUC_{0-\infty}$ (± SD) (μg/mL/hour)
Aspergum®	0.57 (± 0.02)	97.58 (± 12.37)
Asagum®	0.59 (± 0.04)	61.36 (± 9.37)
ASA tablets	1.14 (± 0.19)	165.82 (± 11.94)

that intersubject variation in the absolute bioavailability of salicylamide from the chewing gum was small.

2. *Acetylsalicylic Acid*

Woodford and Lesco [4] compared the bioavailability of acetylsalicylic acid (ASA) in chewing gum (Aspergum; 226.8 mg/piece) and an ASA tablet (324 mg/tablet). Volunteers chewed 3 pieces of gum for 15 minutes followed by a washout period of 7 days followed by the administration of two tablets with 120 mL of water. The amount of ASA absorbed was estimated from measurements of salicylic acid in the urine over a 24 hour period. 63.7% of the administered dose was released from the chewing gum after 15 minutes, 98.2% of which was recovered in the urine. The rate of absorption was fastest for the chewing gum formulation which lead the authors to conclude that chewing gum may be a useful dosage form for acetylysalicylic acid as its rate of onset may be faster than when administered in tablets.

In a second study the relative bioavailability of two formulations of acetylsalicylic acid chewing gums Aspergum® and Asagran® were compared with acetylsalicylic acid tablets (500 mg ASA) [60]. In the study the chewing gum (2 pieces) was chewed for 15 minutes. Table 7 shows the pharmacokinetic data reported in the study.

Table 7 shows a more rapid absorption for the gums than for the tablet. Whether the reason is absorption via the membranes that line the oral cavity, a more rapid absorption from the gastrointestinal tract due to swallowed acetylsalicylic acid reaching the gastrointestinal tract in a more readily available form i.e., dissolved in saliva, or both, was not investigated. The residual quantity of ASA in the chewing gum after the 15 minutes of chewing was not determined, however, using the average value for release of 64.9% ASA when chewing Aspergum® for 15 minutes [4], it can be estimated that the amount of acetylsalicylic released from the gum would be about 310 mg. Thus the relative AUC of Aspergum® to ASA tablet corrected for the amount of ASA released would be about 100%. There was a significant difference in

AUC between the two chewing gum formulations. This highlights the great importance of the chewing gum formulation in relation to the release of incorporated drugs.

3. *Verapamil*

The calcium blocker verapamil is susceptible to extensive first pass metabolism in the liver [61]. It is known that the metabolism is stereospecific and the more active L-isomer is converted to norverapamil. Comparison was made between the bioavailability of verapamil administered perorally in tablets (80 mg) and chewing gum (approximately 25 mg). The AUC mean ratio of verapamil:norverapamil was 0.8 following peroral administration and 1.5 following oral administration. This difference was statistically significant ($p<0.05$). Following administration in chewing gum, measurable concentrations of verapamil could be detected in plasma after 5 minutes, in contrast to 15 minutes when administered as tablets. The results indicate that following administration in chewing gum verapamil shows a more rapid absorption and a reduced first pass metabolism compared to a tablet [62]. A reduction in dose size is another advantage.

4. *Nicotine*

The quantity of nicotine in chewing gum sufficient to provide a sense of smoking sensation varies from person to person, but generally it is between 1-10 mg calculated as nicotine base [63]. Mastication of the nicotine chewing gum described by Lichtneckert [6] resulted in a salivary pH of between 3 and 5 during the release period. The argument for impelling this pH value was that the released nicotine should elicit a burning sensation, which the smoker was supposed to react to in a positive way. In clinical trials it was, however, later discovered that the bioavailability of nicotine was low, and the burning effect when using the acidic nicotine chewing gum formulation was too strong [37]. The low bioavailability was probably the result of a large fraction of nicotine being swallowed and therefore being subjected to first pass metabolism before entering the systemic circulation [64]. The addition of water soluble buffering agents such as alkali carbonates, hydrocarbonates or phosphates, resulted in a salivary pH value of above 7.5 (usually between 8-10). This improved the bioavailability of nicotine by a factor of 2.5, the taste was improved and the irritating burning sensation was reduced without eliminating the pungent taste [37].

The currently marketed nicotine containing chewing gum, Nicorette®, is based on nicotine polacrilex and has been described previously. It is a sugar

Table 8. The Composition of Methadone Chewing Gum.

Ingredients	Weight (mg)
Methadone hydrochloride	25
Gum base	332
Sugar	584
Glucose	39
Glycerol	2.8
Aroma	17
Total chewing gum weight	1000

free chewing gum containing 2 mg or 4 mg of nicotine. The efficacy of Nicorette® has been investigated in more than 60 different clinical studies in more than 20 countries (for references see Christen et al [65]).

B. Drugs not Subject to High First-pass Metabolism

1. Methadone

The absorption of methadone given as chewing gum and tablets has been studied in 7 patients suffering from chronic pancreatitis and one from thyroid cancer [66]. The composition of the chewing gum is given in Table 8.

The relative bioavailability of methadone chewing gum to tablet was 83.6%. The difference was not significant. The absorption of methadone from the oral cavity is known to be pH-dependent [67]. Thus the addition of a basic buffering agent to the chewing gum may have increased the absorption and reduced the intersubject variation in bioavailability. From these initial studies it might be possible to optimize the chewing gum formulation and develop a methadone chewing gum which gives a faster pain relief than the tablet does. This optimization process would have to include masking of the bitter taste of methadone.

2. Ascorbic Acid

A known side-effect of chewing vitamin C tablets is the damage to dental enamel caused either by over use or a build up of high local concentrations of the vitamin due to fragments lodging between teeth. Indeed, in some cases chewing tablets has caused erosion of the teeth [68]. Ascorbic acid in chewing gum is a potentially useful and easy method to administer vitamin C. In a clinical trial the quantity of excreted ascorbic acid in urine measured over 12 hours after administration of vitamin C following the chewing of gum or tablets indicated a recovery of 91.2% and 71.3%, respectively of the dose [69]. Vitamin C chewing gum has been evaluated in the *"Safe for teeth test"* and was found safe [70]. The test itself evaluates the pH levels of saliva in the oral cavity to make sure that it does not fall below pH 5.7 during or after the administration of food, medicines etc. The favorable results obtained from this test for vitamin C suggest that its incorporation into chewing gum is a superior method of administration to chewing tablets since the possibility of fragments of active ingredient becoming stuck between the teeth is less likely.

X. SAFETY ASPECTS

Very few accidents with chewing gum and none concerning medicated chewing gum have been reported in the literature. Different commercial chewing gums have been shown to adhere to different degrees to dentures, fillers, crowns etc., and hard chewing gum has caused broken teeth. Over-chewing causes painful jaw muscles. Chewing gum appears to offer a smaller risk of overdosing by mistake or misuse than flavored chewing tablets or lozenges, which can be consumed within a short period of time in a greater number than pieces of gum. The extensive chewing of sorbitol containing chewing gums has caused diarrhea as a consequence of a high osmotic pressure in the gastrointestinal tract.

The safety aspects of fluoride-containing chewing gums has been investigated. Hatteb et al [71] found that the effect of chewing two sticks (a dose of 0.226 mg of fluoride) on blood plasma levels was negligible (a rise from 16 ng/mL to 24 ng/mL) and the concentration returned to the prechewing value after 2 hours. Oliveby et al [72] measured the influence of chewing two pieces of fluoride gum 10 times a day, a total dose of 5 mg fluoride, on the fluoride plasma concentration. They concluded from their results that even such a frequent use of fluoride gum was acceptable from a toxicological point of view.

If a piece of Nicorette® is swallowed, some of the incorporated nicotine will be released in the gastrointestinal tract. However, the release will take place very slowly and since nicotine is metabolized by a high first pass metabolism in the liver [26] this will not result in adverse effects. It should be realized that Nicorette® has a much firmer consistency than regular chewing gum and, as a result, it might produce occlusal stress in denture wearing individuals when it is erroneously chewed vigorously or for long periods [73].

Medicated chewing gum should, like all other medicaments, be kept out of reach of children and it would be wise to advise people prone to allergic responses to check the flavoring and sweetening agents included in the chewing gum formulation.

XI. FUTURE APPLICATIONS

Chewing gum offers the potential to release drugs over a longer period of time than those delivery systems conventionally used in the oral cavity. The results of clinical investigations using chewing gum as a drug delivery system indicate that it is a viable alternative to traditional dosage forms for drugs intended to cure or relieve diseases in the oral cavity. It probably has limited application for the systemic delivery of drugs but chewing gum may be a potential dosage form for the systemic delivery of drugs used to treat diseases where a rapid onset of action is needed, such as travel sickness, nausea and headache (provided the drug is easily absorbed through the oral mucosa) or drugs that are subject to extensive metabolism when administered orally. It should be remembered, however, that a fraction of the drug will always be swallowed and pass into the gastrointestinal tract during chewing.

If the release of the pure drug is poor due to its inherent physicochemical properties, it may be possible to include a release promoting agent in the formulation to give the desired release pattern. In this respect the addition of a buffering substance for an acidic or a basic drug, or inclusion of a surfactant could be the first approach. If there is the need to reduce the rate of release of drug from chewing gum, e.g., for a water soluble drug, then the coating or embedding methods experienced from working with flavors and sweeteners could be considered. For ionic drugs the principle of complexation with an ion exchange resin might be an approach worth considering.

It should be remembered that the taste of the drug is a important factor to consider during formulation. Although much know-how has been obtained in the pharmaceutical industry of how to mask the taste of a drug with a very bitter taste it is an insurmountable obstacle to overcome in the formulation of a medicated chewing gum.

Finally, in the future, we may see the concept of chewing gum as a drug delivery system used more often in preference to other oral mucosal drug delivery systems for the local and systemic delivery of certain drugs. The reason is that chewing gum has controlled release properties, prolonged release properties, is convenient and easy to administer, is acceptable to the patient and can be taken discreetly without water.

REFERENCES

1. R. Hendrickson, *The Great American Chewing Gum Book*, Clinton Book Company, Radnor, Pennsylvania, 1976.

2. L. A. Cloys, A. G. Christen, and J. A. Christen, The development and history of chewing gum, *Bull. Hist. Dent. 40*:57 (1992).
3. W. F. Semple, U.S. Patent 98, 304. Improved chewing gum, *Dent. Stud. Mag. 47*:626 (1969).
4. W. Woodford, and L. J. Lesco, Relative bioavailability of aspirin gum, *J. Pharm. Sci. 70*:1341 (1981).
5. Commission of the European Communities (1991) CPMP list of allowed terms for pharmaceutical dosage form, route of administration, container, closure and administration devices, III/3593/91.
6. S. Lichtneckert, C. Lundgren, and O. Fernö, Smoking substitutes and method of producing same, London Patent 1,325,011 (1973).
7. S. P. Synosky, and M. Greenberg, Improved wax-free chewing gums with controlled sweetener release, PCT Patent WO 93/17577 (1993).
8. C. Bruun, and H. Givskov, Release of fluoride from fluoride-containing chewing gum, *Commun. Dent. Oral Epidemiology 6*:27 (1978).
9. S. E. Zibell, and K. B. Broderick, Granulation of active ingredients using polyvinyl acetate and alcohol, Eur. Patent 0 492 980 A1 (1992).
10. C. J. Kleber, R. G. Schimmele, M. S. Putt, and J. C. Muhler, A mastication device designed for evaluation of chewing gums, *J. Dent. Res. 60*:109 (1981).
11. A. A. Kassem, S. A. Zaki, and M. F. El-Miligi, Effect of drug solubility on its rate of release from masticates, *Bull. Fac. Pharm. Cairo Univ. 12*:2 (1973).
12. R. L. Liljewall, Methods and apparatus for mechanical processing of a sample and a member of such an apparatus, PCT Patent WO 89/05970 (1989).
13. L. L. Christrup, and N. Møller, Chewing gum as a drug delivery system I. In vitro simulation of human mastication and influence of formulation upon the release rate of a water soluble drug, *Arch. Pharm. Chem. Sci. Ed. 14*:30 (1986).
14. C. Andersen, personal communication 1994.
15. J. N. Rider, E. L. Brunson, W. G. Chambliss, R. W. Cleary, A. H. Hikal, P. H. Rider, L. A. Walker, C. M. Wyandt, and A. B. Jones, Development and evaluation of a novel dissolution apparatus for medicated chewing gum products, *Pharm. Res.* 9:255 (1992).
16. R. Barabolak, K. Hoerman, N. Kroll, and D. Record, Chewing gum profiles in U.S. population, *Commun. Dent. Oral. Epidemiol. 19*:125 (1991).
17. R. Nemeth-Coslett, N. L. Benowitz, N. L. Robinson, and J. E. Henningfield, Nicotine gum: Chew rate, subjective effects and plasma nicotine, *Pharmacol. Biomed. Behav. 29*:747 (1988).

18. L. N. Jensen, L. L. Christrup, N. Menger, and H. Bundgaard, Chewing gum and lozenges as delivery systems for noscapine, *Acta Pharm. Nord. 3*:219 (1991).
19. M. R. Rassing, L. L. Christrup, and J. Møller-Sonnergaard, Absorption of progesterone through the oral mucosa, Proceedings of the 47th International Congress of Pharmaceutical Sciences, Amsterdam, 1987, p. 69.
20. R. D. Emslie, N. Veall, and R. Duckworth, Chewing gum as a vehicle for the administration of fluoride: studies with 18-F, *Br. Dent. J. 110*:121 (1961).
21. C. Bruun, and H. Givskov, Fluoride concentrations in saliva in relation to chewing of various supplementary fluoride preparations, *Scand. J. Dent. Res. 87*:1 (1979).
22. J. Ainamo, and H. Etemadzadeh, Prevention of plaque growth with chewing gum containing chlorhexidine acetate, *J. Clin. Periodontol. 14*:524 (1987).
23. N. Fox, R. G. Kesel, E. R. Neary, and R. H. Herbine, Effect of sulfathiazole in chewing gum in certain oropharyngeal infections, *Arch. Otolaryngol. 41*:278 (1945).
24. L. L. Christrup, and M. R. Rassing, Chewing gum as a drug delivery system. II. Influence of the formulation upon the rate of release of salicylamide, *Farmaci Sci. Ed. 16*:1 (1988).
25. T. Andersen, M. Gram-Hansen, M. Pedersen, and M. R. Rassing, Chewing gum as a drug delivery system for nystatin - influence of solubilizing agents upon the release of water insoluble drugs, *Drug. Dev. Ind. Pharm. 16*:1985 (1990).
26. N. L. Benowitz, P. Jacob, and C. Savanapridi, Determinants of nicotine intake while chewing nicotine polacrilex gum, *Clin. Pharmacol. Ther. 41*:467 (1987).
27. R. Nemeth-Coslett, J. E. Henningfield, M. K. O' Kneeffe, and R. R. Griffiths, Nicotine gum: Dose-related effects on cigarette smoking and subjective ratings, *Psychopharmacol. 92*:424 (1987).
28. A. G. Pack, and M. E. Thomsen, Effects of topical and systemic folic acid supplementation on gingivitis in pregnancy, *J. Clin. Periodontol. 7*:402 (1980).
29. A. G. Pack, Folate mouthwash: Effect on established gingivitis in periodontal patients, *J. Clin. Periodontol. 11*:619 (1984).
30. M. R. Rassing, Chewing gum as a buccal delivery system for folic acid, Proceedings of the World Congress of Pharmacy and Pharmaceutical Sciences, OA-6 (1993).
31. F. Witzel, J. P. Wayne, C. Warren, A. Donald, and M. Mackay, Chewing gum capable of releasing finely divided water-insoluble materials therefrom, U.S. Patent 4,238,475 (1980).

32. M. Pedersen, and M. R. Rassing, Miconazole chewing gum as a drug delivery system. Test of release promoting additives, *Drug Dev. Ind. Pharm. 17*:411 (1991).
33. E. Jensen, K. B. Lokind, M. Pedersen, and M. R. Rassing, Chewing gum as a drug delivery system. Influence of additives upon the rate of release of metronidazole and propranolol hydrochloride from chewing gum, *Farmaci Sci. Ed. 16*:94 (1991).
34. J. Rindum, P. Holmstrup, M. Pedersen, M. R. Rassing, and K. Stoltze, Miconazole chewing gum for treatment of chronic oral candidosis, *Scand. J. Dent. Res. 101*:386 (1993).
35. M. Pedersen, and M. R. Rassing, Miconazole chewing gum as a drug delivery system. Application of solid dispersion technique and lecithin, *Drug Del. Ind. Pharm. 16*:2015 (1990).
36. D. A. M. Mackay, K. W. Clark, F. Witzel, and D. Schoenholtz, Long-lasting flavored chewing gum including chalk-free gum base, U.S. Patent 4,064,274.
37. O. Fernö, The development of a chewing gum containing nicotine and some comments on the role played by nicotine in the smoking habit, Proceedings of the Third World Conference on Smoking and Health, Washington, D. C. US Department of Health, Education and Welfare, 1977, p. 569.
38. R. Cappellary, Chewing gum, Eur. Patent 0,217,109 (1986).
39. M. A. Meyers, Improved high intensity sweetener ingredient, PCT Patent WO 93/22939 (1993).
40. A. I. Bakal, F. Witzel, A. M. Mackay, and D. Schoenholz, Long-lasting flavored chewing gum including sweetener dispersed in ester gums and method, U.S. Patent 4,087,557 (1978).
41. S. C. Sharma, and K. Y. Yang, Chewing gum compositions containing novel sweetener delivery systems and methods for preparation, U.S. Patent 4,597,970 (1986).
42. J. H. Song, and C. M. Copper, Gradual release structures for chewing gum, U.S. Patent 5,165,944 (1992).
43. K. B. Broderick, and D. W. Record, Gum composition containing dispersed porous beads containing active chewing gum ingredients and method, U.S. Patent 5,139,787 (1992).
44. M. R. Rassing, Chewing gum as a drug delivery system, *Adv. Drug Del. Rev. 13*:89 (1994).
45. J. H. Song, and S. B. Courtright, Flavor releasing structures for chewing gum, U.S. Patent 5,128,155 (1992).
46. R. H. Manning, and W. M. Edgar, Salivary stimulation by chewing gum and its role in the remineralization of caries-like lesions in human enamel in situ, *J. Clin. Dent. 3*:71 (1992).

47. S. Fröhlich, H. J. Maiwald, and G. Flowerdew, Effect of gum chewing on the pH of dental plaque, *J. Clin. Dent. 3*:75 (1992).
48. S. A. Leach, G. T. R. Lee, and W. M. Edgar, Remineralization of artificial caries-like lesions in human enamel in situ by chewing sorbitol gum, *J. Dent. Res. 68*:1064 (1989).
49. L. Fløtra, P. Gjermo, G. Rølla, and J. Waerhaug, Side-effects of chlorhexidine mouthwashes, *Scand. J. Dent. Res. 79*:119 (1972).
50. L. Glavind, T. Karring, and J. Heidmann, Effect of chlorhexidine acetate delivered in chewing gum, *J. Dent Res. 71*:584 (1992).
51. J. Ainamo, and H. Etemadzadeh, Prevention of plaque growth with chewing gum containing chlorhexidine acetate, *J. Clin. Periodontol. 14*:524 (1987).
52. D. Birkhed, Plaque pH recovery of sugar-free chewing gum with and without urea, *J. Dent. Res. 68*:1027 (1989).
53. C. C. Pfeiffer, and H. H. Holland, Salivary sulfonamide levels after chewing paraffin and chicle vehicles, *Am. J. Pharm. 44*:695 (1945).
54. J. Ekstrand, D. Birkhed, L. E. Lindgren, A. Oliveby, S. Edwardson, and G. Frostell, Effect of repeated intake of a sugar free fluoride-containing chewing gum on acidogenicity and microbial composition of dental plaque, *Scand. J. Dent. Res. 93*:309 (1985).
55. W. J. Lamb, R. E. Corpron, F. G. More, E. D. Beltran, D. S. Strachan, and C. J. Kowalski, In situ remineralization of subsurface enamel lesions after the use of a fluoride Chewing gum, *Caries Res. 27*:111 (1993).
56. L. Holmen, and A. Thylstrup, Natural caries development and its arrestment, *Factors Relating to Demineralization and Remineralization of the Teeth* (S. A. Leach, ed.), IRL Press, Oxford, 1986, p. 139.
57. L. L. Christrup, J. Bonde, H. Eriksen, S. N. Rasmussen, M. R. Rassing, and K. Simonsen, Chewing gum as a drug delivery system. III. Bioavailability of salicylamide administered in tablets and chewing gum, *Farmaci Sci. Ed. 16*:6 (1988).
58. L. Fleckenstein, G. R. Mundy, R. A. Horovitz, and J. M. Mazullo, Sodium salicylamide: Relative bioavailability and subjective effects, *Clin. Pharmacol. Ther. 19*:451 (1975).
59. A. G. de Boer, D. D. Breimer and J. M. Gubbens-Stubbe, and A. Bosma, First pass elimination of salicylamide in man following oral and rectal administration, *Biopharm. Drug Dispos. 4*:321 (1983).
60. E. Bousquet, S. Tirendi, F. P. Bonina, L. Montenegro, A. Bianchi, and N. Ciampini, Bioavailability of two formulations of acetylsalicylic acid gums, *Pharmazie 47*:607 (1992).
61. M. Eichelbaum, A. Somogyi, G. E. von Unruh, and H. J. Dengler, Simultaneous determination of intravenous and oral pharmacokinetic parameters of D, L, verapamil using stable isotope-labeled verapamil, *Eur. J. Clin. Pharmacol. 19*:133 (1981).

62. L. L. Christrup, J. Bonde, S. N. Rasmussen, and M. R. Rassing, Relative bioavailability of (±)-verapamil hydrochloride administered in tablets and chewing gum, *Acta Pharm. Nord. 2*:6, 371 (1990).
63. N. L. Benowitz, B. L. Lee, and P. Jacob, Toxicity of nicotine. Implications with regard to nicotine replacement therapy, *Prog. Clin. Biol. Res. 261*:217 (1989).
64. D. P. L. Sachs, Nicotine Polacrilex: Practical use requirements, *Curr. Pulmonal. 10*:141 (1989).
65. A. G. Christen, Jr. J. L. McDonald, B. L. Olsen, A. C. Drook, and G. K. Stookey, Efficacy of nicotine chewing gum in facilitating smoking cessation, *J. Am. Dent. Assoc. 108*:595 (1984).
66. L. L. Christrup, H. R. Angelo, J. Bonde F. Kristensen, and S. N. Rasmussen, Relative bioavailability of methadone hydrochloride administered in chewing gum and tablets, *Acta Pharm. Nord. 2*:83 (1990).
67. D. S. Weinberg, C. E. Inturrisi, B. Reidenberg, D. E. Moulin, T. J. Nip, S. Wallenstein, R. W. Houde, and K. M. Foley, Sublingual absorption of selected opioid analgesics, *Clin. Pharmacol. Ther. 44*:335 (1988).
68. J. L. Giunta, Dental erosion resulting from chewable tablets, *J. Am. Dent. Assoc. 107*:253 (1983).
69. L. L. Christrup, S. N. Rasmussen, and M. R. Rassing, Chewing gum as a drug delivery system. IV. Excretion of ascorbic acid in urine after administration of chewing gum and chewing tablets, *Farmaci Sci. Ed. 16*:44 (1988).
70. T. N. Imfeld, In vivo evaluation of the carcinogenic potential of food in man, *Identification of Low Caries Risk Dietary Components* (H. M. Meyers, ed.), S. Karger AG, Basel, 1983, p. 4.
71. F. N. Hatteb, R. M. Gren, K. M. Pang, and Y. C. Mok, Effect of fluoride-containing chewing gum on the remineralization of carious lesions and on fluoride uptake in man, *Clin. Prevent. Dent. 11*:6 (1989).
72. A. Oliveby, J. Ekstrand, and F. Lagerløf, Effect of saliva flow rate on the salivary fluoride clearance after use of fluoride-containing chewing gum, *Caries Res. 21*:393 (1987).
73. A. G. Christen, J. M. Young, B. B. Beiswanger, R. D. Jackson, and R. H. Potter, Effects of nicotine chewing gum on complete dentures and their soft-tissue-bearing areas, *Int. J. Prosthodontol. 2*:155 (1989).

14

Intra-periodontal Pocket Drug Delivery Systems

W. Aubrey Soskolone
Hebrew University-Haddassah Faculty of Dental Medicine, Israel

Michael Freidman
Hebrew University Faculty of Medicine, Israel

I. INTRODUCTION

Concepts of the etiology of the periodontal diseases and their treatment have varied over the years [1, 2]. Today it is well accepted that they are a group of diseases caused by bacterial accumulations, termed dental plaque, on the tooth surfaces in close approximation to the gingival and periodontal tissues. The nature of the disease resulting from dental plaque appears to depend to a large extent on the interaction between the bacterial plaque and the response of the host defense mechanisms. In general the earliest form of periodontal disease is termed gingivitis which is an inflammatory process affecting the marginal gingiva directly adjacent to the bacterial accumulations on the tooth surfaces. The gingiva appear red and swollen and bleed easily on gentle pressure. Pain is not usually present. This process is reversible by simply eliminating the bacterial plaque using mechanical or chemical means. However, as a result of the interactions between the plaque and the host defence mechanisms the untreated gingivitis may develop into periodontitis.

Periodontitis is a destructive process resulting in the breakdown of the periodontal attachment apparatus including the periodontal ligament and the alveolar bone. The junctional epithelium migrates along the exposed root surface and the result is the formation of a periodontal pocket. The continuing loss of the periodontal attachment of the tooth to the alveolar bone results in the loosening of the tooth and its eventual loss. The periodontal pocket (Figure 1), a result of the disease process, provides an anatomical site for the accumulation of bacteria. With increasing depth the pocket and its subgingival bacterial plaque becomes more and more inaccessible to accepted oral hygiene practices. Beyond a depth of 4-5 mm tooth brushing and bacterial mouth rinses [3, 4] which are normally effective in treating gingivitis can no longer reach the base of the pocket [5, 6] and the bacteria which are causing the disease. According to recent studies at least one pocket, measuring 4 mm or more, occurs in 14% of the adult American working population with each person averaging 2 to 3 pockets [7]. In other less developed populations this incidence may be higher.

Therefore once periodontal disease with pocket formation has occurred therapy must be directed at controlling the interactions between the plaque bacteria and the host response. Conventional therapy is directed almost entirely towards controlling the bacteria. It relies on the use of mechanical plaque control including routine oral hygiene procedures, mechanical debridement of the root surfaces and surgical techniques. The surgical procedures are directed

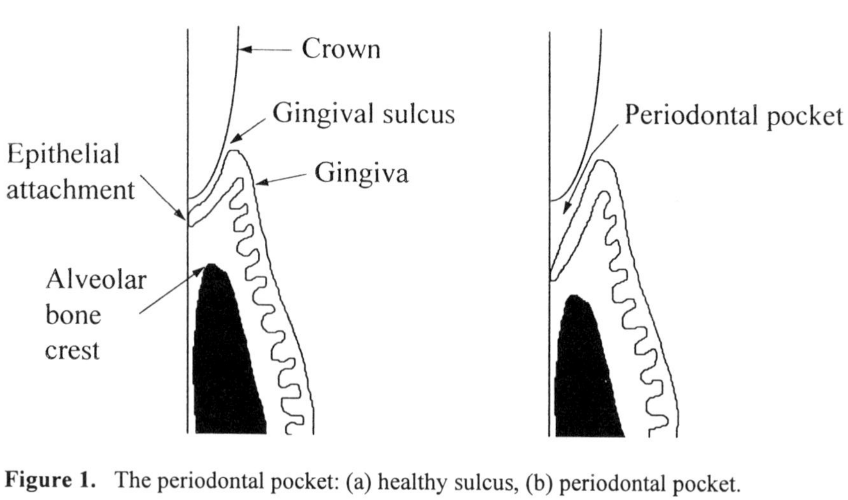

Figure 1. The periodontal pocket: (a) healthy sulcus, (b) periodontal pocket.

either at providing easier access for oral hygiene procedures to previously unaccessible sites, or to regenerate lost periodontal attachment. These regenerative procedures, in addition to regenerating lost periodontal support, eliminate the inaccessible periodontal pocket.

These procedures are time consuming, require highly trained personnel to carry them out and result in varying amounts of discomfort to the patients. Therefore the use of chemotherapeutic agents to control the plaque is an attractive alternative. In addition the use of chemotherapeutic agents can be used to influence the host response. There is evidence that systemic administration of antibiotics [8, 9] and non-steroidal anti-inflammatory drugs (NSAIDs) [10, 11] are effective in altering the progression of certain forms of periodontitis. However, the routine use of antibiotics over long periods of time is contraindicated because of the development of resistant bacterial strains and possible systemic side-effects. Local delivery of chemotherapeutic agents into the pockets via a syringe or irrigating device has been shown to have an effect on the subgingival flora but clinically it has not been effective in halting the progression of periodontal attachment loss [12]. The lack of clinical efficacy is probably because of the short time the irrigating solution remains in contact with the pocket environment. The development of other, more sophisticated, subgingivally placed delivery systems has taken big strides forward over the last decade and it is the purpose of this article to discuss these developments.

II. PATHOGENESIS OF HUMAN PERIODONTAL DISEASES

Periodontal disease is defined as the pathologic destruction and loss of the tissues supporting the teeth. The association of periodontal disease with bacteria and plaque accumulation has been firmly established [13]. The microbial flora associated with periodontal diseases is comprised of Gram-negative bacteria, and some of the bacteria, such as *Porphyromonas gingivalis* and *Actinobacillus actinomycetemcomitans* have been identified as potential periodontal pathogens. However, although a Gram-negative infection is a prerequisite to periodontal destruction, the host response plays an important role in determining the outcome of the process. Early inflammatory lesions of the gingival tissue are associated with a predominantly granulocyte infiltration, while chronic disease and sites with active disease exhibit a predominantly mononuclear cell infiltrate. Lymphocytes constitute the major cell type while monocytes and macrophages constitute a minor component [14].

Once microorganisms have colonized the gingival crevice, LPS derived from periodontal pathogens have the ability to penetrate the root cementum and gingival tissues [15, 16]. LPS derived from periodontal pathogens can stimulate the minor cell population of monocytes and macrophage to secrete cytokines [17]. These cytokines have the ability to stimulate other cell types associated with the inflammatory infiltrate, such as lymphocytes and fibroblasts, to secrete additional inflammatory mediators [18], amplifying the inflammatory response. This cascade of events suggests an important role for LPS-induced inflammatory mediators in the tissue destruction, characteristic of periodontitis. High levels of pro-inflammatory mediators such as TNFα, IL-1β and PG-E_2 with the potential to induce bone resorption have been documented at periodontal disease sites [19-23]. Furthermore, IL-1β and PG-E_2 have been correlated to active phases of periodontal breakdown [22, 24].

Periodontal diseases commonly affects adults over the age of 35 and the incidence increases with age. This type of presentation is termed Adult-type Periodontitis. Young people below 35 years are rarely affected by periodontal disease but when they are it is referred to as Early Onset Periodontitis (EOP).

EOP is a group of heterogeneous diseases whose classification, etiology and diagnostic criteria are still debated. Prepubertal Periodontitis is a condition in which there is periodontal breakdown around the primary teeth of prepubertal children. A more clearly defined form of EOP is Localized Juvenile Periodontitis (LJP) which is confined primarily to the first molars and incisors. Minimal bacterial plaque deposits are usually associated with LJP, although some authors suggest otherwise [25]. The age of LJP affected patients is typically 12 to 26 years of age, and abnormalities in neutrophil function have been described in the affected population. Another less defined disease is referred to as Severe Generalized Periodontitis (SGP), Rapidly Progressive Periodontitis (RPP), or Generalized Juvenile Periodontitis (GJP). Compared to LJP, this condition(s) is a more generalized form of periodontal destruction affecting most of the permanent dentition. SGP patients are usually 12 to 35 years of age.

A specific Gram-negative flora has been found to be associated with the various EOP diseases. *Actinobacillus actinomycetemcomitans* has been associated with LJP and *Porphyromonas gingivalis* is considered a primary etiologic factor in the initiation and progression of SGP [26-28].

III. SPECIAL ASPECTS OF POCKET ANATOMY

The periodontal pocket is a result of the progression of periodontal disease. It is a space, virtual or potential, which results from the pathological detachment of the periodontal tissues from the dental tissues. It is usually confined by the pocket epithelial lining covering the soft tissue walls of the pockets, and by the cementum and dentin of the root surface. The anatomy of the pocket varies extensively and can be tortuous [29]. At one end of the spectrum, when inflammation in the pocket wall is minimal or absent a complete epithelium lining covering the soft tissues exists. In most successful post-treatment circumstances the epithelium attaches to the root surface (long epithelial attachment) and the pocket exists as a potential space only. At the other end of the spectrum the pocket is an easily accessible space, occupied by bacterial plaque, calculus and other debris with an incomplete epithelial lining. The degree of ulceration of the epithelial lining is dependent on the degree of inflammation in the pocket wall. The pocket is constantly washed by the gingival crevicular fluid (for a comprehensive review see [30]). The direction of flow of the crevicular fluid is from the gingival tissues, through the gingival pocket, into the oral cavity. This flow could result in a 40 fold turnover of the pocket volume per hour [31]. The flow rate and volume of the crevicular fluid is dependent on the degree of inflammation in the pocket wall and the volume of the pocket [31, 32].

IV. RATIONAL FOR THE USE OF INTRA-POCKET DELIVERY SYSTEMS

Local application is one way of targeting a drug to a desired site. However, to prolong the therapeutic levels of the drug at the site, a local sustained release device is required.

The periodontal pocket is a defined site surrounded by hard and soft tissues forming a natural reservoir with easy access for inserting a delivery device. The presence of the gingival crevicular fluid bathing the device provides a leaching media for the release of a drug from a solid dosage form. These features, together with the fact that the periodontal diseases are localized to the immediate environment of the pocket make the periodontal pocket a natural site for treatment with local sustained release delivery systems.

The goals to be achieved in using an intra-pocket delivery device are the release of the therapeutic agent into the pocket and the achievement and maintenance of therapeutic levels of the drug for the required period of time.

Although the delivery system and the drug it releases are an integral unit, and most discussions on the subject relate to them as such, it is important to bear in mind that they are in fact two distinct entities. A single drug may be delivered by different delivery systems or alternatively a specific delivery system can be used to deliver different drugs. However there is a strong interdependence between the two which determines (at least in part) the release kinetics of the drug and thus its efficacy in treating the disease.

V. SUSTAINED RELEASE DELIVERY DEVICES

A. Considerations in Designing a Sustained Release Delivery Device

There are a number of considerations to be taken into account when designing a sustained release device for insertion into a periodontal pocket. Important amongst these are (i) the drug to be delivered by the subgingival delivery system, (ii) the release profile of the active agent from the device and (iii) the morphology of the device.

1. Drugs Used in Subgingival Delivery Systems

Garant and Cho [33] and Waerhaug [34, 35] described the limits of action of subgingival plaque bacteria and the substances they release into the periodontal pocket to a radius of up to 2 mm. The concept was further elaborated by Page and Schroeder [36]. This concept may also be applied when considering the use of intra-pocket sustained release delivery systems. The required radius of action of the chemotherapeutic agent from the device would depend on the target. For example, an antibacterial agent directed at the intra-pocket flora would preferably be an agent that acts locally in the environment of the pocket without penetrating the pocket lining into the gingival tissues. On the other hand if one was intent on eliminating bacteria that had penetrated into the pocket wall, affecting inflammatory mediators released from cells of the inflammatory infiltrate or influencing osteoclasts at the resorbing bone surface, a chemotherapeutic agent that can penetrate into the tissues to reach the target would be required. The required radius of action of the drug would depend on the distance of the target from the delivery device.

Highly charged cationic antiseptics such as chlorhexidine would adsorb to both the cementum/dentine as well as the surface of the soft tissue wall of the periodontal pocket without penetrating into the soft tissues [37, 38]. Tetracycline, a strong chelating agent, would attach to the calcified hard tissue wall of the pocket but it would also penetrate into the tissues with detectable levels occurring in the systemic circulation [39]. Other antibiotics such as Metronidazole and the NSAIDs would probably be absorbed rapidly from the pocket into the gingival tissues and on into the systemic circulation [40, 41]. Traditionally the choice of antimicrobial agents for use in local delivery systems has been based on drugs used for systemic drug delivery to the periodontium or drugs used in mouthwashes for supragingival plaque control. There is indeed logic to this approach as the efficacy of these drugs in treating periodontal diseases and in controlling putative periodontal pathogens is well established. However, it is limiting in that there are numerous antibacterial agents, including antibiotics, that are very effective topically but because they lack substantivity or because they cannot be used systemically are not considered. Such agents may prove to be very useful when used in a sustained release formulation in the subgingival environment and further studies using such drugs are necessary.

2. *Release Profile*

One of the most important considerations is achieving and maintaining therapeutic levels of the particular drug in the pocket. The concentration of the drug in the crevice is dependent on a balance between the rate of release of the drug from the device into the gingival crevicular fluid (GCF) and the rate the drug is depleted from the pocket by loss via the GCF into the oral cavity and absorption of the drug through the pocket lining into the systemic circulation. The periodontal pocket is naturally irrigated by the GCF. As mentioned previously the flow rate of the GCF is proportional to the severity of the gingival inflammation and in subjects with periodontal diseases, the mean rate of GCF flow at individual sites has been estimated at between 20 to 30 mL/hour [31, 32]. As the release of a drug from a controled release reservoir is dependent on both diffusion and dissolution mechanisms, the flow rate of GCF will directly influence the release rate of the drug from the delivery device. Consequently, a high flow rate of GCF will result in rapid release of the drug from the reservoir and cause a fast evacuation of the already released drug from the pocket into the mouth thereby depleting the concentration of the drug in the pocket. Therefore, the rate of release of the drug from the reservoir should be high after the initial placement of the device, to achieve and maintain a therapeutic level of the drug in the pocket. As the GCF flow decreases due to the effect of the drug on the gingival inflammation a slower release rate is required to maintain the therapeutic level in the pocket. Another parameter influencing the release of the drug from the device is the rate at which the drug is absorbed from the GCF via the pocket epithelium into the connective tissues and systemic circulation. A poorly absorbing drug enables drug levels in the periodontal pocket to reach higher concentrations and prolongs their retention in the pocket.

Therefore the device should be designed to provide an initial burst of drug into the pocket to achieve therapeutic levels and then a reduced release rate sufficient to maintain the therapeutic levels in the environment of a decreasing GCF flow rate; the nature of the drug having an influence on the design.

3. *Device Morphology*

For the purpose of patient acceptance it is preferable that the local delivery device should have physical characteristics that facilitate a swift atraumatic insertion into the pocket, minimizing pain and discomfort to the patients during and after its placement. A device, once placed, should not be exposed beyond the gingival margin so as not to cause any interference with normal daily oral hygiene procedures, including toothbrushing and interdental cleaning. It should also have as little an influence on the patients eating habits as possible.

B. Types of Devices That Have Been Tested

Intra-pocket devices can be divided into two broad categories depending on whether they are degradable or not. Non-degradable devices have the advantage that the therapist controls the removal of the device and therefore has greater control over the time of exposure of the pocket environment to the drug. However, a non-degradable device left in situ beyond its period of therapeutic efficacy is a potential hazard in that it could result in a foreign body response. The degradable devices have the great advantage of requiring the patient to pay only a single visit to the therapist for inserting the device. This minimizes patient visits and assures compliance in that the patient does not have to return to have the device removed.

1. Fibers

The use of fibers, or thread like devices, for the sustained release of drugs into the periodontal pocket was first introduced by Goodson et al [42] using cellulose acetate dialysis tubing to deliver tetracycline hydrochloride into the periodontal pocket. Although the system showed some clinical effect it was concluded that it was unable to sustain therapeutic levels of the drug for sufficient time to be clinically useful [43]. Using the same delivery system studies were done on the release of chlorhexidine gluconate [44] and metronidazole [45] with similar conclusions. These initial studies were followed by a series of further studies by Goodson and his co-workers [42, 43, 46-50] which have led to the development of a commercially available delivery system (Actisite®, Alza Corporation, Palo Alto, California) based on a monolithic ethylene vinyl acetate fibre that delivers tetracycline hydrochloride. Published data from two multicenter studies [49, 51] show that the treatment of periodontal pockets with this system resulted in significant reductions in pocket probing depths and bleeding on probing and significant increases in attachment levels compared to the other treatment modalities tested.

Clinically the placement of fibers into a periodontal pocket is well within the ability of the dental practitioner being similar to the standard dental technique of placing retraction cord into the gingival crevice prior to taking an impression of a crown preparation. The fiber can be placed around the circumference of the tooth to the depth of the pocket and folded back on itself repeatedly to completely fill the pockets. Its disadvantages are the relatively long time it takes to place the fibre (7-10 minutes/tooth) [52] and the need to use either a periodontal pack or a cyanoacrylate glue to retain the device within the pocket for the duration of the treatment. Because they are not degradable they have the added disadvantage of needing at least two visits to the therapist, one for insertion and one for removal of the device. A fairly high risk of 23% has been reported for extrusion of these fibers from the pockets during the 10 days of treatment [51]. There is also the possibility of lack of compliance with the patient not returning to remove the device.

2. *Films*

A far more widely used form of intra-pocket delivery device has been in the shape of a film. This dosage form has several advantageous physical properties for intra-pocket use. The dimensions and shape of the film can be easily controlled to correspond to the dimensions of the pocket to be treated. It can be rapidly inserted into the pocket with minimal discomfort to the patient. It can be inserted to the base of the pocket and be totally submerged. If the thickness of the film does not exceed approximately 400 μm, and its physical properties provide it with sufficient adhesiveness, it will remain submerged without any noticeable interference to the patient's eating and oral hygiene habits.

Both degradable and non degradable forms of films have been developed and therefore the discussion will relate to these two forms under separate headings.

a. Non-degradable Films

The first descriptions of film intra-pocket delivery devices appeared in 1982 [53, 54]. Addy and coworkers [53] described the use of films of methylmethacrylate for the intra-pocket delivery of tetracycline, metronidazole and chlorhexidine. A self polymerizing mixture of the polymer, monomer, and the appropriate drug were cured, as sheets, under high pressure and then cut into suitable sized films. Studies showed that the release of drugs from acrylic films measuring 10 x 1 x 0.5 mm was dependent on the nature of the drug and its concentration in the delivery device. They described formulations which delivered, in-vitro, therapeutic levels of all three drugs over a 14 day period. In later studies [55-57] they showed various degrees of clinical efficacy but this system has not been developed for clinical use.

In the same year an ethylcellulose film for intra-pocket drug delivery was described [54]. These films were made by casting ethanol or chloroform solutions of the polymer into molds and allowing the solvent to evaporate. The appropriate drug and plasticizing agent were incorporated into the solution prior to casting. The dried films (200-300 μm thick) were then cut into the required shapes. Films containing chlorhexidine [54, 58-60], metronidazole [61] minocycline [62] and tetracycline [63, 64] have been developed and tested to varying degrees. The release of the therapeutic agent from these films is dependent on the solvent used, the presence of a plasticizer, the nature and concentration of the drug in the film and on the physical dimensions of the film. The most extensive, published, clinical studies have been carried out using films that release 80% of their chlorhexidine content over a three day period. Using this formulation clinical efficacy, compared to no treatment, was demonstrated for up to 12 weeks post treatment for pockets exposed to the device for three consecutive three day periods [59]. This formulation has also been shown to be significantly better than routine therapy in the maintenance of periodontal pockets over a two year period [60]. A formulation releasing tetracycline over a 7 day period was developed [64] and the results of a clinical trial indicated that as an adjunct to scaling and root planing it produced significantly better results than scaling and root planing alone over the 12 weeks of the study [63]. The published data was analyzed by assessing each individual pocket as the experimental unit however when the data were re-analyzed using the patient as the experimental unit the tetracycline formulation resulted in significantly greater improvements in pocket depths at 4 weeks post treatment than the controls. This difference became more obvious at 12 weeks when the experimental treatment gave a mean improvement in probing pocket depth of 2.4 mm (± 0.2) compared to 0.9 mm (±0.4) in the control group

b. Degradable Devices

Many degradable devices in the form of a film have been tested experimentally. Resorbable hydoxypropylcellulose based devices for the delivery of tetracycline and chlorhexidine [65] and ofloxacin [66, 67] have been tested clinically. The first report on a degradable intra-pocket sustained release delivery system was the study of Noguchi et al [65] using hydoxypropylcellulose films. In this study a rapid release of the drugs from the film within 2 hours was demonstrated in vitro with maximum dissolution of the film occurring after 3 hours. In vivo, retention of tetracycline in the pockets could be detected 24 hours after insertion of the device and significant clinical and microbiological advantages over the control group were described. Although this was a pioneering study in the development of a degradable system, the rapid degradation of the device and the short duration of drug exposure were distinct disadvantages. Using a modification of this system by incorporating slowly soluble methacrylic acid copolymer particles into the hydoxypropylcellulose films [66, 67], the release of the drug ofloxacin from the device was prolonged such that 70% was released in the first 8 hours in vitro. In vivo levels above 2 μg/mL of ofloxacin were maintained for 7 days after treatment with the device. Two applications of this device one week apart resulted in significant reductions in the number of spirochetes and motile organisms in the pockets as identified by dark field microscopy. Similar shifts were not seen in the placebo treated or untreated control pockets. Re-treatment of these same pockets with films after scaling and root planing showed further reductions in the pathological flora but the changes were not significantly different from controls.

Deasy et al [68] studied the effects of tetracycline hydrochloride and metronidazole released from 0.5 mm thick films formed by compacting a 15 mg mixture of the drug and polyhydroxybutyric acid in an infrared press. The in vitro release rate of the drug depended on the drug load, and the drug used. In vitro the films, although intact after 5 days in a buffer solution, became progressively more fragile with loss of mechanical strength. Clinically, films containing 25% of either drug were placed into pockets at 4 day intervals for 16 days and their effect compared to untreated control pockets. In general improvement in the clinical and microbiological parameters measured were noted over the 16 days of treatment with a return to control levels on cessation of treatment. No information was provided on the in vivo survival time of the film.

The biodegradable polyester poly(ε-caprolactone) has been tested in vitro as a matrix for sustained release delivery both as a fiber for the delivery of tetracycline [42, 69] and as a film for the delivery of chlorhexidine [70]. Clinically the fibers released their tetracycline content very rapidly with a half life of 11 hours [42]. No clinical studies could be found in which the films containing chlorhexidine had been tested in periodontal pockets.

Different types of collagen based membranes have also been tested as degradable devices for local drug delivery. A degradable controlled release device based on a formaldehyde crosslinked Byco protein matrix containing chlorhexidine has been described by Steinberg et al [71]. Byco protein is a hydrolyzed gelatin of bovine origin. The release of chlorhexidine from this device and its dissolution in vitro were shown to be dependent on the degree of protein cross-linking. The nature of the chlorhexidine salt used also affected the release rate. Based on this study the Perio Chip® (Perio Products Ltd., Jerusalem, Israel) has been developed for the controlled delivery of chlorhexidine subgingivally. This is a 5 mm x 4 mm x 0.3 mm film containing 2.5 mg of chlorhexidine gluconate. When the Perio Chip is placed subgingivally it releases its chlorhexidine content and degrades over a 7-10 day period. Clinical trials have been carried out to examine the efficacy of the chip for the treatment of periodontal pockets. Using a cross over 4 arm study the effect of a single Perio Chip was compared to the effect of 2 Perio Chips placed 1 week apart, a placebo chip and no treatment. When a combined analysis was carried out on the results from 60 patients from 2 different centers (USA and Germany) using the same protocol, greater improvements in probing pocket depths and attachment levels were seen in the Perio Chip treated pockets at 3 and 6 months post treatment. These differences were significant for pocket depth measurements at 3 months (0.57 mm $\pm$ 0.21, $p<0.01$) with the attachment level difference approaching significance at 6 months (unpublished data submitted to the Israel Ministry of Health and the Federal Drug Administration of the USA).

Using a 2% glutaraldehyde cross-linked atelocollagen film (atelocollagen is a pepsin digested preparation of insoluble bovine skin collagen), Minabe et al [72] developed a degradable delivery system to deliver tetracycline. Intra-pocket levels of tetracycline greater than 8 μg/mL were reported 10 days after insertion of the film into pockets. Two clinical studies were carried out to test the efficacy of the system. Four applications of these films to pockets with probing depths of 4 mm or more, at one week intervals, were compared to the effect of placebo films. The tetracycline containing films resulted in a significant improvement in bleeding on probing and a reduction in the percentage of spirochetes and black pigmented bacteroides species one and four weeks after the last application. The placebo treated pockets showed no change [73]. A seven week follow up of pockets treated with a single application showed significant improvements in plaque index, gingival index, pocket depth and bleeding on probing, at various time points, compared to the baseline measurements and to the results obtained with placebo films [74]. The device was reported to dissolve in the pocket in about 1 week.

A collagen film containing 5% metronidazole was evaluated as an adjunct to scaling and root planing in a three month clinical trial [75]. Beside the dimension of the device (5 mm x 5 mm) no information was provided about the nature of the matrix, the release kinetics of the device or its degradability. These authors reported a significant adjunctive effect for the local metronidazole therapy on gingival index, bleeding on probing, probing pocket depth and attachment level measurements, compared to scaling and root planing alone.

3. *Injectable Devices*

The possibility of injecting a delivery system into the pocket has a number of advantages. It is a relatively simple procedure with little or no discomfort associated with the insertion of the dose form. The initial fluid nature of the formulations, which is necessary for its use with a syringe, would theoretically allow the formulation to gain access to the entire pocket. In order to be retained in the pocket the formulation would need to undergo a change into a sticky semi-solid or solid phase so as to prevent it from being washed out of the pocket by the GCF flow.

Two different systems have been described in the literature, both of which are commercially available. The first, a 2% Minocycline containing ointment (Dentomycin®, Cyanamid International, Lederle Division, Wayne, NJ and SunStar, Osaka, Japan), does not appear to have any sustained release properties. In a study using this ointment as an adjunct to scaling and root planing [76], 4 applications of the ointment into the pocket were made at two weekly intervals starting immediately after completion of the scaling and root planing. This resulted in a significant, 0.3 mm greater improvement in pocket depth than did the placebo gel at 12 weeks post scaling and root planing and 6 weeks after the last application of the gel. The changes in the bleeding index and probing attachment levels were not significantly different. In the minocycline treated pockets there was a significant increase in the number of pockets with undetectable levels of *Porphyromonas gingivalis* and *Porphyromonas intermedius* compared to the controls, throughout the study. The minocycline effect on *Actinobacillus actinomycetemcommitans* only became significant after the 3rd application of the ointment and remained significant 6 weeks after the last application.

The second system (Elyzol®, Dumex, Copenhagen, Denmark) is a bona-fide controlled release delivery system. The liquid phase of this formulation consists of a water free mixture of melted glycerol mono-oleate and metronidazole benzoate to which a triglyceride, sesame oil, has been added to lower the melting point in order to improve the flow properties of the gel in the syringe. When the mixture comes into contact with water it sets in a liquid crystalline state. The formulation contains 25% metronidazole as 40% w/w metronidazole benzoate. The solubility of the drug and its concentration in the formulation influences its release profile. The matrix is degraded by neutrophil and bacterial lipases present in the GCF [77]. Concentrations of 103-1297 μ g/mL of metronidazole were recorded in inflamed pockets treated with this device with effective doses being maintained for 24-36 hours [78]. Systemic levels of metronidazole between 0.2-1.3 μg/mL were measured after the administration of 29-103 mg of the gel [40]. The recommended therapy is two separate applications into each pocket, one week apart [79]. The results of clinical studies comparing this therapeutic approach alone, to scaling and root planing, indicate that the metronidazole gel results in a reduction in probing pocket depth and bleeding on probing which is not significantly different from the results obtained with scaling and root planing [80, 81].

VI. DISCUSSION

The periodontal pocket is the result of the apical migration of the epithelial attachment along the root surface and loss of the supporting periodontal structures caused by periodontal disease. The importance of the pocket is that it is still one of the best predictors (but never the less inadequate) of further periodontal breakdown and that it presents a nidus for bacterial colonization which is difficult to control or eradicate using the oral hygiene procedures that are conventionally used for infection control in the oral cavity [82-84]. Therefore until we have more reliable methods for predicting periodontal attachment loss we will continue to treat all periodontal pockets as our primary means of controlling the infection and the resultant inflammatory processes that cause periodontal disease. The nature of the studies that have been carried out to date using subgingival sustained release delivery devices vary considerably in their aims as well as in the thoroughness and care of their execution. However in general the conclusions are that the use of intra-pocket delivery devices beneficially affect the pocket flora as well as the clinical parameters associated with periodontal disease. The devices have been used as adjunctive therapy to routine scaling and root planing, instead of scaling and root planing and as an alternative to routine maintenance of periodontal pockets after definitive therapy. Some reports indicate that the sustained subgingival release of antimicrobial agents alone approaches the effectiveness [80, 81], or are as effective as [49], subgingival scaling and root planing in improving the measured clinical parameters. However it would seem that substantially more evidence is required, especially over the long term, before the dental profession could be persuaded to discard the established therapy of scaling and root planing, and to leave subgingival deposits of calculus, for these new treatment forms. At this early stage in the development of strategies for local subgingival periodontal therapy, a much more conservative, and therefore generally acceptable approach, is the use of these devices as adjuncts to thorough subgingival scaling and root planing. Evidence for the effect-

Table 1. List of 4 Subgingival Delivery Systems Available on the World Markets.

Trade name	Manufacturer	Drug	Matrix	Degradable
Perio Chip®	Perio Products, Jerusalem, Israel	Chlorhexidine	Film	Yes: 7-10 day dissolution time
Actisite®	Alza Corp., Palo Alto, CA, USA	Tetracycline		Non-degradable
Elyzol®	Dumex, Copenhagen, Denmark	Metronidazole	Gel	Yes: no data on dissolution time
Dentomycin®	Lederle Div., Wayne, NJ, USA	Minocycline	Ointment	No solid phase

iveness of this approach is beginning to become available [76, 85, 86]. There is also evidence that local delivery of the antimicrobial chlorhexidine, provides a more effective means of maintaining periodontal pockets than regular maintenance therapy [60]. It would seem that the approach of maintenance of periodontal pockets provides one of the most practical strategies for using devices for subgingival sustained release delivery of antibacterial agents. For this to be an acceptable and viable alternative, the use of sustained release delivery devices need to be more effective than accepted maintenance therapy, simple to apply by therapists who usually carry out maintenance therapy and effective after a single application.

Today there are at least 4 products available on the world markets for subgingival delivery of antibacterial agents (Table 1). They represent the initial steps that have been taken in the field of topical sustained release chemotherapy for the treatment and control of periodontal disease. With time and clinical experience the dental community will learn how best to put these devices to clinical use for the benefit of their patients. Although the road is difficult and time consuming there is a need for developing, refining and testing new and more effective delivery systems that will not only deliver antibacterial agents to the subgingival environment but also anti-inflammatory and immune modulating drugs which may well prove useful in the treatment of periodontal diseases.

REFERENCES

1. S. Schluger, R. Yuodelis, R. C. Page, and R. H. Johnson, *Periodontal Diseases*, Lea and Febiger, Philadelphia, London, 1990.
2. L. Abrahams, and S. R. Patashnick, *Contemporary Periodontics* (R. J. Genco, H. M. Goldman, and D. W. Cohen, eds.), C V Mosby Company, St. Louis, Baltimore, Philadelphia, Toronto, 1990, p. 194.
3. L. Flotra, P. Gjermo, G. Rolla, and G. Waerhaug, A 4 - month study on the effect of a chlorhexidine mouthwash on 50 soldiers, *Scand. J. Dent. Res. 80*:10 (1972).
4. N. P. Lang, P. Holtz, H. Graf, A. H. Geering, U. P. Saxen, O. P. Sturzenberg, and A. H. J. Merckel, Effects of supervised chlorhexidine mouthrinses in children, *J. Periodont. Res. 17*:101 (1982).
5. G. R. Pitcher, H. N. Newman, and J. D. Strahan, Access to subgingival plaque by disclosing agents using mouthrinsing and direct irrigation, *J. Clin. Perio. 7*:300 (1980).
6. L. Flotra, Different modes of Chlorhexidine application and related local side effects, *J. Periodont. Res. 8*:41 (1973).
7. A. J. Miller, J. A. Brunelle, J. P. Carlos, L. J. Brown, and H. Loe, *Oral Health of United States Adults*, U. S. Department of Health and Human Services, NIH Publication #87-2868, Washington, 1987.

8. R. J. Genco, Antibiotics in the treatment of human periodontal diseases, *J. Periodont. 52*:545 (1981).
9. W. H. Van Palastein Helderman, Is antibiotic therapy justified in the treatment of human chronic inflammatory periodontal disease?, *J. Clin. Perio. 13*:932 (1986).
10. R. C. Williams, M. K. Jeffcoat, M. L. Kaplan, P. Goldhaber, H. G. Johnson, and W. J. Wechter, Flurbiprofen: a potent inhibitor of alveolar bone resorption in beagles, *Science 227*:640 (1985).
11. R. C. Williams, M. K. Jeffcoat, and T. H. Howell, Altering the progression of human alveolar bone loss with the non-steroidal anti-inflammatory drug flurbiprofen, *J. Periodont. 60*:486 (1989).
12. G. Greenstein, Effects of subgingival irrigation on periodontal status, *J. Periodont. 58*:827 (1987).
13. J. Lindhe, *Textbook of Clinical Periodontology*, Munksgaard, Copenhagen, 1989.
14. U. Zappa, M. Reinling-Zappa, H. Graf, and M. Espeland, Cell populations and episodic periodontal attachment loss in humans, *J. Clin. Perio. 18*:508 (1991).
15. J. J. Aleo, F. A. DeRenzio, P. A. Farber, and A. P. Varboncoeur, The presence and biological activity of cementum bound endotoxin, *J. Periodont. 45*:672 (1974).
16. J. Schwartz, M. L. Stinson, and R. B. Parker, The passage of tritiated bacterial endotoxin across intact gingival epithelium, *J. Periodont. 43*:270 (1972).
17. L. Shapira, S. Takashiba, S. Amar, and T. E. Van Dyke, Porphyromonas gingivals lps stimulation of human monocytes: dependence on serum and CD14 receptor, *Oral Microbiol. Immunol. 9*:112 (1994).
18. K. Takahashi, M. Takigawa, S. Takashiba, A. Nagai, M. Miyamoto, H. Kurihara, and Y. Murayama, Role of cytokines in the induction of adhesion molecules on cultured human gingival fibroblasts, *J. Periodont. 65*:230 (1994).
19. J. Honig, C. Rordorf-Adam, C. Siegmund, W. Wiedermann, and F. Erard, Increased interleukin-1 beta concentration in gingival tissue from periodontitis patients, *J. Periodont. Res. 24*:362 (1989).
20. M. P. Masuda, R. Persson, J. S. Kenney, S. W. Lee, R. C. Page, and A. C. Allison, Measurements of interleukin-1 alpha and interleukin-1 beta in gingival crevicular fluid: implications of pathogenesis of periodontal disease, *J. Periodont. Res. 25*:156 (1990).
21. E. F. Rossomando, J. E. Kennedy, and J. Hadjimichael, Tumor necrosis factor alpha in gingival crevicular fluid as a possible indicator of periodontal disease in humans, *Arch. Oral Biol. 35*:431 (1990).

22. P. Stashenko, P. Fujiyoshi, M. N. Obernesser, L. Prostak, A. D. Haffajee, and S. S. Socransky, Levels of interleukin-1 beta in tissue from sites of active periodontal disease, *J. Clin. Perio. 18*:548 (1991).
23. P. Stashenko, J. J. Jundinski, P. Fujiyoshi, J. Rynar, and S. S. Socransky, Tissue levels of bone resorptive cytokines in periodontal disease, *J. Periodont. 62*:504 (1991).
24. S. Offenbacher, B. M. Odle, and T. E. van Dyke, The use of crevicular fluid PG-E2 levels as a predictor of periodontal attachment loss, *J. Periodont. Res. 21*:101 (1986).
25. J. A. Burmeister, A. M. Best, K. G. Palcanis, and R. R. Ranney, Localized juvenile periodontitis and generalized severe periodontitis: clinical findings, *J. Clin. Perio. 11*:181 (1984).
26. J. J. Zambon, Actinobacillus actinomycetemcomitans in human periodontal disease, *J. Clin. Perio. 12*:1 (1985).
27. J. Slots, J. Bragd, M. Wikstrom, and G. Dahlen, The occurrence of Actinobacillus actinomycetemcomitans, Bacteroides gingivalis and Bacteroides intermedius in destructive periodontal disease in adults, *J. Clin. Perio. 13*:570 (1986).
28. A. J. van Winkelhoff, T. M. J. Van Steenbergen, and J. de Graaff, The role of black-pigmented Bacteroides in human oral infections, *J. Clin. Perio. 15*:145 (1988).
29. J. W. Krayer, and T. D. Rees, Histologic observations on the topography of a human periodontal pocket viewed in transverse step-serial sections, *J. Periodont. 64*:585 (1993).
30. G. Cimasoni, *Crevicular Fluid Updated, Monographs in Oral Science,* Volume 12, Krager, Basel, 1983.
31. J. Hattingh, and E. Ho, The concentration of proteins in human gingival crevicular fluid, *J. Periodont. Res. 15*:90 (1980).
32. J. M. Goodson, Pharmacokinetic principles controlling efficacy of oral therapy, *J. Dent. Res. 68*:1625 (1989).
33. P. R. Garant, and M. I. Cho, Histopathogenesis of spontaneous periodontal disease in conventional rats. I Histometric and histologic study, *J. Periodont. Res. 14*:297 (1979).
34. J. Waerhaug, The angular bone defect and its relationship to trauma from occlusion and down growth of subgingival plaque, *J. Clin. Perio. 6*:61 (1979).
35. J. Waerhaug, The infrabony pocket and its relationship to trauma from occlusion and subgingival plaque, *J. Periodont. 50*:355 (1979).
36. R. C. Page, and H. E. Schroeder, *Periodontitis in Man and Other Animals, A Comparative Review*, Krager, Basel, New York, 1982, p. 266.

37. P. Germo, P. Bonesvoll, and G. Rolla, Relationship between plaque-inhibiting effect and retention of chlorhexidine in the human oral cavity, *Arch. Oral Biol. 19*:1031 (1974).
38. M. J. Winrow, Metabolic studies with radiolabeled chlorhexidine in animals and man, *J. Periodont. Res. 8*:45 (1973).
39. J. W. Rapley, C. M. Cobb, W. J. Killoy, and D. R. Williams, Serum levels of tetracycline during treatment with tetracycline containing fibers, *J. Periodont. 63*:817 (1992).
40. K. Stoltze, and M. Stellfeld, Systemic absorption of metronidazole after application of a metronidazole 25% dental gel, *J. Clin. Perio. 19*:693 (1992).
41. M. J. Doyle, W. Buchanan, G. R. Kelm, M. P. Meredith, S. L. Nelson, T. T. Charles, K. R. Wehmeyer, J. G. Collins, and S. Offenbacher, Inhibition of PGE2 with Ketorolac rinses, *J. Dent. Res. 73*:117 (1994).
42. J. M. Goodson, D. Holborow, R. L. Dunn, P. Hogan, and S. Dunham, Monolithic tetracycline-containing Fibers for controlled delivery to periodontal pockets, *J. Periodont. 54*:575 (1983).
43. J. M. Goodson, S. Offenbacher, D. H. Farr, and P. E. Hogan, Periodontal disease treatment by local drug delivery, *J. Periodont. 56*:265 (1985).
44. J. Coventry, and H. N. Newman, Experimental use of a slow release device employing chlorhexidine gluconate in areas of acute periodontal inflammation, *J. Clin. Perio. 9*:129 (1982).
45. W. Z. A. Wan Yusof, H. N. Newman, J. D. Strahan, and J. F. Coventry, Subgingival metronidazole in dialysis tubing and subgingival chlorhexidine irrigation in the control of chronic inflammatory periodontal disease, *J. Clin. Perio. 11*:166 (1984).
46. M. Tonetti, M. A. Cugini, and J. M. Goodson, Zero-order delivery with periodontal placement of tetracycline-loaded ethylene vinyl acetate Fibers, *J. Periodont. Res. 25*:243 (1990).
47. L. Heijl, G. Dahlen, Y. Sundin, A. Wenander, and J. M. Goodson, A 4-quadrant comparative study of periodontal treatment using tetracycline-containing drug delivery fibers and scaling, *J. Clin. Perio. 18*:111 (1991).
48. J. M. Goodson, M. A. Cugini, R. L. Kent, G. C. Armitage, C. M. Cobb, D. Fine, M. E. Fritz, E. Green, M. J. Imoberdorf, W. J. Killoy, C. Mendieta, R. Niederman, S. Offenbacher, E. J. Taggart, and M. Tonetti, Multicentre evaluation of tetracycline fiber therapy: I. Experimental design, methods, and baseline data, *J. Periodont. Res. 26*:361 (1991).
49. J. M. Goodson, M. A. Cugini, R. L. Kent, G. C. Armitage, C. M. Cobb, D. Fine, M. E. Fritz, E. Green, M. J. Imoberdorf, W. J. Killoy, C. Mendieta, R. Niederman, S. Offenbacher, E. J. Taggart, and M. Tonetti,

Multicenter evaluation of tetracycline fiber therapy. II. clinical response, *J. Periodont. Res. 26*:371 (1991).
50. J. M. Goodson, A. Tanner, S. McArdle, K. Dix, and S. M. Watanabe, Multicentre evaluation of tetracycline fiber therapy: III. Microbiological response, *J. Periodont. Res. 26*:450 (1991).
51. M. G. Newman, K. S. Kornman, and F. M. Doherty, A 6 month multicenter evaluation of adjunctive tetracycline fiber therapy used in conjunction with scaling and root planning in maintenance patients: Clinical results, *J. Periodont. Res. 65*:685 (1994).
52. J. M. Goodson, Antimicrobial strategies for treatment of periodontal diseases, *Perio. 2000 5*:142 (1994).
53. M. Addy, L. Rawle, R. Handley, H. N. Newman, and J. F. Coventry, The development and in vitro evaluation of acrylic resin strips and dialysis tubing for local drug delivery, *J. Periodont. 53*:693 (1982).
54. M. Friedman, and G. Golomb, New sustained release dosage form of chlorhexidine for dental use, *J. Periodont. Res. 17*:323 (1982).
55. F. I. S. Yeung, H. N. Newman, and M. Addy, Subgingival metronidazole in acrylic resin vs. chlorhexidine irrigation in the control of chronic periodontitis, *J. Periodont. 54*:651 (1983).
56. M. Addy, and M. Langeroudi, Comparison of the immediate effects on the sub-gingival microflora of acrylic strips containing 40% chlorhexidine, metronidazole or tetracycline, *J. Clin. Perio. 11*:379 (1984).
57. M. Addy, H. Hassan, J. Moran, W. Wade, and R. Newcombe, Use of antimicrobial containing acrylic strips in the treatment of chronic periodontal disease. A three month follow-up study, *J. Periodont. 59*:557 (1988).
58. W. A. Soskolne, G. Golomb, M. Friedman, and M. N. Sela, New sustained release dosage form of chlorhexidine for dental use II. use in periodontal therapy, *J. Periodont. Res. 18*:330 (1993).
59. A. Stabholz, M. N. Sela, M. Friedman, G. Golomb, and W. A. Soskolne, Clinical and microbiological effects of sustained release chlorhexidine in periodontal pockets, *J. Clin. Perio. 13*:783 (1986).
60. A. Stabholz, W. A. Soskolne, M. Friedman, and M. N. Sela, The use of sustained release delivery of chlorhexidine for the maintenance of periodontal pockets: 2-year clinical trial, *J. Periodont. 62*:429 (1991).
61. G. Golomb, M. Friedman, W. A. Soskolne, A. Stabholz, and M. N. Sela, Sustained release device containing metronidazole for periodontal use, *J. Dent. Res. 63*:1149 (1984).
62. R. Elkayam, M. Friedman, A. Stabholz, W. A. Soskolne, M. N. Sela, and L. Golub, Sustained release device containing minocycline for local treatment of periodontal disease, *J. Control. Rel. 7*:231 (1988).
63. A. Stabholz, R. Elkayam, M. Friedman, M. N. Sela, R. Azoury, and W. A. Soskolne, Clinical and microbiological evaluation of sustained

release device of tetracycline in periodontal pockets, *Proceed. Int. Conf. Pharm. Tech. 2*:336 (1989).

64. R. Elkayam, M. Friedman, A. Stabholz, W. A. Soskolne, and R. Azoury, Sustained release device of tetracycline for dental use, structure and kinetics of drug release in vitro and in vivo, *Proceed. Int. Conf. Pharm. Tech. 2*:346 (1989).
65. T. Noguchi, K. Izumizawa, M. Fukuda, S. Kitamura, Y. Suzuki, and H. Ikura, New method for local drug delivery using resorbable base material in periodontal therapy, *Bull. Tokyo Med. Dent. Univ. 31*:145 (1984).
66. K. Higashi, K. Morisaki, S. Hayashi, M. Kitamura, N. Fujimoto, S. Kimura, S. Ebisu, and H. Okada, Local ofloxin delivery using a controlled-release insert (PT-01) in the human periodontal pocket, *J. Periodont. Res. 25*:1 (1990).
67. S. Kimura, H. Toda, Y. Shimabukuro, M. Kitamura, N. Fujimoto, Y. Miki, and H. Okada, Topical chemotherapy in human periodontitis using a new controlled release insert containing ofloxacin. 1. Microbiological observations, *J. Periodont. Res. 26*:33 (1991).
68. P. B. Deasy, A. E. M. Collins, D. J. MacCarthy, and R. J. Russell, Use of strips containing tetracycline hydrochloride or metranidazole for the treatment of advanced periodontal disease, *J. Pharm. Pharmacol. 41*:694 (1989).
69. R. L. Dunn, B. H. Perkins, and J. M. Goodson, Controlled release of tetracycline from biodegradable Fibers, *J. Dent. Res. 62*:289 (1983).
70. N. J. Medlicott, D. S. Jones, I. G. Tucker, and D. Holborow, Preliminary release studies of chlorhexidine (base and diacetate) from poly(ε-caprolactone) films prepared by solvent evaporation, *Int. J. Pharm. 84*:85 (1992).
71. D. Steinberg, M. Friedman, W. A. Soskolne, and M. N. Sela, A new degradable controlled release device for treatment of periodontal disease: In vitro release study, *J. Periodont. 61*:393 (1990).
72. M. Minabe, A. Uematso, K. Nishijima, E. Tomomatsu, T. Tamura, T. Hori, T. Umemoto, and T. Hino, Application of a local drug delivery system to periodontal therapy: 1. Development of collagen preparations with immobilized tetracycline, *J. Periodont. 60*:113 (1989).
73. M. Minabe, K. Takeuchi, E. Tomomatsu, T. Hori, and T. Umemoto, Clinical effects of local application of collagen film-immobilized tetracycline, *J. Clin. Perio. 16*:291 (1989).
74. M. Minabe, K. Takeuchi, T. Tamura, T. Hori, and T. Umemoto, Subgingival administration of tetracycline on a collagen film, *J. Periodont. 60*:552 (1989).
75. C. Hitzig, Y. Charbit, C. Bitton, T. Fosse, M. Teboul, L. Hannoun, and R. Varonne, Topical metronidazole as an adjunct to subgingival

debridement in the treatment of chronic periodontitis, *J. Clin. Perio. 21*:146 (1994).

76. D. van Steenberghe, P. Bercy, J. Kohl, J. de Boever, P. Adriaens, A. Vanderfaeillie, C. Andriaenssen, E. Rompen, H. de Vree, F. McCarthy, and G. Vandenhoven, Subgingival minocycline hydrochloride ointment in moderate to severe chronic adult type periodontitis: A randomized, double blind, vehicle-controlled, multicenter study, *J. Periodont. 64*:637 (1993).

77. T. Norling, P. Lading, S. Engstrom, K. Larsson, N. Krog, and S. S. Nissen, Formulation of a drug delivery system based on a mixture of monoglycerides and triglycerides for use in the treatment of periodontal disease, *J. Clin. Perio. 19*:687 (1992).

78. K. Stoltze, Concentration of metronidazole in periodontal pockets after application of a metronidazole 25% dental gel, *J. Clin. Perio. 19*:698 (1992).

79. B. Klinge, R. Attstrom, T. Karring, J. Kisch, B. Lewin, and K. Stoltze, 3 regimens of topical metronidazole compared with subgingival scaling on periodontal pathology in adults, *J. Clin. Perio. 19*:708 (1992).

80. V. Pedrazzoli, M. Kilian, and T. Karring, Comparative clinical and microbiological effects of topical subgingival application of metronidazole 25% dental gel and scaling in the treatment of adult periodontitis, *J. Clin. Perio. 19*:715 (1992).

81. J. Ainamo, T. Lie, B. H. Ellingsen, B. F. Hansen, L. A. Johansson, T. Karring, J. Kisch, K. Paunio, and K. Stoltze, Clinical responses to subgingival application of a metronidazole 25% gel compared to the effect of subgingival scaling in adult periodontitis, *J. Clin. Perio. 19*:723 (1992).

82. J. D. Beck, G. G. Koch, and S. Offenbacher, Attachment loss trends over 3 years in community-dwelling older adults, *J. Periodont. 65*:737 (1994).

83. M. G. Newman, K. S. Kornman, and S. Holtzman, Association of clinical risk factors with treatment outcomes, *J. Periodont. Res. 65*:489 (1994).

84. E. E. Machtei, J. Norderyd, G. Koch, R. Dunford, S. Grossi, and R. J. Genco, The rate of periodontal attachment loss in subjects with established periodontitis, *J. Periodont. 64*:713 (1993).

85. B. Pihlstrom, C. Michalowicz, J. Cob, J. Caton, M. Goodson, and M. Encarnacion, Maintenance response to tetracycline periodontal fiber therapy, *J. Dent. Res. 73*:306 (1994).

86. W. A. Soskolne, P. A. Heasman, A. Stabholz, G. J. Smart, M. Palmer, M. Flashner, and H. N. Newman, submitted for publication.

15

The Intraoral Delivery of Fluoride

Bernadette K. Drummond
University of Otago, New Zealand

John C. Rodda
University of Otago, New Zealand

I. INTRODUCTION

The recognition of a relationship between fluoride and the health of teeth in the 1930s has resulted in over 60 years of comprehensive research. After the confirmation of the relationship between mottling of dental enamel (dental fluorosis) and high levels of fluoride in domestic water supplies, Dean [1] in 1936 reported the results of several comprehensive surveys on the relationship between the levels of fluoride in the water and the presence or absence of dental mottling. He showed that water levels of fluoride at 1 parts per million fluoride (ppmF) or below had no public health significance [2]. Ainsworth [3] in 1933 had already reported that there was less dental caries (tooth decay) in the higher water fluoride areas, and in 1942 after further investigation, Dean et al [4] reported that a maximum reduction in caries occurred with a concentration of 1ppmF in the drinking water with a low prevalence of the mildest forms of enamel fluorosis. In 1945, Grand Rapids, Michigan was the first city to adjust the fluoride levels in its water supply as a public health measure to reduce dental caries. The effects of 10 and 15 years of fluoridation were reported by Arnold et al [5] in 1956 and Arnold et al [6] in 1962. Their findings of a 50% reduction in dental caries have subsequently been supported by many other studies. Following on from these early studies, research has focused on looking at how fluoride affects the process of dental caries, when it is best used, and how the protective effects can be optimized by the way it is applied directly to the teeth and placed within their immediate environment within the mouth.

Fluoride is the charged ion of fluorine which has an atomic weight of 19 and is the most electronegative and reactive of all the elements. Fluorine reacts with metallic elements to form compounds which are usually ionic and many are soluble in water. These fluoride compounds are widely present in rocks and mineral soils mainly as fluorspar (CaF_2), apatite ($3Ca_3(PO_4)_2.Ca(F.OH.Cl)_2$), and cryolite ($3NaF.AlF_3$). Sodium fluoride and magnesium fluoride are also found as natural minerals. The fluoride content of soils may be increased by phosphate-containing fertilizers, pesticides and by deposition of gaseous and particulate emissions from manufacturing premises. Fluoride is present in both surface and ground water. The concentrations vary widely from less than 0.01 ppmF to over 25 ppmF. The fluoride content of sea water is slightly higher. In areas which choose to have fluoride in the water at an optimal level to prevent dental caries, it is either added or removed to reach a level of around 1.0 ppmF. Traces of fluoride may appear in the air from volcanic activity, dust from soils, or sea water droplets. Other sources of airborne fluoride are from industries such as aluminum, steel, superphosphate, and ceramic production.

Because of the presence of fluoride in soil, water and air, it is inevitably present in foods, notably fish, some green leafy vegetables and tea. If bone fragments are left in meat products such as ground beef or chicken, higher fluoride levels may also be found. The fluoride content of foods may also be increased by its incorporation during food preparation. Food prepared with fluoridated water contains higher amounts of fluoride. This is particularly seen in beverages [7]. The fluoride content of adult diets was reviewed by Burt in 1992 [8] and was found to vary depending on the fluoride content of the water. Substitutes for human milk and infant foods have been reported to have variable levels of fluoride depending on where they are processed [8-11] Where the level of fluoride is not controlled, infant formulae and milk may contribute to the risk of dental fluorosis (mottling) at least in the anterior adult teeth as it is now known that these teeth are most at risk of developing fluorosis during their formation from about 18 months to 3 years of age [12, 13]

Fluoride as already mentioned is widely present in nature and is also a by product of many industrial processes which use raw materials which contain fluoride. There are two health areas where fluoride compounds are used. The first is in preventing or decreasing the severity of dental caries and the second less major use has been in the treatment of osteoporosis. It was originally thought that to have an effect on dental caries, fluoride needed to be incorporated in the enamel during the development of teeth. Therefore, initially research concentrated on the best systemic ways of giving fluoride during tooth development in children. These beliefs have continued to a certain extent although it is now well understood that the predominant effect of fluoride is via a topical presence, that is on the surface of the teeth. Furthermore it is most effective in altering the severity of dental caries if it is present and available in ionic form while the caries process is actively occurring. The emphasis has now shifted to achieving effective delivery of fluoride via topical vehicles which result in raising the fluoride levels on the surface of the enamel, high enough to interfere with the caries process. The topical vehicles which are used and/or have been investigated are toothpastes, rinses, gels, varnishes, chewing gums, dental floss, dental restorative materials, slow release polymers and glasses which are attached to teeth, and slow release mucosal patches which temporarily adhere to the mucosa of the mouth. Other vehicles which provide a substantial topical effect but which also result in ingestion of fluoride are water, food and chewable tablets or lozenges. While the fluoride is swallowed some remains in the mouth and some re-enters the mouth via the saliva.

This chapter reviews the effects that fluoride has in altering the process of dental caries and examines the methods for measuring fluoride in the oral cavity, including the different tissues and fluids which are present such as dental enamel, dentine, saliva, and dental plaque. It also reviews the vehicles for fluoride delivery and current knowledge of the success of the various vehicles in delivering appropriate amounts of fluoride to reduce the effects of dental caries.

II. DENTAL CARIES

Dental caries is initiated when bacteria present in the plaque on the surface of teeth enamel produce acids such as proprionic, acetic, lactic and formic acids as part of their metabolism of fermentable carbohydrates. The relationship of these three essential components is illustrated in Figure 1. Demineralization can only occur when all three components are present at the same time. If the acids result in a pH drop below the critical pH (range 5.2-5.5), demineralization (dissolving) of enamel begins. If acids are produced frequently such as when food is eaten more than 5-6 times per day, the amount of demineralization increases until the crystals collapse and a cavity is seen. Enamel, the outer layer of the tooth crown is the most dense biologic material. By weight, enamel is made up of 92-94% hydroxyapatite ($Ca_{10}(PO_4)_6(OH)_2$), 2-4% CO_3^{2-}, about 1% Na, Mg, K, Cl, Zn, 0.01-0.05% F, 2-3% water and about 1% protein and lipid. Enamel is porous with the water and organic content making up about 15% of the volume. Enamel hydroxyapatite is soluble in acid under some conditions as are the related phosphates dicalcium phosphate dihydrate, tricalcium phosphate and octacalcium phosphate which may be present or may form depending on the local conditions such as the pH, or calcium and phosphate concentrations.

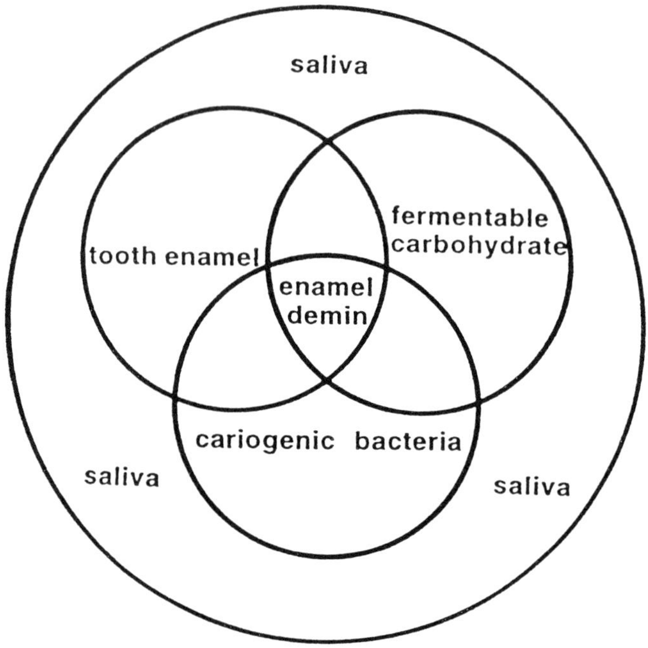

Figure 1. Relationships of the components of the dental caries process. (Adapted from Keyes [87] and Nikiforuk [23]).

The dissolution of the hydroxyapatite crystals results in a loss of calcium and phosphates from the surface of the crystals but as the pH increases above the critical pH, the crystals may also remineralize. This is also related to the conditions in the local environment especially the concentrations and compounds of calcium and phosphate present in plaque and saliva [14].

Bacteria in plaque, implicated in dental caries initiation and progression have specific properties which allow them to adhere to teeth and survive in the oral environment. They metabolize fermentable carbohydrate, producing acid as a by-product (acidogenic) they are aciduric allowing survival in the very low pHs which occur in dental plaque, and they can produce and store polysaccharides which allow them to survive between supplies of substrate. The main species of bacteria involved in dental caries of the crowns of teeth are *Streptococcus mutans* and *Lactobacillus mutans.*

The other part of the dental caries triad is fermentable carbohydrate. The bacteria which produce dental caries can metabolize any fermentable carbohydrate and not just sucrose as is commonly believed. When the bacteria are present in plaque in the mouth, each time fermentable carbohydrate enters the mouth the pH in the plaque drops below the critical pH from 20 minutes to over an hour [15, 16]. The newly demineralized enamel can remineralize after these attacks if the time period in between eating is long enough and there is enough saliva present. However when the number of eating occasions increases and especially when this is at night when there is a low salivary flow, the demineralization exceeds the remineralization and a cavity eventually forms.

Saliva plays a critical role in whether the demineralization of the enamel crystals progresses, is halted, or is reversed by remineralization. Saliva influences the process of dental caries in several ways including by clearing fermentable carbohydrates that the bacteria use, by buffering systems which effectively buffer the bacterial acids to raise the pH above the critical pH, by the enzyme amylase which breaks down carbohydrate to allow the bacteria to use it more effectively and by the fact that it is saturated with respect to calcium and phosphate which makes it an effective source of these minerals for remineralization. It also contains fluoride, antibacterial substances and proteins which play a role in the caries process [17, 18]. Although the crystals of enamel can begin to demineralize as soon as the plaque bacteria become active, it takes time for the demineralization to become great enough for the surface of the tooth to collapse and form a cavity. In adult enamel this may take up to three years but is considerably shorter in primary teeth where the enamel is much thinner. In the early stages of dental caries the lesion appears as an opaque white spot with a shiny surface when the tooth is dried. With the loss of tooth mineral the enamel becomes very porous, especially beneath the enamel surface, and this is associated with a loss in translucency. The paradox of an apparent intact surface with underlying subsurface demineralization occurs as a result of preferential deposition of mineral within the surface, a process that is enhanced by fluoride. Surface layers up to 88 μm thick have been shown in individuals living in areas with water fluoridation [19]. Furthermore this surface layer is more resistant to acid demineralization when compared to the surrounding normal enamel.

III. FLUORIDE EFFECT ON THE PROGRESSION OF DENTAL CARIES

A. Theories

Two major theories exist for the cariostatic mechanism of fluoride. The first supposes that increased enamel resistance is due to a high concentration of fluoride in the enamel apatite imparting a lower solubility. However because fluoride needs to be in solution to affect both the demineralization and remineralization processes, it theoretically can only affect these processes once apatite is dissolved. The second theory of decreasing enamel solubility is based on the presence of fluoride in solution. When the fluoride concentration in the aqueous phase of enamel is high, the concentrations of calcium and phosphate only need to rise slightly for the formation of fluorhydroxyapatite which stops further dissolution of the crystals. To achieve this, fluoride needs to be maintained on the surface and in the enamel fluid in some way. This theory has the most support, hence the need to develop vehicles for fluoride which will ensure that the concentration remains high enough to protect the enamel during acidic challenge.

Fluoride also has been shown in in vitro studies to interfere with plaque bacteria metabolism including the metabolism of carbohydrate with resulting decrease in acid production. It is not clear at the present time how significant this is in caries reduction in the oral environment because the concentration of fluoride needed to achieve this appears to be much higher than the fluoride concentration which affects demineralization or remineralization [20, 21]. There has been some indication of a decrease in the amount of plaque formed with fluoride treatments in the mouth [22]. However, the decrease appears to be short term and there is some suggestion that the bacteria may adapt to the increased fluoride in the environment.

B. Fluoride Effect on Demineralization and Remineralization

When the pH in plaque on the surface of enamel is lowered from the physiological level of about pH 7.0 to below 5.5, the critical pH, the solubility of enamel increases about 100 times. Fluoride in concentrations as low as 0.1 ppmF appear to significantly decrease the mineral loss from enamel at these lower pHs. The concentration range of fluoride which is required to decrease the degree of demineralization and increase remineralization has been extensively investigated. This has been done using artificially created enamel lesions in human or bovine enamel. These enamel blocks are then cycled in solutions with different pHs, different concentrations of minerals, and different degrees of buffering. Ten Cate [20] summarized the studies of effects of fluoride under different conditions. When the pH decreases in the absence of fluoride there is significant loss of calcium from enamel. When fluoride is added, the loss of calcium is significantly decreased. The concentration of fluoride needed to significantly decrease demineralization and increase remineralization has been reported to be between 1.5 and 250 mmol/L. In experiments designed to look at the net effect of daily fluoride solution treatments on the demineralization and remineralization of dental enamel, Featherstone et al [21] demonstrated that the relative mineral loss was dependent on the logarithm of the fluoride concentration. A fluoride concentration of 9.4 mmol/L (178 ppmF) gave a 90% protection in their in vitro experiments. Although the results of this work cannot be directly translated to the oral environment, they suggest that significant fluoride effects on dental caries may be achieved with low concentrations in a daily application. The conditions present in the mouth cannot be completely modeled in in vitro conditions and it is clear from studies using daily fluoride mouthrinses that while significant reductions in dental caries can be achieved the reductions reported have generally been less than 50% [23].

C. Enamel Fluoride

Fluoride may be permanently bound in the enamel apatite and only lost if the apatite is dissolved. It may also be loosely bound in the enamel adsorbed to the apatite crystals, or in the aqueous environment or as calcium fluoride formed during demineralization or after topical fluoride has been applied to the teeth under acid conditions. During development, fluoride is taken up during three stages - secretion of the enamel matrix, during transition when the major mineralization is occurring and during maturation [24]. The concentration of fluoride in the subsurface enamel reflects fluoride which is incorporated during enamel development and this remains fairly constant during the life of the tooth unless the enamel is subsequently demineralized due to dental caries or acid erosion. When measuring fluoride in enamel, the depth at which the samples are taken, how long the teeth have been erupted in the mouth, which part of the crown the sample is taken from, whether the crown has wear, and whether the teeth have suffered demineralization due to dental caries must all be taken into account.

Subsurface enamel fluoride concentrations in low fluoride areas are usually around 40 ppmF while in optimally fluoridated areas (1.0 ppmF in the drinking water), the concentration is usually about 100 ppmF. The fluoride concentration in the surface enamel however, changes after the tooth erupts. Because tooth enamel is not fully mineralized on eruption, the surface enamel accumulates fluoride as further mineralization or maturing of the enamel occurs. In low fluoride areas the surface enamel fluoride concentration varies from 500-1000 ppmF. In optimally fluoridated areas the surface enamel fluoride concentration may be as high as 2500 ppmF [25]. The fluoride concentrations in different types of teeth in the mouth also vary and possibly reflect how mature the teeth are when they erupt. This means it is important to realize that a sample of the enamel of one tooth will not necessarily reflect all the teeth or the whole fluoride history of the individual. The fluoride concentration in the surface enamel may also vary in teeth at different sites in the mouth because the distribution of fluoride is different throughout the mouth [26, 27].

As well as becoming incorporated into enamel either after dissolution and reprecipitation of the crystals or by ionic exchange, fluoride may also be adsorbed onto the enamel mineral. At neutral pH fluoride reacts with acid phosphates to form calcium fluoride. At low pH calcium fluoride may form during enamel dissolution. Under electron microscopy, fluoride is observed on the surface of the enamel as spherical globules of calcium fluoride which are insoluble in saliva at neutral pH and may persist on the tooth surface for months after topical fluoride application [28, 29].

Salivary proteins and phosphates bind to the CaF_2 surface inhibiting dissolution. At pH less than 5.2 these coatings are lost and the calcium fluoride dissolves providing F^-. As the pH rises again, the coatings reestablish on the remaining CaF_2. This pH dependent mechanism provides for the bioavailability of the fluoride ion (F^-) during enamel demineralization either within plaque or within the rough topography of the enamel surface.

This fluoride contributes to supersaturation of the plaque fluid with respect to fluorapatite or fluorhydroxyapatite as calcium and phosphate ions are dissolved from the enamel surface. The supersaturated plaque fluid induces re-precipitation of mineral in the form of fluorapatite or fluorhydroxyapatite into the enamel surface which appears to be more resistant to subsequent dissolution. Therefore one important approach to maintaining adequate fluoride for caries inhibition appears to be the delivery of fluoride which will encourage the formation of calcium fluoride on the surfaces of the enamel [30].

D. Plaque Fluoride

Generally the concentrations of fluoride in plaque are much high than those in saliva [31]. The fluoride exists in both ionic form and bound forms complexed to organic material. Plaque fluoride concentration may be 100-10 000 times that in saliva. The concentrations reported over several studies were summarized by Tatevossian [32]. He reported a range of 0.3-5.1 mmol/L in wet plaque and 0.7-70.1 mmol/L in dry plaque depending on whether it was mineralized or not. Fluoride in plaque is derived from saliva, crevicular fluid, diet and fluoride products such as toothpastes and mouthrinses [33]. Since the concentration of fluoride in plaque is usually much higher than in saliva, some research has focused on trying to raise and sustain the fluoride in plaque to improve the effect on caries. It is thought that the more important effect on caries is that fluoride in plaque acts as a reservoir for ionic fluoride which is released from fluoride compounds when the pH in the plaque drops. Jenkins and Edgar [31] have reported that plaque with higher levels of fluoride shows a smaller pH drop when exposed to sucrose than plaque with lower levels of fluoride.

E. Fluoride in Saliva

Investigation of fluoride in saliva has been directed towards determining concentrations which provide the maximum decrease in dental caries. This has covered the concentrations achieved after systemic ingestion of fluorides, or after using various fluoride concentrations in different topical vehicles such as toothpaste and mouthwashes. The main aim of this work has been to achieve a sustained increase in the fluoride concentration in saliva in order to maintain higher levels at the tooth surface as demineralization starts and to retard or reverse the progression of dental carious lesions. Many of these studies have examined vehicles which would result in an increase in the fluoride concentrations in both saliva and dental plaque [34].

There have been some problems in correlating the levels of fluoride in saliva reported in early studies with those more recently reported. This has been because of the difficulties in determining the physiologically very low levels of fluoride present in saliva, the methods employed and the nature of the saliva sample. The concentration of fluoride in saliva is related to whether it is measured in whole saliva from all of the salivary glands or ductal saliva from one gland only. Whole saliva contains other debris such as food and plaque which may also contain fluoride. Saliva collected from the ducts will give a much clearer picture of the actual amounts of fluoride being excreted. Salivary concentrations of fluoride were reported as 0.13 ppmF by Carlson et al [35] using a radiofluoride method and 0.1 ppmF by McClure [36] who measured salivary fluoride levels in low fluoride water areas. In later studies after the development of the fluoride ion specific electrode by Frant and Ross [37], Grøn [38] used a known addition technique to measure the fluoride in saliva after acidification of the samples to avoid interference between the electrode crystal and salivary phosphate ions which occur at neutral pH. He reported fluoride concentrations between 0.01 and 0.04 ppmF. The concentrations were correlated with the fluoride concentrations in the drinking water and are similar to levels reported in later studies including those of Shannon and Edmonds [39], after diffusion of the fluoride from the samples, Ekstrand [40] using a direct determination technique, and Drummond et al [41] who determined the fluoride levels after prior diffusion of the fluoride with hexamethyldisiloxane hydrochloric acid. This latter method of Taves [42] is used most commonly at the present time.

Fluoride in saliva is related both to the systemic ingestion of fluoride and the fluoride in the mouth from topical fluorides. The levels of fluoride in mixed whole saliva are higher than in ductal saliva because of the contamination from plaque, foods, or toothpastes and other fluoride products [43]. Salivary levels of fluoride have also been shown to be related to the concentrations of fluoride in the drinking water. Bruun and Thylstrup [44] found that the mean salivary fluoride level was 0.03 ppmF in individuals drinking water with a fluoride concentration of 0.36 ppmF and 0.05 ppmF in individuals drinking water with 2.6 ppmF. They noted that fluoride levels in the early morning samples were higher than in the midday samples. This has been shown also by Zero et al [45] suggesting that the rate of fluoride clearance from saliva in the mouth may be lower during the night when the flow rate of saliva is reduced. The levels of fluoride in saliva may also vary if the saliva is sampled from different sites in the mouth. It is now clear that substances do not spread uniformly around the mouth and the concentrations of fluoride have been shown in several studies to vary from site to site [26, 27].

The fluoride concentration curves in saliva after the ingestion of fluoride follow those in plasma very closely but at lower concentrations. The ratio between fluoride in saliva and fluoride in plasma has been reported to be around 0.6 by Ekstrand [40] and Oliveby [46, 47]. Variation in the ratios reported previously, may be due to the sampling from ducts or whole saliva or due to the methods of measurement. Most investigators have found the ratios to be stable within individuals and once established for an individual, salivary fluoride concentrations appear to be an accurate indicator of fluoride in plasma for that individual. Collecting saliva is less invasive than collecting plasma and while not fully proven, saliva may also be a safer fluid to collect as it does not appear to always contain viruses present in plasma.

Attempts to sustain an increase in fluoride in saliva have used several approaches. Earlier studies investigated if the amounts of systemic fluoride ingested would increase the fluoride in saliva and sustain the increase. Shannon et al [48] showed a ten fold increase in salivary fluoride 40-50 minutes after the ingestion of 10 mg of fluoride. However this was reduced to a 2.3 times increase by eight hours after the original ingestion. Grøn [38] found the ingestion of 1.0 mg fluoride produced a salivary fluoride peak of 0.08 ppmF, 5 mg produced a peak of 0.18 and 10.0 mg produced a peak concentration of 0.24 ppmF. Further studies investigated whether the different fluoride compounds ingested resulted in different concentration profiles of fluoride in saliva. While the concentration of fluoride produced in saliva has been shown to be related to the solubility of the fluoride compound ingested, none of the compounds (Na_2PO_3F, NaF, SnF_2 AlF_3) have shown a sustained increase in the salivary fluoride beyond about 0.1 ppmF [49].

The early results were considered disappointing because it was believed that to provide significant caries protection, the salivary concentration of fluoride would need to be much higher. Now that it is understood that plaque has higher levels of fluoride than in saliva and that the plaque fluoride and the tooth surface enamel fluoride can be increased by intermittent applications of fluoride, it is considered that even the small increase in salivary fluoride found in fluoridated areas compared with non fluoridated areas plays a significant role in maintaining higher levels of fluoride at the tooth surface. In 1987 [50] a study of two groups of children - one with no dental caries and the other with a high level of dental caries found mean salivary fluoride concentrations of 0.04 ppmF in the caries-free children and 0.02 ppmF in the children with a high level of dental caries. There is no doubt that there are other major factors which differ between groups and play a role in caries prevention, but it is now understood that the fluoride levels in saliva may not need to be as high as once believed.

IV. VEHICLES FOR DELIVERY OF FLUORIDE

Since the recognition that fluoride does have a role in the prevention of dental caries, it has been used in many forms. Initially the systemic and topical forms were used to increase the amount of fluoride in developing teeth. Systemic vehicles for fluoride include drinking water, either as public supplies or school supplies, tablets, drops, milk, salt and there has been some investigation of incorporating fluoride in sugar. All systemic vehicles, except tablets if swallowed without chewing or sucking, have a topical effect during ingestion and all contribute to increasing the fluoride content of saliva. Consequently they still have a role when the use of topical vehicles is impractical. However as the main effect of fluoride is a topical effect which decreases demineralization of enamel during an acid attack and enhances remineralization after the acid attack is over, the emphasis has shifted away from developing further systemic vehicles. There are now clear indications that vehicles which result in sustained higher levels of fluoride at the plaque-enamel interface by the deposition of calcium fluoride on the surface of the enamel under acid conditions are the most effective vehicles.

A. Water Fluoridation

When the amount of fluoride in drinking water was first adjusted to 1.0 ppmF as a public health measure, this concentration was chosen after extensive population investigations by Dean [1] to determine the maximum reduction in dental caries with the minimum appearance of enamel fluorosis. The numerous extensive global studies of fluoridated populations compared with populations without fluoridated water supplies have shown caries reductions in the primary dentitions of 40-49% and in the permanent dentitions of 50-59%. These global results were reviewed by Murray [51] in 1991 who concluded that the studies showed that the caries reductions in these populations was both from a systemic and topical effect. As already discussed, the fluoride levels in saliva and plaque in individuals drinking optimally fluoridated water are higher than in individuals living in areas with low concentrations of <0.3 ppmF fluoride in the water.

B. Tablets and Drops

Many studies comparing the use of fluoride tablets over the last five decades have lead researchers to believe that although there is some effect from the systemic use either by the fluoride being excreted in the saliva or by incorporation in developing teeth, the most important effect is most likely from the topical effect of the tablet itself, especially if it is sucked or chewed before being swallowed. The fluoride supplement caries-preventive studies up to 1988 as reviewed by Murray [51] showed that the level of prevention for the primary dentition was between 40 and 93% in studies of varying length and design. For the permanent dentition the reductions reported were mostly around 40%. The main problem as perceived by many clinicians and researchers is that the compliance of tablet taking is low. To combat this problem some trials have been conducted giving the tablets on school days under supervision. Tablets or drops may be most effective when sucked before swallowing or when dissolved in water to make a concentration of 1.0 ppmF. When sucked or chewed tablets may also contribute to the reservoirs of calcium fluoride on the teeth. This may be a useful way of protecting the teeth of frail elderly.

Systemic fluorides have some limitations in very young children while their tooth enamel is forming. If the systemic intake at this time is too high, the enamel of the forming teeth may erupt hypomineralized (without the crystals fully formed) which appears as white lines and marks on the teeth and is known as fluorosis. Many other factors can cause the same problem although the pattern of hypomineralization in fluorosed teeth is quite distinctive. In areas with 1 ppmF in the drinking water the maximum caries benefit is gained with the minimum fluorosis of the teeth. It has been shown that fluorosis is more likely to occur when fluoride supplements are given, when baby foods or formulae do not have their amount of fluoride controlled during manufacture and when young children ingest fluoride containing toothpastes [52, 53].

C. Milk, Salt and Sugar

Künzel [54] reviewed the effect of adding fluoride to domestic salt, milk or sugar. Several countries have introduced fluoride for systemic consumption in domestic salt. These include Switzerland, Spain, Colombia, Hungary and France. Caries reductions of 36.4 to 79.3% have been reported in studies ranging from 4 to 24 years. The designs of the studies varied widely and other preventive agents were in place or introduced during these studies. However there is no doubt that fluoridated salt is an effective delivery system. Marthaler [55] reported that the reduction in caries due to salt fluoridation is comparable to water fluoridation over a long time period. Studies of the effect of adding fluoride to milk have reported caries reductions between 17-82%. Most studies have been short term and focused on children only. While drinking fluoridated milk may well provide a significant caries reduction, it has difficulties in determining the amount of milk which is drunk and in the handling and delivery. Similar results have been found in studies which have examined the effect of drinking high-fluoride beverages such as tea and mineral waters.

Adding fluoride to sugar has been investigated on the basis that fluoride is present with the sugar at the time when acid is being produced and thus should have optimal effect. In in vitro experiments, the addition of fluoride reduced the demineralization of the enamel. In animal studies the addition of fluoride to sugar in the diets resulted in significant reductions in dental caries. In a dietary study over three years where fluoride was added to several sugar products of the diet of children in institutions, the reduction in caries between the test and control groups was 42% [56]. This study suggests that further research should be conducted over longer periods. Another source of fluoride in foods is that which is inadvertently incorporated during processing or during reconstitution with fluoridated water. The levels have not been shown to be of significance except for those in baby formulae and some baby foods. Children who have been given these foods containing higher levels of fluoride, have been shown to have a higher risk of dental fluorosis of their permanent teeth [53].

D. Prenatal Supplementation

Several papers have claimed significant reductions in dental caries in the primary dentition when fluoride supplements were given during pregnancy. However none of these studies were double blind and other factors such as the use of fluoride after the teeth erupted, the diet and oral hygiene procedures were not included [57].

E. Topical Fluorides - General

When topical fluorides are used they usually result in raised salivary fluoride levels at least for a short period. There is also evidence that they contribute to the fluoride content of enamel and of plaque especially where demineralization and remineralization are occurring. Fluoride from toothpaste and other topical agents such as gels and varnishes also contributes to the formation of calcium fluorides or to their maintenance on the enamel surfaces of teeth. It is now accepted that topical fluorides when used appropriately have the most significant effect on the dental caries process.

F. Topical Fluorides - Toothpastes

The investigations of using fluoride in toothpastes began in the 1940s. Of all the fluoride vehicles used, toothpaste is the only one which is used as a routine part of personal hygiene habits - that is teeth cleaning. In terms of importance in caries preventive strategies, fluoride toothpaste is the only vehicle that is common to all countries which have shown a reduction in the amount of dental caries [58]. There is good evidence to show that fluoride from toothpaste is taken up by enamel - especially enamel that has already been partially demineralized. The fluoride compounds which have been most commonly tested in toothpastes are sodium monofluorophosphate, sodium fluoride, stannous fluoride, acidulated phosphate fluoride, and amine fluoride. An allied development is that of compatible abrasive systems which will not interfere with the uptake of fluoride. This was reviewed by von der Fehr and Møller in 1978 [59]. Clinical trials of fluoride toothpastes have shown caries reductions of up to 48% over 1-11 year periods [51].

The concentration of fluoride added to toothpastes has generally been about 1000 parts per million. Studies comparing both lower and higher amounts were reviewed by Murray et al in 1991 [51]. There is still debate as to whether toothpastes with lower concentrations of fluoride are as effective and, although there is some further reduction in caries when more fluoride is added to toothpaste, this has not always been statistically significant. The effective concentration is probably related to the effective fluoride levels that are achieved in plaque and at the enamel surface during tooth demineralization. At the present time this appears to be in the 1000 ppmF range.

A further consideration of the fluoride concentration in toothpastes is related to the tendency of preschool children to swallow toothpaste either inadvertently or deliberately while brushing. Prior to 3-4 years-of-age, it has been shown in many studies that a third or more of the toothpaste put on the brush is swallowed [60]. The fluoride in toothpaste is absorbed effectively despite the type of paste or the age of the person swallowing it [41, 61]. If the toothpaste is squeezed across the brush head this is equivalent to about 1 g of toothpaste containing 1 mg of fluoride. One third of this, swallowed twice daily is double the recommended systemic intake of fluoride for preschool children. Consequently as a result of the fluoride in food or water or a fluoride tablet, fluorosis can be increased in this age group. The preschool years represent the time of highest risk for fluorosis during tooth development. Because the benefits of fluoride toothpaste are very important, the current recommendation is to continue to use fluoride toothpaste in preschool children under adult supervision and only use a smear of paste on the brush so that the systemic intake is reduced to a minimum.

Toothpastes (prophylaxis pastes) used for professional cleaning by dentists, dental hygienists or dental therapists contain considerably higher levels of fluoride than toothpastes which are available over the counter. Most commonly used are prophylaxis pastes with varying levels of abrasives containing 1.23% F-acidulated phosphate fluoride (APF). Some studies have shown reductions in dental caries when patients in low fluoride area have their teeth cleaned with these prophylaxis pastes as part of a professional tooth cleaning program [62]. The caries reduction probably is related to the uptake of fluoride by enamel and the formation of calcium fluorides. The degree of protection depends on the frequency of application and the time interval between applications.

G. Topical Fluorides - Rinses

Mouthwashes containing fluoride are either formulated for home use or for rinsing programs in schools. Home-use fluorides are either used daily (0.05% neutral sodium fluoride or 0.4% stannous fluoride) or weekly (0.2% sodium fluoride). The fluorides may also be incorporated in gels to use in trays which fit over the teeth. The school rinsing programs usually occur weekly or every two weeks. Fluoride mouthrinses have been shown to be of benefit both in low fluoride communities and to have an added benefit when used in communities with optimum fluoride in the water [63, 64]. Fluoride mouthrinses raise the levels of fluoride in saliva for several hours [65, 66] and Rølla and Saxegaard [67], Ögaard [29] and Cruz [68] have all shown that fluoride rinses can also result in higher fluoride in enamel and the formation of calcium fluoride on the teeth. Undoubtedly fluoride rinses also contribute to the remineralization of early carious lesions in enamel.

H. Topical Fluorides - Gels

Acidulated phosphate fluoride (1.23% F), stannous fluoride (8.0% F) and more recently introduced neutral sodium fluoride gels (2.0% F) are used in professional preventive treatments of dental caries. They are applied to the teeth in trays which surround the teeth for periods of one to four minutes. Gels designed for home use have lower concentrations of fluoride. The effectiveness of the neutral sodium fluoride gels has not been widely investigated but they have been introduced because of the concern that the APF gels might etch the glass filler particles and the porcelain of many of the newer dental restorative materials. In studies of the application of 1.23% APF gel in low fluoride communities either once or twice yearly the caries rate was reduced in school children by between 3 and 41% [69]. Because of the high levels of fluoride it is generally recommended that these fluoride vehicles be used only for patients at higher risk of caries. Apart from those patients at high risk of caries because of their diets, other groups which should be targeted for these treatments are patients who have head and neck radiation, patients who are immunocompromised, elderly individuals at risk of tooth root caries and perhaps patients with physical disabilities. Many of these patients and others on drugs which affect salivary flow have xerostomia (dry mouth).

I. Topical Fluorides - Varnishes

Two varnishes containing fluoride are currently available. The first is a neutral colophomium base with 5% sodium fluoride by weight and the second is a polyurethane base with 0.9% fluorsilane. Varnishes have been developed to try to improve the duration of contact of the fluoride with the enamel and provide a waterproofing after a fluoride treatment. Increases in the enamel and in salivary fluoride concentrations have been demonstrated. Various studies have shown that fluoride varnishes effectively inhibit demineralization and several studies have shown that children at higher risk of dental caries have significant decreases in caries. However in individuals with low caries no significant improvements have been shown [63, 70].

J. Topical Fluorides - Slow Release Delivery Systems

Slow release fluoride delivery systems have been designed to stay in the oral environment for prolonged periods of time in order to maintain higher levels of fluoride in saliva, plaque and on the enamel surface. The various devices may be bonded to tooth tissue using composite resins, be incorporated in dental appliances such as dentures or orthodontic appliances or adhere temporarily to oral mucosa. Mirth [71], reported on a study of the fluoride release profiles from a copolymer device which could be attached to the buccal surfaces of teeth. The device developed by Cowsar et al [72] was made up of an inner core of a hydrogel: a copolymer of hydroxyethylmethacrylate (HEMA) and methylmethacrylate (MMA) in a 50:50 ratio containing NaF. This was surrounded by an outer membrane of HEMA/MMA in a ratio of 30:70. This device with a reservoir of 200-485 mg fluoride, was demonstrated in in vitro studies to have linear release characteristics of 0.02 to 1.0 mg fluoride per day. for 30-180 days. Consideration was also given to the problem of the device detaching from the tooth surface and being swallowed. Because of the hydrogel the fluoride was only released slowly even if the device was ruptured.

Friedman [73], described a fluoride containing film which could be used to coat orthodontic bands and chewing gums. The film made up of polydimethylsiloxane (silicone), ethylcellulose (EC) and ethylcellulose with polyethylene glycol (PEG) had fluoride embedded during polymerization. Fluoride was released from this film in a non linear fashion at 0.06-0.5 mg/day for 304 days.

Bottenberg et al [74], investigated the concentrations of fluoride in saliva with the use of conventional fluoride tablets, either swallowed directly or dissolved before swallowing, and bioadhesive slow release tablets. The bioadhesive tablets consisted of polyethylene glycol polymers. They found that the fluoride release from the conventional tablets when sucked was nearly complete after 30 minutes and 100% was released after one hour. Only a slight rise in the saliva fluoride was seen after 30 minutes when the tablets were ingested. The bioadhesive tablets showed a more gradual release of fluoride and reached complete release after 8 hours. The retention time was unrelated to the flow rate of saliva. These tablets were well tolerated by the subjects although some noticed increased salivary viscosity which was thought to be due to the slow erosion of the tablet surface with polymer particles spreading throughout the mouth.

Slow release delivery systems offer much potential for contributing to sustained release fluoride delivery and may be especially useful for individuals who are at high risk of dental caries but who may not cooperate to allow fluoride to be applied in other ways. There is also extra safety in that the fluoride is not swallowed in one dose which may be important in very young children to avoid fluorosis of developing teeth. The time of day to apply the fluoride may be chosen and the tablet may be placed in the mouth nearest to teeth which are most caries active.

Toumba and Curzon [75] reviewed the concept of slow release fluoride. They pointed out that some devices can produce an increase in salivary fluoride in humans for up to two years and that clinical trials were underway to look at the caries reduction with fluoride releasing copolymer or glass devices. Fluoride releasing glass was developed from a similar glass designed for the slow release of trace elements in cattle. The glass devices are attached to the teeth with composite resin and the glass dissolves slowly in saliva resulting in an increase in salivary fluoride.

All the devices currently available have been shown to increase fluoride concentration in adjacent enamel. Mirth et al [76] found 63% less caries in rats using a copolymer device. However at the present time there are unanswered questions. The first is; "do these devices result in a decrease in caries in humans?" The second is; "what are the optimal sites for placement of the devices?" This is important in view of the fact that substances in saliva do not spread evenly in the mouth and the profile of fluoride release from these devices needs to be better understood (see Chapter 8). Finally, in individuals who have problems with salivary flow or the components of saliva which are also important in maintaining teeth; "can these devices also be used to provide other appropriate minerals along with the fluoride?"

K. Topical Fluorides - Dental Materials

Some materials used to restore teeth after they have become damaged by dental caries may also act as slow release vehicles for fluoride. The material itself, however, needs to remain intact as the fluorides are released. A material used in the past, silicate cement based on a fluorosilicate glass, was very effective in preventing further caries in developing around the margins of fillings because of the continuous fluoride release as the filling slowly dissolved [77]. High fluoride concentrations in excess 4000 ppmF were found in enamel adjacent to silicate restorations.

Newer materials such as the glass ionomer cements based on customized fluorosilicate glasses, as well as fluoride ion exchange resins, provide prolonged fluoride release, adhesion to enamel and dentine and greater stability in the mouth [78-81]. Recent clinical studies indicate that tooth surfaces adjacent to glass ionomer cement have reduced caries susceptibility [82, 83] and this may be partially attributable to an inhibitory effect on the growth of *Streptococcus mutans* in the plaque [83, 84]. After placement of these materials, Hatibovic-Kofman and Koch [85] demonstrated that salivary fluoride levels also remained elevated. Recent in vitro tests [86] found that glass ionomer cements could absorb fluoride from APF solutions and release it slowly. This approach offers a means of replenishing or boosting the fluoride content of older glass ionomer restorations without removing them.

V. FUTURE PERSPECTIVES

It has become more difficult to investigate the efficacy of different fluoride compounds or different vehicles because of the wide range of fluorides available and being used together with the presence of fluoride in many products including food and beverages. For most individuals there will already be a fluoride effect and the new fluoride concentration or method of delivery being tested has to be effective enough to be detected against the other fluorides already influencing the dental caries activity.

Current and future investigations of fluoride vehicles in particular may center around several aims. One is to improve the delivery of fluoride to the sites on the teeth that are most at risk of caries. At the present time one method is the deliberate precipitation of calcium fluoride layers on the surface of the teeth which act as a type of slow release when the pH at the surface of the enamel drops. Another aim is to increase the ability of fluorides to decrease demineralization and enhance remineralization of early carious lesions. This requires the fluoride levels to be maintained at the sites on teeth where acid is most likely to be produced. The effectiveness of fluoride may be improved by incorporation into different vehicles or by delivery with other synergistic compounds. These aspects require ongoing investigation.

Another aspect to fluoride delivery is determining the most effective vehicles related to different ages and different needs of various groups with different clinical problems. One example would be to find the most effective way to maintain effective levels of fluoride in the mouths of elderly patients after a stroke who are at high risk for dental caries because of poor oral hygiene and changed dietary habits. The possibilities here are to attach a mucosal slow release device that delivers fluoride and simultaneously an antibacterial agent effective against caries producing bacteria. However the safety factors need to be taken into consideration - especially in young children where prolonged fluoride administration is required for caries control, however, simultaneously there is a need to keep ingestion to a minimum.

Some of these research projects require the development of teams to manage the different aspects. It appears that pharmaceutical scientists working in conjunction with enamel chemists and dental clinicians could together answer some of the remaining difficulties related to effective and cost effective fluoride delivery.

VI. CONCLUSIONS

Fluoride in the many different vehicles currently available has drastically altered the level of dental caries in individuals and population groups. Recently a better understanding of the mechanisms by which fluoride acts has led researchers to consider and devise different delivery systems to effectively maintain the necessary concentrations of fluoride needed at the tooth surface to interfere with the dental caries process. Today there is a focus on placing delivery systems at specific sites within the mouth capable of providing selective and improved means of controlling dental caries.

REFERENCES

1. H. T. Dean, Chronic endemic dental fluorosis (mottled enamel), *J. Am. Med. Assoc. 107*:1269 (1936).
2. H. T. Dean, and E. Elove, Some epidemiological aspects of chronic endemic dental fluorosis, *Am. J. Pub. H. 26*:567 (1936).
3. N. J. Ainsworth, Mottled teeth, *Brit. Dent. J. 60*: 233 (1933).

4. H. T. Dean, F. A. Arnold (Jun), and E. Elove, Domestic water and dental caries. V. Additional studies of the relation of fluoride domestic waters to dental caries experience in 4,425 white children aged 12-14 years, of 13 cities in 4 states, *Pub. Health Rep. 57*:1155 (1942).
5. F. A. Arnold (Jun), H. T. Dean, P. Jay, and J. W. Knutson, Effect of fluoridated public water supplies on dental caries prevalence. 10th year of the Grand Rapids-Muskegon study, *Pub. Health Rep. 71*:652 (1956).
6. F. A. Arnold, R. C. Likens, A. L. Russel, and D. B. Scott, Fifteenth year of the Grand Rapids fluoridation study, *J. Am. Dent. Assoc. 65*:780 (1962).
7. J. G. Stannard, Y. S. Shim, M. Kritsineli, P. Labropoulou, and A. Tsamtsouris, Fluoride levels and fluoride contamination of fruit juices, *J. Clin. Ped. Dent. 16*:38 (1991).
8. B. A. Burt, The changing patterns of systemic fluoride intake, *J. Dent. Res. 71*:1228 (1992).
9. A. Vlachou, B. K. Drummond, and M. E. J. Curzon, Fluoride concentrations of infant foods and drinks in the United Kingdom, *Caries Res. 26*:29 (1992).
10. N. G. Chowdhury, R. H. Brown, and M. G. Shepherd, Fluoride intake of infants in New Zealand, *J. Dent. Res. 69*:1828 (1990).
11. J. Johnson, and J. W. Bawden, The fluoride content of infant formulas available in 1985, *Pediatr. Dent. 9*:33 (1987).
12. O. Fejerskov, F. Manji, and B. Baelum, The nature and mechanisms of dental fluorosis in man, *J. Dent. Res. 69*:692 (1990).
13. R. W. Evans, and J. W. Stamm, An epidemiological estimate of the critical period during which human maxillary central incisors are most susceptible to fluorosis, *J. Publ. Health Dent. 51*:251 (1991).
14. A. Thylstrup, and O. Feyerskov, *Textbook of Cariology*, Munksgaard, Copenhagen, (1994).
15. A. J. Rugg-Gunn, W. M. Edgar, D. A. M. Geddes, and G. N. Jenkins, The effect of different meal patterns on plaque pH in human subjects, *Brit. Dent. J. 139*:351 (1975).
16. M. E. Jensen, and C. F. Schachtele, The acidogenic potential of reference foods and snacks at interproximal sites, *J. Dent. Res. 62*:889 (1983).
17. C. Dawes, Inorganic constituents of saliva in relation to caries, *Cariology Today* (B. Guggenheim ed.) Basel, Karger (1984).
18. F. Lagerlöf, Effects of flow rate and pH on calcium phosphate saturation in human parotid saliva, *Caries Res. 17*:403 (1983).
19. V. Patanapiradez, and J. C. Rodda, Impregnation of early carious lesions in enamel with dental resins, *J. Dent. Res. 64*:250 Abstract 682 (1985).
20. J. M. ten Cate, In vitro studies on the effects of fluoride on de- and remineralization, *J. Dent. Res. 69*:614 (1990).

21. J. B. D. Featherstone, R. Glena, M. Shariati, and C. P. Shields, Dependence of in vitro demineralization of apatite and remineralization of dental enamel on fluoride concentration, *J. Dent. Res. 69*:620 (1990).
22. C. van Loveren, The antimicrobial action of fluoride and its role in caries inhibition, *J. Dent. Res. 69*:676 (1990).
23. G. Nikiforuk, *Understanding Dental Caries. 2. Prevention Basic and Clinical Aspects,* Karger, Basel, (1985).
24. C. Robinson, and J. Kirkham, The effect of fluoride on the developing mineralized tissues, *J. Dent. Res. 69*:685 (1990).
25. R. Aasenden, E. C. Moreno, and F. Brudevold, Fluoride levels in the surface enamel of different types of human teeth, *Arch. Oral. Biol. 18*:1403 (1973).
26. J. A. Weatherell, M. Strong, C. Robinson, and J. P. Ralph, Fluoride distribution in the mouth after fluoride rinsing, *Caries Res. 20*:111 (1986).
27. R. E. Primosch, J. A. Weatherell, and M. Strong, Distribution and retention of salivary fluoride from a sodium fluoride tablet following various intraoral dissolution methods, *J. Dent. Res. 65*:1001 (1986).
28. A. G. Dijkman, P. Deboer, and J. Arends, In vivo investigation on the fluoride content in and on human enamel after topical applications, *Caries Res. 17*:392 (1983).
29. B. Ögaard, Effects of fluoride on caries development and progression in vivo, *J. Dent. Res. 69*:813 (1990).
30. G. Rølla, B. Ögaard, and R. De Almeida Cruz, Topical application of fluorides on teeth. New concepts of mechanism of interaction, *J. Clin. Periodontol. 20*:105 (1993).
31. G. N. Jenkins, and W. M. Edgar, Distribution and forms of F in saliva and plaque, *Caries Res. 11*:226 (1977).
32. A. Tatevossian, Fluoride in dental plaque and its effects, *J. Dent. Res. 69*:645 (1990).
33. W. M. Edgar, G. S. Ingram, and S. N. Morgan, Fluoride in saliva and plaque in relation to fluoride in drinking water and in dentifrices, *Clinical and Biological Aspects of Dentifrices* (G. Embery, and G. Rolla eds.) Oxford University Press, Oxford, 1992, p. 157.
34. C. Bruun, D. Lambrou, M. J. Larsen, O. Fejerskov, and A. Thylstrup, Fluoride in mixed human saliva after different topical fluoride treatments and possible relation to caries inhibition, *Comm. Dent. Oral Epidemiol. 10*:124 (1982).
35. C. H. Carlson, W. D. Armstrong, and L. Singer, Distribution and excretion of radiofluoride in the human, *Proc. Soc. Expt. Biol. Med. 104*:235 (1960).
36. F. J. McClure, Domestic water and dental caries. III. Fluorine in human saliva, *Am. J. Dis. Child. 62*:512 (1941).

37 M. S. Frant, and J. W. Ross, Electrode for sensing fluoride ion activity in solution, *Science 154*:1553 (1966).

38. P. Grøn, H. G. McCann, and F. Brudevold, The direct determination of fluoride in human saliva by a fluoride electrode, *Arch. Oral Biol. 3*:203 (1968).

39. I. L. Shannon, and E. J. Edmonds, Effect of fluoride dosage on human parotid saliva fluoride levels, *Arch. Oral Biol. 17*:1303 (1972).

40. J. Ekstrand, A micromethod for the determination of fluoride in blood plasma and saliva, *Cal. Tiss. Res. 23*:225 (1977).

41. B. K. Drummond, M. E. J. Curzon, and M. Strong, Estimation of fluoride absorption from swallowed fluoride toothpastes, *Caries Res. 24*:211 (1990).

42 D. R. Taves, Separation of fluoride by rapid diffusion using hexamethyldisiloxane, *Talanta 15*:969 (1968).

43. C. Bruun, H. Givskov, and A. Thylstrup, Whole saliva fluoride after toothbrushing with NaF and MFP dentifrices with different fluoride concentrations, *Caries Res. 18*:282 (1984).

44. C. Bruun, and A. Thylstrup, Fluoride in whole saliva and dental caries experience in areas with high or low concentrations of fluoride in the drinking water, *Caries Res. 18*:450 (1984).

45. D. T. Zero, R. F. Raubertas, J. Fu, A. M. Pedersen, A. L. Hayes, and J. B. D. Featherstone, Fluoride concentrations in plaque, whole saliva, and ductal saliva after application of home-use topical fluorides, *J. Dent. Res. 71*:1768 (1992).

46 A. Oliveby, F. Lagerlöf, J Ekstrand, and C. Dawes, Studies on fluoride concentrations in human submandibular/sublingual saliva and their relation to flow rate and plasma fluoride levels, *J. Dent. Res. 68*:146 (1989).

47. A. Oliveby, F. Lagerlöf, J Ekstrand, and C. Dawes, Studies on fluoride excretion in whole saliva and its relation to flow rate and plasma fluoride levels, *Caries Res. 23*:243 (1989).

48. I. L. Shannon, R. P. Feller, H. H. Chauncey, Fluoride in human parotid saliva, *J. Dent. Res. 55*:506 (1976).

49. F. Brudevold, Y. Bakhos, and P. Grøn, Fluoride in human saliva after ingestion of aluminum chloride, and sodium fluoride or sodium monofluorophosphate, *Arch. Oral. Biol. 18*:699 (1973).

50. C. P. Shields, D. H. Leverett, S. M. Adair, and J. B. D. Featherstone, Salivary fluoride levels in fluoridated and non-fluoridated communities, *J. Dent. Res. 66*:141 Abstract 277 (1987).

51. J. J. Murray, A. J. Rugg-Gunn, and G. N. Jenkins, *Fluorides in Caries Prevention*, Butterworth-Heinemann, Oxford, 1991

52. O. Fejerskov, F. Manji, V. Baelum, The nature and mechanisms of dental fluorosis in man, *J. Dent. Res. 69*: 692 (1990).

53. D. G. Pendrys, and R. V. Katz, Risk of enamel fluorosis associated with fluoride supplementation, infant formula, and fluoride dentifrice use, *Am. J. Epidemiol. 130*:199 (1989).
54. W. Künzel, Systemic use of fluoride-other methods: salt, sugar, milk, etc., *Caries Res. 27*:16 (1993).
55. T. M. Marthaler, Cariostatic efficacy of the combined use of fluorides, *J. Dent. Res. 69*:797 (1990).
56. H. Luoma, A. Nyman, A. Toivonen, S. Söderholm, T. Nuuja, R. L. Kantero, M. L. Hassinen, M. Jokela, P. Nummikoski, R. Ranta, and I. Thesleff, Effect on caries in mentally handicapped children of addition of fluoride and bicarbonate-phosphate to dietary sugar products, *Scand. J. Dent. Res. 87*:197 (1979).
57. W. S. Driscoll, A review of the clinical research on the use of prenatal fluoride administration for prevention of dental caries, *J. Dent. Child. 48*:109 (1981).
58. G. Rølla, B. Ögaard, and R. de Almeida-Cruz, Clinical effect and mechanism of cariostatic action of fluoride-containing toothpastes: A review, *Int. Dent. J. 41*:171 (1991).
59. F. R. von der Fehr, and I. J. Møller, Caries-preventive fluoride dentifrices, *Caries Res. 12*:31 (1978).
60. W. E. Barnhart, L. K. Hiller, G. T. Leonard, and S. E. Michaels, Dentifrice usage and ingestion among four age groups, *J. Dent. Res. 53*:1317 (1974).
61. B. K. Drummond, and M. E. J. Curzon, Fluoride absorption from swallowed fluoride toothpaste in infants, *J. Dent. Res. 64*:1145 (1985).
62. S. Poulsen, N. Agerbaek, B. Melsen, D. C. Korts, L. Glavind, and G. Rølla, The effect of professional tooth cleansing on gingivitis and dental caries in children after one year, *Comm. Dent. Oral Epidemiol. 4*:195 (1976).
63. L. G. Petersson, Fluoride mouthrinses and fluoride varnishes, *Caries Res. 27*:35 (1993).
64. L. W. Ripa, Rinses for the control of dental caries, *Int. Dent. J. 42*:263 (1992).
65. U. Heintze, and L. G. Peterson, Accumulation and clearance of fluoride in human mixed saliva after different topical fluoride treatments, *Swed. Dent. J. 3*:141 (1979).
66. L. G. Petersson, N. Ludvigsson, C. Ullbro, A. Gleerup, and G. Koch, Fluoride clearance of whole saliva in young children after topical application, *Swed. Dent. J. 11*:95 (1987).
67. G. Rølla, and E. Saxegaard, Critical evaluation of the composition and use of topical fluorides with emphasis on the role of calcium fluoride in caries inhibition, *J. Dent. Res. 60*:780 (1990).

68. R. Cruz, G. Rølla, and B. Ögaard, Formation of fluoride on enamel in vitro after exposure to fluoridated mouthrinses, *Acta. Odontol. Scand. 4 9*:329 (1991).

69 S. H. Y. Wei, and C. K. Y. Yiu, Evaluation of the use of topical fluoride gel, *Caries Res. 27*:29 (1993).

70. D. C. Clark, A review on fluoride varnishes: an alternative topical fluoride treatment, *Comm. Dent. Oral Epidemiol. 10*:117 (1982).

71. D. B. Mirth, The use of controlled and sustained release agents in dentistry: a review of applications for the control of dental caries, *Pharmacol. Ther. Dent. 5*:595 (1980).

72. D. Cowsar, O. Tarwater, and A. Tanquaery, Controlled release of fluoride from hydrogels for dental applications, *Hydrogels for Medical and Related Applications* (J. D. Andrade ed.) Washington. American Chemical Society, 1976, p. 180.

73. M. Friedman, Fluoride prolonged release preparations for topical use, *J. Dent. Res. 59*:1392 (1980).

74. P. Bottenberg, R. Cleymaet, C. De Muynck, J. P. Remon, D. Coomans, and D. Slop, Comparison of salivary fluoride concentrations after administration of a bioadhesive slow-release tablet and a conventional fluoride tablet, *J. Pharm. Pharmacol. 44*:684 (1992).

75. K. J. Toumba, and M. E. J. Curzon, Slow-release fluoride, *Caries Res. 27*:43 (1993).

76. D. Mirth, D. Adderly, and S. Amsbaugh, Inhibition of experimental dental caries using an intra-oral device for the controlled release of fluoride, *J. Am. Dent. Assoc. 107*:55 (1983).

77. A. S. Hallsworth, and J. A. Weatherell, The microdistribution, uptake and loss of fluoride in human enamel, *Caries Res. 3*:109 (1969).

78. M. L. Swartz, R. W. Phillips, and H. E. Clark, Long-term release from glass ionomer cements, *J. Dent. Res. 63*:158 (1984).

79. L. Skartveit, A. B. Tveit, B. Totdal, R. Ovrebo, and M. Raadal, In vivo fluoride uptake in enamel and dentine from fluoride containing materials, *J. Dent. Child. 58*:97 (1990).

80. L. Forsten, Short- and long-term fluoride release from glass ionomer liners, *Scan. J. Dent. Res. 93*:340 (1991).

81. K. J. Donly, Enamel and dentin demineralization inhibition of fluoride-releasing materials, *Am. J. Dent. 7*:275 (1994).

82. M. Svanberg, Class II amalgam restorations, glass-ionomer tunnel restorations, and caries development on adjacent tooth surfaces: A 3-year study, *Caries Res. 26*:315 (1992).

83. E. M. Benelli, M. C. Serra, A. L. Rodrigues, and J. A. Curry, In situ anticariogenic potential of glass ionomer cement, *Caries Res. 27*:280 (1993).

84. M. Svanberg, B. Krasse, and H. -O. Örnerfeld, mutans streptococci in interproximal plaque from amalgam and glass ionomer restorations, *Caries Res. 24*:133 (1990).
85. D. Hatibovic-Kofman, and G. Koch, Fluoride release from glass ionomer cements in vivo and in vitro, *Swed. Dent. J. 15*:253 (1991).
86. A. Kupietzky, M. Houpt, J. Mellberg, and J. Shey, Fluoride exchange from glass ionomer preventive resins restorations, *Pediatr. Dent. 116*:340 (1994).
87. P. H. Keyes, The infectious and transmissible nature of experimental dental caries, *Archs. Oral Biol. 1*:304 (1960).

Author Index

A

Aasenden, R., 387, *401*
Abbs, E. T., 205, *217*
Abernathy, J. L., 36, *47*
Abraham, W., 33, 35, *45*
Abrahams, L., 359, *373*
Abrams, K., 31, *43*
Achari, R., 253, *277*
Acosta, E., 103, *115*
Adair, S. M., 390, *402*
Adams, D., 56, *61*, 96, *100*
Adderly, D., 397, *404*
Addy, M., 135, *155*, 312, *316, 376,* 367, *377*
Adjenpon-Yamoah, K. K., 134, *154*, 253, *278*
Adkins, E. L., 16, *25*, 58, *62*, 86, *98*, 135, 136, 138, *155*, 253, *278*, 297, *314*
Adriaens, P., 370, 372, *378*
Adson, A., 106, 107, *118*
Agerbaek, N., 395, *403*
Aguirre, A., 198, 202, *215*, 207, *219*
Ainamo, J., 329, *354*, 344, *356*, 371, *379*
Ainsworth, N. J., 381, *399*
Al-Hashimi, I., 192, *211*, 192, 198, *212*, 223, *236*
Al-Sayed-Omar, O., 58, *62*, 253, *278*
Aladib, W., 209, *220*
Albanese, E., 114, *119*
Albery, W. J., 30, *42*
Aleo, J. J., 361, *374*
Alfano, M. C., 10, *22*, 56, *61*, 86, 93, *98*, 255, *279*, 256, *280*
Allen, A., 204, *217*, 223, *236*, 224, *237*
Allenby, C. F., 40, *48*
Allison, A. C., 361, *374*
Alvares, O. F., 2, *19*
Amar, S., 361, *374*
Amsbaugh, S., 397, *404*
Anders, R., 67, *80*, 123, *153*, 233, *239*, 261, 263, *280*, 274, *284*, 287, 297, *313*, 311, *315*, 312, *316, 317*
Anderson, B., 103, *116*
Andersen, C., 326, *353*
Andersen, T., 332, 333, 338, 339, *354*
Anderson, W. F., 209, *220*

Andersson, T. F., 33, *45*
Andriaenssen, C., 370, 372, *378*
Angelo, H. R., 271, *281*, 350, *357*
Anguiano-Igea, S., 272, 273, *283*
Anlar, S., 273, *283*
Apicella, A., *238*
Appleton, J., 13, *23*
Araki, M., 70, 72, *81*
Aramaki, Y., 205, *218*
Arbab, A. G., 134, *155*, 253, *278*
Arends, J., 388, *401*
Arenholt-Bindslev, D. D., 104, 110, 111, 113, *116*, 101, 102, *114*, *117*
Arglebe, C., 246, 271, *275*
Armitage, G. C., 366, 371, *376*
Armstrong, W. D., 389, *401*
Arnold, Jr., F. A., 381, *400*
Aronson, P. S., 58, *63*
Artursson, P., 205, *217*
Arvidson, K., 103, 104, 113, *115*, 104, 111, 112, 113, *117*
Ashburn, M. A., 269, *280*
Atkinson, J. C., 195, *213*
Attenborough, D., 28, *41*
Attstrom, R., 371, *378*
Aubert, J. P., 196, 197, *214*
Audie, J. P., 196, 197, *214*
Audus, K. L., 76, *82*, 102, 103, 105, 106, 107, *114*, 104, 108, 109, 110, 112, 113, *117*, *118*, 111, *119*
Augustinsson, K. B., 247, *276*
Aumonier, P., 272, *282*
Aungst, B. J., 16, *24*, 68, 71, 77, 78, *80*, 70, 74, 76, *82*, 79, *83*, 86, *98*, 123, *152*, *153*, 274, *284*, 297, *315*, 308, *315*
Austin, D. F., 14, *23*
Autrup, H., 104, 110, 111, 113, *116*
Autrup, J. L., 104, 111, 112, 113, *116*
Awata, N., 69, 74, *81*, 123, *152*
Awazu, S., 59, *63*
Aya, N., 123, *151*
Azoury, R., 367, *377*

B

Baelum, B., 382, *400*
Baelum, V., 392, *402*
Baig, M. M., 198, *215*
Bajocchi, G., 209, *219*
Bakal, A. I., 342, *355*
Bakhos, Y., 390, *402*
Bandrua, J. P., 134, *154*, 253, *277*
Banks-Schlegel, S. P., 103, *115*
Barabolak, R., 328, *353*
Bargon, J., 209, *220*
Barkhaus, J. K., 291, 292, *314*, 312, *316*
Barkvoll, P., 14, *24*
Barlage, B., 176, *188*
Barlow, Y., 111, *118*
Barnhart, W. E., 394, *403*
Barry, B. W., 76, *83*, 205, *217*
Barsuhn, C. L., 16, *25*, 58, *62*, 86, *98*, 106, 107, *118*, 135, 136, 138, *155*, 253, *278*, 297, *314*, 311, *315*
Bartel, R. L., 102, 103, 104, 105, 106, 107, 108, 109, *114*
Bartkiewicz, A., 111, *119*
Bartsch, H., 104, 111, 112, 113, *117*
Basbaum, C. B., 204, *217*
Bass, P., 79, *83*
Bates, S., 32, *44*
Baum, B. J., 207, *219*, 209, *220*
Bawden, J. W., 382, *400*
Baybrooks, M. P., 205, *217*
Bayley, D. L., 70, 72, *82*
Beall, P. T., 87, *98*, 123, 124, *151*
Beck, J. D., 371, *379*

Beckett, A. H., 57, *61, 62,* 134, *153, 154,* 253, *276, 277*
Becks, H., 158, *186*
Beg, Z. H., 32, *44*
Beiswanger, B. B., 351, *357*
Belinsky, A., 104, 105, 106, 110, 111, 113, *117*
Bell, R. M., 33, *44*
Beltran, E. D., 345, *356*
Ben-Amor, A., 272, *282*
Benelli, E. M., 398, *404*
Benes, L., 288, *313*
Bennick, A., 195, *213*
Benowitz, N. L., 271, *281,* 328, *353,* 332, 351, *354,* 349, *357*
Benz, L., 79, *83*
Bercy, P., 370, 372, *378*
Berenson, G. S. 31, *43*
Bergey, E. J., 192, *211,* 198, *212,* 194, 195, *213,* 200, *215,* 203, 204, 205, *217,* 223, *236*
Bergman, S., 68, *80,* 86, *97,* 123, *151*
Berman, D., 112, *119*
Bernabei, M. T., 228, *238*
Berner, B., 123, 124, *150,* 228, 234, *238,* 234, *239,* 273, *283*
Bernheim, A., 196, *214*
Bernstein, L., 14, *23*
Bertolero, F., 104, 105, 106, 113, *117*
Bertram, U., 207, *219*
Best, J. S., 164, 165, 167, 168, 174, 181, 183, *187*
Best, A. M., 361, *374*
Bhandary, K. K., 194, 195, *212,* 194, *213*
Bhat, M., 66, *80*
Bhatt, P. I. P., 312, *316*
Bianchi, A., 348, *356*
Bickel, M. H., 134, *154,* 253, *277*
Biesbrock, A. R., 193, 200, *212,* 196, 200, 202, *214,* 202, *215,* 203, *216*
Bikales, N. M., 226, *238*
Birkhed, D., 172, *188,* 344, 345, *356*
Bitton, C., 369, *378*
Blackett, A. N., 134, *155,* 253, *278*
Blanco-Fuente, H., 272, 273, *283*
Blanco-Méndez, J., 272, 273, *283*
Bland, C. R., 123, *153*
Blank, I. H., 28, *41*
Blom, C., 196, *213*
Bloomfield, A. L., 166, 176, 181, 183, *187*
Blot, W. J., 14, *23, 24*
Blumberg, B. M., 203, *217*
Bobek, L. A., 193, 200, *212,* 195, 202, *213,* 196, *214,* 207, *219*
Boddé, H. E., 10, *22,* 30, *42,* 51, *60,* 56, *61,* 57, *62,* 76, *82,* 78, *83,* 86, 88, *98,* 108, *118,* 221, *236,* 225, *237,* 242, 245, 246, 247, 261, *274,* 256, 261, 262, *280,* 273, *283,* 296, 297, *314*
Bolton, S., 232, *239,* 268, 273, *283*
Bonde, J., 271, *281,* 347, *356,* 349, 350, *357*
Bonesvoll, P., 364, *375*
Bonina, F. P., 348, *356*
Borchardt, R. T., 102, 103, 105, 106, 107, *114, 118*
Bosma, A., 347, *356*
Bothwell, J. W., 40, *48*
Bottenberg, P., 206, *218,* 397, *404*
Bouchier, I. A., D. 4, 7, *19,* 36, *47*
Bouckaert, S., 223, *236,* 232, *238*
Bourekis, G., 103, *115*
Bousquet, E., 348, *356*
Bouwstra, J. A., 76, *82,* 207, *218,* 225, *237*

Bowen, W. H., 166, *187*
Bowser, P. A., 35, *46*
Boyce, E. N., 111, 112, 113, *119*
Bradway, S. D., 192, *211,* 203, 204, 205, *217,* 207, *219*
Bragd, J., 362, *374*
Brandtzag, P., 256, *280*
Braquet, P., 58, *62*
Brassart, D., 103, *115*
Braun, P. E., 32, *44*
Breathnach, A. S., 6, *19,* 38, *48*
Breckenridge, A. M., 134, *154,* 253, *278*
Breimer, D. D., 66, *80,* 347, *356*
Brewer, Jr. H. B., 32, *44*
Bridges, J. F., 206, *218*
Brion, N., 134, *155,* 253, *278*
Britse, A., 168, 171, 184, *187*
Broderick, K. B., 323, *353,* 342, *355*
Broich, G., 195, *213*
Brookes, L. G., 77, *83*
Brown, B. E., 34, *46*
Brown, L. J., 360, *373*
Brown, R. H., 382, *400*
Brudevold, F., 387, *401,* 389, 390, *402*
Brunelle, J. A., 360, *373*
Brunson, E. L., 326, 327, 329, *353*
Brussee, J., 76, *82,* 78, *83*
Bruun, C., 176, *188,* 322, 345, *353,* 329, *354,* 389, *401, 402*
Buchanan, W., 364, *375*
Buhe, H., 176, *188*
Bundgaard, H., 123, *152,* 271, *281,* 329, 330, 331, *354*
Burch, G. E., 28, *41,* 31, *43*
Burggraaf, K., 66, *80*
Buri, P. A., 222, 223, *236*, 272, *282,* 296, *314*
Burke, F. M., 123, *150*
Burmeister, J. A., 361, *374*
Burnette, R. R., 92, *99*
Burnside, B. A., 123, *153,* 268, 270, 272, *281*
Burr, G. O., 33, *44*
Burr, M. M., 33, *44*
Burstone, M., S., 247, *276*
Burt, B. A., 382, *400*
Burton, P. S., 106, 107, *118,* 311, *315*
Buscard, D., 103, *115*
Busscher, H. J., 273, *283*
Büttner, W., 176, *188*
Byrd, J. C., 196, *214*

C

Cadoni, A., 114, *119*
Cancedda, R., 114, *119*
Cannon, C. L., 10, *22*
Cannon, M., 195, *213*
Cantieri, J. S., 6, *19*
Capan, Y., 273, *283*
Cappellary, R., 342, *355*
Cardinal, J. R., 228, *238*
Carlos, J. P., 360, *373*
Carlson, E. R., 195, *213*
Carlson, C. H., 389, *401*
Carlstedt, I., 205, *217*
Carnoy, C., 199, *215*
Carpenter, B., 225, *237*
Cassidy, J. P., 16, 18, *25,* 123, 124, *150,* 228, 234, *238, 239,* 273, *283,* 297, 302, *315*
Caston, A. J., 207, *218*
Castonguay, A., 104, 105, 106, 110, 111, 113, *117*
Caton, J., 372, *379*
Caughman, G. B., 103, 105, 108, *115*
Celebi, N., 272, 273, *282*
Ch'ng, H. S., 224, *237,* 288, *313*
Challacombe, S. J., 14, *24*

Chambliss, W. G., 326, 327, 329, *353*
Chan, K., 134, *154*, 203, *216*, 234, *238*, *277*, 273, *283*
Chandler, S. G., 78, *83*
Chandran, V. R., 302, *315*
Chandrasekaran, S. K., 30, *42*
Chang, F., 34, *46*, 36, *47*
Chapkin, V. R. S., 33, *45*
Charbit, Y., 369, *378*
Charles, P., 196, *214*
Charles, T. T., 364, *375*
Chasen, A. E., 10, *22*
Chasens, A. I., 86, 93, *98*, 256, *280*
Chauncey, H. H., 95, *100*, 247, *276*, 390, *402*
Cheema, M. S., 123, *153*
Chen, S, -Y., 2, *19*, 16, *25*, 36, *47*, 96, *100*
Chen, J. L., 206, *218*, 223, 225, *236*
Chen, W. -G., 272, 273, *282*
Chen, W., 312, *316*
Cherrick, H. M., 106, *117*
Chesters, J., 13, *23*
Chien, Y., 274, *284*
Chien, Y. W., 312, *315*, *316*
Cho, E. S., 34, *45*
Cho, M. -I., 203, *217*, 363, *375*
Chowdhury, N. G., 382, *400*
Christen, A. G., 320, *353*, 350, 351, *357*
Christen, J. A., 320, *353*
Christophers, E., 28, *42*
Christrup, L. L., 123, *152*, 271, *281*, 324, 325, 326, 339, *353*, 328, 329, 330, 331, 332, 334, 343, *354*, 347, *356*, 349, 350, 351
Chulia, D., 272, *282*
Ciampini, N., 348, *356*
Ciancio, S., 68, *80*, 86, *97*, 123, *151*
Cid, M. C., 209, *219*
Cimasoni, G., 362, *375*
Clark, D. C., 396, *404*
Clark, H. E., 398, *404*
Clark, K. W., 341, *355*
Clausen, H., 103, *115*, *116*
Cleary, R. W., 326, 327, 329, *353*
Cleymaet, R., 206, *218*, 397, *404*
Cline, W. S., 79, *83*
Cloys, L. A., 320, *353*
Cob, J., 372, *379*
Cobb, C. M., 364, *375*, 366, 371, *376*
Cohen, J. S., 209, *220*
Cohen, R. E., 192, 193, 194, 202, *211*, 192, 198, *212*, 198, *215*, 223, *236*
Collins, A. E. M., 123, *150*, 368, *378*
Collins, A. R., 203, *217*
Collins, J. G., 364, *375*
Collins, L. M. C., 4, *19*, 158, 163, *186*, 224, *237*, 244, 247, *275*
Collins, P., 18, *25*
Collins, W. J. N., 158, *186*
Conine, W. J., 268, 274, *284*
Coomans, D., 206, *218*, 397, *404*
Copper, C. M., 342, *355*
Coppi, G., 228, *238*
Corpron, R. E., 345, *356*
Courtright, S. B., 343, *355*
Coutel-Egros, A., 70, 72, *81*
Coventry, J. F., 366, 367, *376*
Cowell, V. M., 112, *119*
Cowsar, D., 396, *404*
Cox, P., 14, *24*, 18, *26*, 31, 32, 34, 36, 38, *43*, 40, *44*, *46*, *47*, 86, *97*, 103, 108, *115*
Cox, P. S., 244, *275*
Craane, W. I. H. M., 86, 88, *98*, 256, *280*
Cruchley, A. H., 4, *19*, 12, *22*, 40, *48*, 86, 93, *98*

Cruchley, A. T., 40, *48*
Cruz, R., 395, *404*
Crystal, R. G., 209, *219, 220*
Csako, G., 202, *215*
Cugini, M. A., 366, 371, *376*
Cullander, C., 56, *61,* 108, *118*
Cumpstone, N. B., 10, *22*
Curry, J. A., 398, *404*
Curzon, M. E. J., 167, *187,* 382, *400,* 389, 394, *402,* 394, *403,* 397, *404*
Cyr, G. N., 206, *218,* 223, 225, *236*

D

Dabelsteen, E., 103, *115, 116*
Dahlen, G., 362, *374,* 366, *376*
Dale, B. A., 6, *20,* 103, *115*
Dalemans, W., 209, *220*
Danel, C., 209, *219, 220*
Danhof, M., 66, *80*
Daskal, E., 196, *214*
Dave, S. C., 312, *316*
Davidson, E. A., 196, 210, *213*
Davies, T. G. H., 176, *188*
Davis, B. J., 253, *278,* 268, 273, *283*
Davis, S. S., 123, *153,* 182, *189,* 207, *218,* 232, *239*
Dawes, C., 4, *19,* 158, 162, 163, *186,* 164, 172, *187,* 173, *188,* 224, *237,* 244, 247, *275,* 385, *400,* 390, *402*
Dawson, D., 301, 306, *315*
de Almeida Cruz, R., 388, *401,* 394, *403*
de Boer, A. G., 207, *218,* 347, *356*
de Boever, J., 370, 372, *378*
de Garreta, A. C., 144, *156*
de Graaff, J., 203, *216*
de Graaff, J., 362, *375*
de Haan, F. H. N., 56, *61*
de Luca, M., 113, *119*
de Muynck, C., 206, *218,* 397, *404*
de Vree, H., 370, 372, *378*
de Vries, M. E., 10, *22,* 51, *60,* 57, *62,* 86, 88, *98,* 221, *236,* 242, 245, 246, 247, 261, *274,* 256, 262, *280,* 273, *283,* 296, 297, *314,* 311, *315*
Dean, D. H., 123, *153*
Dean, H. T., 381, *399, 400*
Dearden, J. C., 134, *154,* 253, *276*
Deasy, P. B., 123, *150,* 232, *239,* 272, 273, *282,* 368, *378*
Deboer, P., 388, *401*
Decoodt, A., 16, *24*
Degand, P., 196, 197, *214*
DeGrande, G., 288, *313*
Dekker, J., 196, 200, *213,* 197, *214*
Delgado-Charro, B., 272, 273, *283*
Dellow, P. G., 123, *151*
Dengler, H. J., 348, *356*
Denis, C., 196, *214*
Denny, P. A., 204, *217*
Denny, P. C., 204, *217*
DeNuzzio, J. D., 234, *239*
DeRenzio, F. A., 361, *374*
Desai, M. A., 205, *218*
Desmarais, A. J., 268, 273, *283*
Devine, P. L., 204, *217*
Dewhurst, F. E., 33, *45*
Dibella, R. J., 7, *20*
Dickinson, D. P., 193, *212*
Diehl, D. L., 14, *24*
Dijkman, A. G., 388, *401*
Dinh, S. M., 234, *239,*
Dirksen, T. R., 103, 105, 108, *115*
DiStefano, J. J., 140, *156,*
Dix, K., 366, *376*
Doherty, F. M., 366, *376,*
Donald, A., 336, *354,*
Donatsky, O., 207, *219*
Donly, K. J., 398, *404*

Douglas, W. H., 194, 195, *212,* 202, *215*
Downing, D. T., 6, *19, 20,* 10, *21,* 31, *43,* 32, 35, *44,* 33, 37, *45* 34, *46,* 36, 38, *47,* 37, 38, 40, *48,* 35 *49,* 244, *275*
Dowty, M. E., 16, *25,* 52, 56, 58, *60, 62,* 59, *63,* 86, 87, 89, 90, 93, 95, 96, *97*
Doyle, M. J., 364, *375*
Dragsted, L., 104, 110, 111, 113, *116*
Driscoll, W. S., 393, *403*
Drook, A. C., 350, *357*
Drummond, J. F., 56, *61,* 86, 93, *98,* 255, *279*
Drummond, B. K., 242, 245, 247, 260, 265, 266, *275,* 286, 287, *313,* 382, *400,* 389, 394, *402,* 394, *403*
Duchateau, A. M. J. A., 269, 270, *281*
Duchene, D., 206, *218,* 223, *236,* 272, 273, *282*
Duckworth, R., 328, 329, 333, 336, 337, 345, *354*
Ducloux, N., 288, *313*
Duell, E. A., 33, *45*
Dufoir, A., 16, *24*
Dufosse, J., 196, 197, *214*
Duijsters, P. P. E., 176, *189*
Duncan, R., 206, *218*
Dunford, R., 371, *379*
Dunham, S., 365, 366, 369, *375*
Dunn, R. L., 365, 366, 368, 369, *375,* 368, *378*
Durandeau, C., 272, *282*
Duxbury, A. J., 207, *219*

E

Eadie, M. J., 134, *154,* 253, *278*
Ebert, C. D., 58, *62,* 70, 79, *82*, 87, *98,* 123, 127, *150,* 124, *151,* 128, *153,* 312, *316*
Ebisu, S., 203, *216,* 358, *377*
Edgar, W. M., 246, 247, *275,* 343, *355,* 344, *356,* 385, *400,* 388, *401*
Edgerton, M. E., 203, *216*
Edie, J., 9, *21*
Edmonds, E. J., 389, *402*
Edwards, G., 134, *154,* 253, *278*
Edwardson, S., 345, *356*
Eggerth, R. M., 86, 87, 90, *98*
Eichelbaum, M., 348, *356*
Ekstrand, J., 345, *356,* 351, *357,* 389, 390, *402*
El-Miligi, M. F., 324, 329, 330, *353*
Elias, P. M., 6, *19,* 27, *41*, 29, 35, 38, *42*, 31, 87, *43*, 34, *46,* 40
Elkayam, R., 367, *377*
Ellen, R. P., 203, *216*
Ellingsen, B. H., 371, *379*
Ellison, J. A., 223, 224, *236*
Ellison, S. A., 96, *100,* 192, *211*, 246, 247, *275*
Elove, E., 381, *399,* 381, *400*
Embery, G., 198, *215*
Emslie, R. D., 328, 329, 333, 336, 337, 345, *354*
Encarnacion, M., 372, *379*
Engstrom, S., 371, *378*
Epstein, E. H., 34, 35, *46*
Epstein, L. G., 203, *217*
Erard, F., 361, *374*
Erbland, J. F., 104, *116,*
Eriksen, H., 271, *281,* 347, *356*
Espeland, M., 361, *373*
Etemadzadeh, H., 329, *354,* 344, *356*
Etherden, I., 203, 208, *216*
Evans, J. C., 224, *237*

Evans, R. W., 382, *400*
Evered, D. F., 134, *154,* 253, *278*

F

Farber, P. A., 361, *374*
Farr, D. H., 365, 366, *375*
Fawzi, M. B., 86, 87, 90, *98*
Featherstone, J. D. B., 176, 177, 178, *189,* 386, *401,* 390, *402*
Feingold, K. R., 31, 87, *43*
Fejerskov, O., 10, *21,* 176, *189,* 382, *400,* 389, *401,* 392, *402*
Feldman, S., 209, *219*
Feller, R. P., 390, *402*
Felton, J., 88, 95, *99*
Ferguson, M. M., 312, *316*
Fernö, O., 321, 323, 334, 342, 349, *353,* 342, 349, *355*
Ferrario, V. F., 163, *186*
Ferry, D. G., 176, 178, *189*
Fetherston, J., 207, *219*
Feyerskov, O., 384, *400*
Fillery, E. D., 203, *216*
Fine, D. H., 8, *21*
Fine, A., 88, 95, *99*
Fine, D., 366, 371, *376*
Fischer, S. J., 203, 208, *216*
Fischer, S. M., 104, *117*
Fleckenstein, L., 347, *356*
Fleming, S. M., 14, *24*
Fløtra, L., 344, *356,* 360, *373*
Flowerdew, G., 343, *356*
Foley, K. M., 350, *357*
Forest, N., 102, 103, *114, 115*
Forget, P., 272, *282*
Forni, F., 228, *238*
Forsten, L., 398, *404*
Forusz, H., 69, *81*, 123, 124, 125, *150*
Fosse, T., 369, *378*
Foster, S. N. E., 224, *237*
Fox, N., 329, 345, *354*
Fox, P. C., 195, 204, *213,* 207, *219,* 209, *220*
Fox, P. L. A., 57, *62,* 86, *98*
Franchebois, P., 14, *23*
Francoeur, M. L., 76, *82*
Franke, W. F., 103, *114*
Franke, W. W., 103, *115*
Frant, M. S., 389, *402*
Franz, T. J., 40, *4*
Franzi, A. T., 114, *119*
Fraumeni, J. F., 14, *24*
Freimann, V., 58, *62*
Freinkel, R. K., 34, 35, *45, 46*
Frelin, C., 58, *63*
Friedman, M., 367, *376,* 372, *377,* 369, *378*, 396, *404*
Friend, D. S., 6, *19,* 29, 35, 38, *42*
Fritz, M. E., 366, 371, *376*
Fröhlich, S., 343, *356*
Frosch, P. J., 28, *42*
Frost, P., 40, *48*
Frostell, G., 345, *356*
Fu, J., 390, *402*
Fu, M. J., 176, 177, 178, *189*
Fujimoto, N., 368, *377*
Fujiyoshi, P., 361, *374*
Fukayama, M., 209, *220*
Fukuda, H., 16, *24,* 123, *152*
Fukuda, M., 368, *377*
Fukuhara, H., 203, *216*

G

Gale, R., 27, *41*
Galey, W. R., 86, 93, *97*
Gandhi, R., 70, 77, 79, *82*, 287, 292, *313*
Garant, P. R., 363, *375*
Garber, A. J., 66, *80*
Garcia-Gonzalez, N., 272, 273, *283*

Gardner, I. D., 103, *115*
Garnham, J. C., 253, *277*
Garren, K. W., 57, *62,* 86, 88, *98,* 95, 95, *99*
Garret, E. R., 302, *315*
Garro, A. J., 14, *23*
Gavel, Y., 197, *214*
Gazzeri, P., 272, *282*
Geddes, D. A. M., 158, *186,* 385, *400*
Geering, A. H., 360, *373*
Geha, R. S., 40, *48*
Geiger, B., 103, *114*
Genco, R. J., 203, *216,* 360, *373,* 71, *379*
Gennissen, A. M. C., 196, *214*
Gerson, S. J., 244, *275*
Ghadially, R., 40, *48*
Gibaldi M., 51, *60*
Gibbons, R. J., 194, 195, *212,* 203, 208, *216*
Gibson, D. M., 32, *44*
Gijsman, H. J., 58, *62,* 123, 127, *150*
Giunta, J. L., 350, *357*
Givskov, H., 322, 345 *353,* 329, *354,* 389, *402*
Gjermo, P., 344, *356*, 360, *373,* 364, *375*
Glass, H. I., 144, *156*
Glavind, L., 344, *356,* 395, *403*
Gleason, D. D., 16, *25,* 58, *62,* 86, *98,* 135, 136, 138, *155,* 253, *278,* 297, *314*
Gleerup, A., 395, *403*
Glena, R., 386, *401*
Glover, D. D., 66, *80*
Gniecko, J., 16, 18, *25*
Golden, G. M., 40, *48*, 76, *82*
Goldhaber, P., 360, *373*
Goldsmith, L. A., 36, *47*
Goldstein, J. C., 104, *117*
Golliard, M., 103, *115*
Golomb, G., 367, *376, 377*
Golub, L., 367, *377*
Goodhart, F. W., 86, 87, 90, *98*
Goodman, T., 6, *19,* 12, *23,* 38, *48*
Goodson, J. M., 33, *45*, 246, *275,* 362, 364, 365, 366, 368, 369, *375,* 371, *376, 378,* 372, *379*
Gordon, H. P., 14, 16, *24,* 68, 72, 73, 79, *80*, 86, 93, *97,* 123, *152,* 255, *279*
Gosselin, F., 103, *115*
Goto, S., 69, *81*, 123, *152*
Graf, H., 360, *373,* 361, *373*
Graffner, C., 271, *281*
Grafström, R. C., 104, 105, 106, 110, 111, 112, 113, *117, 118*
Gram, J., 111, *118*
Gram-Hansen, M., 332, 333, 338, 339, *354*
Grant, P. R., 104, *117*
Grass, G. M., 88, 90, *99*
Gravenmade, E. J., 196, *213,* 207, *219*
Gray, G. M., 31, *43*, 31, *44*, 35, *46*
Grayson, S., 34, 35, *46*
Grech, O., 253, *276*
Green, D. R., 198, *215*
Green, H., 6, 13, *19, 20,* 35, *47* 40, *48*, 103, *115*
Green, E., 366, 371, *376*
Greenberg, M., 321, *353*
Greenberg, R. S., 14, *23*
Greenstein, G., 360, *373*
Gren, R. M., 351, *357*
Grennstein, G., 112, *119*
Grice, R. A., 14, *23*
Griffiths, R. R., 332, *354*
Grøn, P., 389, 390, *402*
Gross, M., 6, *19,* 38, *48*, 196, *214*
Grossi, S., 371, *379*
Grove, D. A., 203, *216*
Grubauer, G., 31, 87, *43*
Grubb, C., 4, *19,* 7, *20,* 36, *47*

Gruenert, D. C., 102, 103, *114*
Gu, J. -M., 222, *236*
Gu, M., 203, *217*
Gubbens-Stubbe, J. M., 347, *356*
Guiggno, W. B., 209, *220*
Gullikson, G. W., 79, *83*
Gum, E., 196, *214*
Gum, J. R., 196, 197, *214*
Gunning, R. R., 66, *80*
Guo, J. -H., 291, 293, 294, 296, *314*
Gupta, P. K., 109, *118*
Gurny, R., 206, *218*, 286, *313*, 292, *314*
Gusterson, B. A., 104, *117*
Guyonnet-Duperat, V., 196, 197, *214*
Guzek, D. B., 10, *22*, 76, *82*

H

Hackemann, M., 4, *19*, 7, *20*, 36, *47*, 51, 52, *60*
Hadgraft, J., 30, *42*, 242, 244, 245, 247, *274*
Hadjimichael, J., 361, *374*
Haffajee, A. D., 361, *374*
Hague, B., 58, *62*
Haidaris, C. G., 203, *216*
Hakomori, S. -I., 103, *116*
Hall, B. K., 13, *23*, 14, *24*, 16, *25*, 29, *42*, 55, *61*, 86, 93, 95, *97*, 88, *99*, 254, *279*
Hallsworth, A. S., 398, *404*
Hamada, C., 16, *25*, 68, *81*, 123, *151*, 123, *152*
Hammarskjold, M. -L., 203, *217*
Hammerstrom, S., 33, *45*
Hanaki, M., 170, 173, *188*
Handley, R., 367, *376*
Hannon, C. S., 10, *22*
Hannoun, L., 369, *378*
Hannun, Y. A., 33, *44*
Hansen, B. F., 371, *379*
Hansen, C. 104, 111, *116*
Hansen, H. S., 33, 34, *45*
Hansen, L. B., 123, *152*
Haraszthy, G. G., 193, 200, *212*, *215*
Hardy, J. G., 182, *189*
Harris, D., 51, *60*, 206, *218*, 244, 245, 247, 256, 260, *275*, 285, 286, *313*
Harris, R. M., 31, 87, *43*
Harrison, M. P., 134, *154*
Hartop, P. J., 40, *48*
Harvell, J. D., 31, *43*
Hase, J. C., 172, *188*, 174
Hashimoto, K., 7, *20*
Hassan, H., 367, *377*
Hassinen, M. L., 393, *403*
Hatibovic-Kofman, D., 398, *405*
Hatteb, F. N., 351, *357*
Hattingh, J., 362, 364, *375*
Hatton, M. N., 202, *215*, 207, *219*
Haugen, E., 56, *61*
Havekes, L., 32, *44*
Haverkort, M., 78, *83*
Hay, D. I., 192, *211*, 194, 195, *212*, *213*
Hayakawa, E., 95, *100*
Hayashi, M., 59, *63*
Hayashi, S., 368, *377*
Hayes, A. L., 176, 177, 178, *189* 390, *402*
Hayes, N. F., 207, *219*
Hayward, A. F., 7, *20*, 34, *46*
Heaney T. G., 18, *25*
Hecht, S. A., 14, *23*
Hecht, S. S., 104, 111, *117*
Hector, M. P., 167, 176, 184, *187*
Hedberg, C. L., 32, 35, *44*
Hefferren, J. J., 111, *119*
Heiber, S. J., 312, *316*
Heiblum, R., 104, 111, *116*

Heidmann, J., 344, *356*
Heijl, L., 366, *376*
Heintze, U., 395, *403*
Helliwell, M., 224, *237*
Hendrickson, R., 320, *352*
Henningfield, J. E., 328, *353,* 332, *354*
Henry, J. A., 134, *155,* 253, *277,* 253, *278*
Herbine, R. H., 329, 345, *354*
Herp, A., 202, *215*
Hicks, D. C., 57, *62,* 134, *154,* 253, *277*
Hicks, J. W., 196, 197, *214*
Hidalgo, I. J., 102, 103, 105, 106, 107, *114*
Higashi, K., 368, *377*
Higuchi, W. I., 253, *278, 279*
Hikal, A. H., 326, 327, 329, *353*
Hilkens, J., 196, *214*
Hill, B. T., 106, *118*
Hill, K. R., 4, *19,* 7, *20,* 36, *47*
Hill, M. W., 12, *22,* 5, *26,* 35, *47* 55, *61,* 254, *279*
Hill, R. L., 36, *47*
Hiller, L. K., 394, *403*
Hillman, R. W., 14, *23*
Hincal, A. A., 273, *283*
Hino, T., 369, *378*
Hirai, S., 76, *82*
Hiramoto, R. N., 123, *153*
Hisaichi, S I., 16, *24,* 16, *25,* 68, 69, 72, 76, 79, *81,* 123, *151,* 123, *152*
Hitzig, C., 369, *378*
Ho, E., 362, 364, *375*
Ho, N. F. H., 58, *62,* 86, *98,* 106, 107, *118,* 135, 136, 138, *155,* 253, *278,* 253, *279,* 286, *313,* 297, *314,* 311, *315*
Ho, S. B., 196, *214*
Hobbes, J., 207, *219*
Hoerman, K., 328, *353*
Hoffman, M. P., 203, *216*
Hogan, M. E., 209, *220*
Hogan, P. E., 365, 366, 368, 369, *375*
Holborow, D. W., 176, 177, 178, *189,* 312, *316,* 365, 366, 368, 369, *375, 378*
Holbrook, K. A., 6, *20*
Holbrook, N. S., 10, *22*
Holland, H. H., 345, *356*
Holloway, P. J., 176, *188*
Holman, R. T., 33, *45*
Holmen, L., 345, *356*
Holmes, E. H., 103, *116*
Holmstrup, P., 207, *219*, 338, 346, *355*
Holroyde, C. P., 32, *44*
Holt, B., 228, 234, *238,* 273, *283*
Holterman, H. J., 196, *213*
Holtz, P., 360, *373*
Holtzman, S., 371, *379*
Holubar, K., 34, *46*
Homalle, A., 28, *41*
Hong, L -Z., 16, *24,* 69, 76, *81*
Hong, S. H., 204, *217*
Honig, J., 361, *374*
Honigsmann, H., 10, *22*
Hoogstraate, A. J., 30, *42,* 56, *61,* 108, *118,* 297, *314*
Hooper, W. D., 134, *154*, 253, *278*
Hoover, C. I., 203, 208, *216*
Hopfenberg, H. B., *238*
Hopps, R. M., 4, *19,* 9, *21,* 12, *23,* 52, *60,* 55, *61,* 244, 245, *275*
Hopwood, D., 4, 7, *19,* 36, *47*
Hori, T., 369, *378*
Horie, T., 59, *63*
Horovitz, R. A., 347, *356*
Horriere, F., 288, *313*
Hortobagyi, I., 134, *155*
Hou, S, Y. E., 40, *48*
Houde, R. W., 350, *357*
Houpt, M., 398, *405*

Houtsmuller, U. M. T., 35, *46*
Howell, T. H., 360, *373*
Howes, C., 70, 72, *82*
Howlett, J. A., 104, 111, *116*
Huebner, R. D., 67, *80*
Hunt, G., 222, 223, *236,* 226, 234, *237*
Hussain, M. A., 86, *98,* 274, *284,* 297, *315*
Hwang, G. C., 272, 273, *282,* 312, *316*
Hybbinette, S. S., 104, 105, 106, 113, *117*

I

Iannuccelli, V., 228, *238*
Ibraheem, J. J., 66, *80*
Ichikawa, K., 76, *82*
Ikura, H., 265, *280,* 368, *377*
Ikuta, Y., 69, *81*, 123, *152*
Illum, L., 78, *83*
Imfeld, T. N., 351, *357*
Imoberdorf, M. J., 366, 371, *376*
Inagaki, K., 95, *100*
Ingelbritsen, T. S., 32, *44*
Ingram, D. L., 18, *25*
Ingram, G. S., 388, *401*
Innes, P. B., 36, *47*
Inové, S., 56, *61*
Inturrisi, C. E., 350, *357*
Irons, B. K., 16, *25,* 52, 56, 58, *60,* 86, 87, 89, 90, 93, 95, 96, *97*
Ishida, M., 16, *25,* 68, 72, *80*, 123, *150, 151, 152,* 227, 231, *238*
Isseroff, R. R., 34, 35, *46*
Itoh, T., 111, *119*
Ivanyi, L., 103, *115*
Izumizawa, K., 368, *377*
Izutsu, K. T., 16, *25,* 57, *62,* 86, 87, 93, *97,* 254, *279*

J

Jabbari, E., 296, *314*
Jackson, R. D., 351, *357*
Jacobs, H., 228, *238*
Jacob, P., 271, *281,* 332, 351, *354,* 349, *357*
Jacobsen, J., 106, 108, *118*
Jacques, Y., 272, *282*
Jaffe, H. A., 209, *216*
Jaffin, R., 112, *119*
Jain, C. P., 265, 268, *280*
Jan, H. S. I., 297, *314*
Jany, B., 204, *217*
Jarvis, M. J., 271, *281*
Jay, P., 381, *400*
Jeffcoat, M. K., 360, *373*
Jenkins, G. N., 164, 166, 167, 172, 176, 180, 181, 183, *187,* 385, *400,* 388, *401,* 391, 392, 394, *402*
Jensen, B., 33, 34, *45*
Jensen, E., 339, *355*
Jensen, L. N., 271, *281,* 329, 330, *354*
Jensen, M. E., 385, *400*
Jepsen, A., 10, *21,* 86, 87, *98,* 101, 102, *114,* 104, 110, 111, 113, *116, 117*
Jespersen, J., 111, *118*
Johansen, J. R., 56, *61*
Johansson, L. A., 371, *379*
John, A., 123, 124, *151*
John, V., 87, *98,* 228, 234, *238,* 273, *283*
Johnsen, T., 207, *219*
Johnson, A. J., 134, *154*
Johnson, D., 12, *22*
Johnson, G. K., 12, *23*
Johnson, H. G., 360, *373*
Johnson, J., 382, *400*
Johnson, M., 194, 195, *213*
Johnson, N. W., 51, 52, *60,* 58, *62*

Johnson, N. W., 4, *19,* 12, *23*, 244, 245, *275*
Johnson, T. P., 312, *316*
Johnson, R. H., 359, *373*
Johnson-Winegar, A. G., 34, 35, *46*
Johnsson, M., 194, 195, *212, 213*
Johnston, A., 253, *278*
Jokela, M., 393, *403*
Jones, A. B., 326, 327, 329, *353*
Jones, P. C., 192, *211,* *1*98, 199, 200, 202, *212, 215,* 204, 205, *217,* 223, *236*
Jones, D. S., 368, *378*
Jones, R. S., 18, *25*
Jonsen, J., 86, *97*
Jørgensen, A., 123, *152*
Juhl, M., 103, *115*
Jundinski, J. J., 361, *374*
Junginger, H. E., 10, *22,* 51, *60,* 56, *61,* 86, 88, *98,* 108, 207, *218,* 221, *236,* 225, *237,* 242, 245, 246, 247, 261, *274,* 256, 261, 262, *280,* 273, *283,* 286, *313,* 296, 297, *314*

K

Kaaber, S., 13, *23,* 40, *49*, 135, *155*
Kajii, H., 59, *63*
Kakumoto, M., 274, *284*
Kane, D., 68, *80*, 86, *97,* 123, *151*
Kanfer, J. N., 32, *44*
Kanig, J. L., 51, *60*
Kantero, R. L., 393, *403*
Kaplan, M. L., 360, *373*
Karlsson, U. L., 14, *24*
Karlsson, J., 205, *217*
Karring, T., 344, *356,* 371, *378,* 371, *379*
Karsenty, H., 288, *313*
Karthigasan, J., 35, *47*
Kashi, S. D., 95, *100*
Kaspi, T., 253, *277, 278*
Kassem, A. A., 324, 329, 330, *353*
Kates, R. E., 134, *154*
Katz, R. V., 392, 393, *403*
Kawamura, S., 76, *82*
Kawata, H., 76, *82*
Kaye, C. M., 134, *155,* 253, *277, 278*
Kearney, A., 86, *98*
Kearney, P., 205, *217,* 222, *236,* 224, *237*
Keith, A. D., 123, *153,* 268, 270, 272, *281*
Kellaway, I. W., 123, 126, 127, *151,* 222, *236,* 224, 226, 234, *237,* 233, 235, *239,* 268, 273, *283,* 291, 292, *314*
Kelly, P., 224, *237*
Kelm, G. R., 364, *375*
Kempenaar, J., 32, *44,* 78, *83*
Kemppainen, B. W., 16, 18, *25,* 86, 93, *98*
Kennedy, A. H., 10, *22*, 76, *82*
Kennedy, J. E., 361, *374*
Kennerley, J. W., 182, *189,* 270, *281*
Kenney, J. S., 361, *374*
Kent, R. L., 366, 371, *376*
Kesel, R. G., 329, 345, *354*
Keyes, P. H., 384, *405*
Khare, A. R., 226, 229, *238*
Kiddie, M. A., 253, *277*
Kilian, M., 371, *379*
Killoy, W. J., 364, *375,* 366, 371, *376*
Kim, K., 106, *117*
Kim, S. H., 228, *238*
Kim, S. W., 228, *238*, 312, *316*
Kim, Y. S., 196, 197, *214*
Kimura, S., 368, *377*

Kimura, T., 16, *24, 25,* 68, 69, 70, 72, 76, 79, *81*, 123, *151,* 126, *152,* 135, 149, *156,* 273, *283*
Kinugawa, M., 59, *63*
Kirkham, J., 387, *401*
Kisch, J., 371, *378,* 371, *379*
Kislal, O., 272, 273, *282*
Kissin, B., 14, *23*
Kitamura, M., 368, *377*
Kitamura, S., 368, *377*
Kitayama, M., 69, *81*, 123, *152*, 273, *283*
Kitko, D. J., 36, 38, *47*
Klauser, D. K., 204, *217*
Klausner, M., 10, *22*
Kleber, C. J., 323, 324, *353*
Klein, A., 199, *215*
Kleinman, H. K., 209, *219*
Klestov, A. C., 207, *219*
Kligman, A. M., 6, *19,* 28, 29, 40, *41*, *48*
Klinge, B., 371, *378*
Klinman, A. M., 28, *42*
Knuth, K. E., 16, *25,* 52, 56, 58, *60,* 86, 87, 89, 90, 93, 95, 96, *97*
Knutson, J. W., 381, *400*
Knutson, K., 273, *283*
Koch, G. G., 371, *379,* 395, *403,* 398, *405*
Koch, P. L., 312, *316*
Koda, R. T., 253, *277*
Koerten, H. K., 56, *61*
Kohl, J., 370, 372, *378*
Kok, W., 207, *218*
Kondo, K., 170, 173, *188*
Konishi, R., 228, 233, *238,* 273, *283,* 286, *313*
Koop, H. M., 203, *216*
Kooyman, D. J., 31, *43*
Kopecek, J., 206, *218*
Kornman, K. S., 366, *376,* 371, *379*
Korsmeyer, R. W., 228, 229, *238*
Korts, D. C., 395, *403*
Koval, C. A., 274, *284,* 297, *315*
Kowalski, C. J., 345, *356*
Kraeling, M., 69, *81*, 123, 124, 125, *150*
Kramer, P. A., 123, 132, 133, *150*
Krasse, B., 398, *405*
Krayer, J. W., 362, *375*
Krebsbach, P. H., 166, 176, 180, 181, 183, *187*
Kremer, M. J., 10, *22,* 31, 32, 34, 36, *43*
Krepler, R., 103, *115*
Kristensen, F., 271, *281*
Kristensen, J. F., 350, *357*
Kritsineli, M., *400*
Krog, N., 371, *378*
Kroll, N., 328, *353*
Kubilus, J., 10, *22*
Kubo, J., 265, *280*
Kulkarni, P., 104, 105, 106, 113, *117*
Künzel, W., 392, *403*
Kuo, W. -L., 196, *214*
Kupietzky, A., 398, *405*
Kurihara, H., 361, *374*
Kurosaki, Y., 16, *24, 25,* 68, 69, 70, 72, 76, 79, *81*, 123, 126, *152,* 135, 149, *156,* 273, *283*

L

Labropoulou, P., 382, *400*
Lacey, C. F., 66, *80*
Lacoste, C., 288, *313*
Lading, P., 371, *378*
Ladoux, A., 58, *63*
Laffoon, J., 18, *25*
Lagace, R. L., 196, *214*
Lagain, D., 288, *313*

Lagas, M., 269, 270, *281*
Lagerlöf, F., 159, 162, *186,* 168, 171, 184, *187,* 174, *188,* 385, *400,* 390, *402,* 351, *357*
Laine, A., 197, *214*
Lamb, W. J., 345, *356*
Lamblin, G., 199, *215,* 389, *401*
Lamkin, M. S., 194, *212*
Lampe, M. A., 31, *43*
Lamport, D. T. A., 196, *214*
Landaw E. M., 140, *156*
Landeen, L. K., 103, 104, 108, 109, *114*
Landmann, L., 6, *20,* 27, 34, *41,* 35, *47*
Landzert, N. M., 234, *239*, 302, *315*
Lane, E. B., 103, *115,* 106, *118*
Lang, N. P., 360, *373*
Langer, R., 228, 229, *238*
Langeroudi, M., 367, *377*
Langley, S., 302, *315*
Larsen, M. J., 176, *189,* 389, *401*
Larsson, K., 371, *378*
Laskiewicz, B., 106, *118*
Latt, D., 207, *219*
Lavker, R. M., 6, *20,* 35, *46*
Lazdunski, M., 58, *63*
Le Brun, P. P. H., 57, *62,* 86, *98*
Leach, S. A., 344, *356*
Lecocq, J. -P., 209, *219, 220*
Lecompte, P., 164, 172, *187*
Lee, B. L., 349, *357*
Lee, E. S., 228, *238*
Lee, G. T. R., 344, *356*
Lee, J. -Y., 203, *216*
Lee, P. I., 228, 229, 230, *238*
Lee, S. W., 361, *374*
Lee, T., 203, 208, *216*
Lee, V. H. L., 58, *63,* 88, 95, *99, 100*, 286, 287, *313*
Lee, Y., 312, *315, 316*
Lefebvre, R. A., 232, *238*
Lehr, C. -M., 207, *218,* 225, *237*
Leigh, I., 103, *115*
Lejoyeux, F., 272, *282*
Lemarchand, P., 209, *219*
Lennard, T. W. J., 204, *217*
Lentner C., 178, *189*
Leonard, G. T., 394, *403*
LeRoy, S., 16, 18, *25*
Lesch, C. A., 16, *19,* 8, *21,* 29, *42* 40, *48*, 86, 93, *98*
Lesco, L. J., 320, 329, 348, *353*
Leung, D. Y. M., 40, *48*
Leung, S. -H. S., 109, *118,* 222, *236,* 312, *315*
Leverett, D. H., 390, *402*
Levine, M. J., 96, *100,* 192, 193, 194, 202, *211,* 195, 198, 199, 200, *212, 213,* 196, *214, 215,* 203, 208, *216,* 204, 205, *217,* 207, *219,* 223, 224, *236,* 246, 247, *275*
Lewin, B., 371, *378*
Lhote, O., 16, *24*
Li, C., 312, *316*
Liau, Y. H., 103, *115*
Lichtneckert, S., 321, 323, 334, 342, 349, *353*
Lie, T., 371, *379*
Lieber, C. S., 14, *23*
Lien, E., 253, *277*
Ligtenberg, A. J. M., 203, *216*
Ligtenberg, M. J. L., 196, *214*
Likens, R. C., 381, *400*
Liljewall, R. L., 324, *353*
Lillie, J. H., 10, *21,* 101, 102, 114, *114,* 104, *117*
Linder, J. E., 55, *61*
Lindgren, J. A., 33, *45*
Lindgren, L. E., 345, *356*
Lindhe, J., 361, *373*
Lindquist, I., 247, *276*

Ling, S. Y., 6, *20*
Lionetti, F., 95, *100,* 247, *276*
Lisanti, V. F., 95, *100,* 247, *276*
Listgarten, M. A., 8, *21*
Little, W. A., 111, *119*
Liu, Y., 103, 104, 113, *115,* 105, 106, 110, 111, 112, *117*
Livingston, T., 302, *315*
Loe, H., 112, *119*, 360, *373*
Logan, K. R., 4, 7, *19,* 36, *47*
Lokind, K. B., 339, *355*
Long, A. D., 253, *277*
Long, S. A., 37, *4*
Long, V. J. W., 31, *43*
Longer, M. A., 16, *25,* 89, *99,* 129, *153,* 206, *218,* 223, *236,* 233, *239,* 268, 274, *284,* 288, *313,* 312, *317*
Lonsdale, H. K., 86, 93, *97*
Loomis, R. E., 192, *211,* 198, 199, 200, 202, *212, 215,* 223, *236*
Lorenzsonn, V., 79, *83*
Ludvigsson, N., 395, *403*
Lundgren, C., 321, 323, 334, 342, 349, *353*
Luoma, H., 393, *403*

M

Ma, J. K. H., 66, *80*
MacCallum, D. K., 88, *99,* 101, 114, *114,* 104, *117*
MacCarthy, D. J., 368, *378*
MacCullum, D. K., 10, *21*
Machida, Y., 16, *25,* 68, 72, *80* 70, 72, *81* 123, *150,* 227, 231, *238,* 297, *314,* 312, *315*
Machtei, E. E., 371, *379*
Mackay, A. M., 342, *355*
Mackay, D. A. M., 341, *355*
Mackay, M., 336, *354*
Mackenzie, I. C., 8, *21,* 28, *42*
Macpherson, L. M. D., 172, 173, *188*
Madapallimattam, G., 195, *213*
Maddox, D. H., 123, *153,* 270, *281*
Madison, K. C., 6, *19, 20,* 10, *21,* 34, 35, *46*, 36, 38, *47*, 38, *48*
Maeno, H., 76, *82*
Mahjour, M., 86, 87, 90, *98*
Maibach, H. I., 31, *43*
Main, C., 158, *186*
Main, D. M. G., 159, 161, 166, 178, 184, *186,* 164, *187*
Main, J. H. P., 104, *116*
Maitani, Y., 70, 72, *81*
Maiwald, H. J., 343, *356*
Majer, J. R., 35, *46*
Majka, J., 103, *115*
Maland, L., 58, *62*
Malanga, C. J., 66, *80*
Mali, J. W. H., 31, *43*
Malkinson, F. D., 1, *18*
Mandel, I. D., 96, *100,* 192, *211, 212,* 198, *215,* 223, 224, *236,* 246, 247, *275*
Mandel, U., 103, *116*
Mangiante, P. E., 114, *119*
Manji, F., 382, *400,* 392, *402*
Manning, A. S., 134, *154*
Manning, R. H., 343, *355*
Marcelo, C., 33, *45*
Marecki, N. M., 291, 292, *314*
Mark, H. F., 226, *238*
Marko, M., 104, *116*
Marrakchi, S., 197, *214*
Marriott, C., 205, *217*
Martens, T. W., 16, *25,* 129, *153,* 233, *239,* 268, 274, *284,* 312, *317*
Marthaler, T. M., 392, *403*
Martin, B. M., 196, *214*
Martin, C. M., 36, *47*
Martin, M. V., 13, *23*

Martinez, I. R., 6, *20*
Marzulli, F. N., 28, *42*
Masada, M., 70, 72, *81*
Mascres, C., 14, *23*
Masi, C. W., 10, *22,* 86, 93, *98,* 256, *280*
Mason, D. K., 207, *219*
Mastrangeli, A., 209, *219,* 209, *220*
Masuda, M. P., 361, *374*
Matheny, J., 12, *22*
Mather, L. E., 302, *315*
Mathison, I. W., 134, *154,* 253, *277*
Matoltsy, A. G., 6, *19,* 36, *47*
May, C. S., 134, *154*
Mazullo, J. M., 347, *356*
Mazzenga, G. C., 234, *239*
McArdle, S., 366, *37*
McCann, H. G., 389, 390, *402*
McCarthy, F., 370, 372, *378*
McClure, F. J., 389, *401*
McCoy, G. D., 14, *23*, 88, *99*
McCrary, B. R., 207, *219*
McDevitt, E., 67, *80*
McDonald, J. L., 350, *357*
McDougall, W. A., 256, *280*
McElnay, J. C., 134, *155*
McJames, S., 58, *62,* 123, 127, *150,* 128, *151*
McKenzie, I. F. C., 204, *217*
McKibben, D. H., 8, *21*
McKie, J. E., 40, *48*, 76, *82*
McLaughlin, J. K., 14, *23*
McMillan, M. D., 112, *119*
McNamara, K., 207, *219*
McNee, S. G., 158, *186*
McNeill, S. C., 10, *22*
McNutt, N. S., 29, 38, *42*
McQuinn, R. L., 291, 292, *314,* 312, *31*
Medlicott, N. J., 176, 177, 178, *189,* 312, *316,* 368, *378*
Meerzaman, D., 196, *214*
Megna, M., 114, *119*
Mehta, M., 16, 18, *25,* 86, 93, *98*
Meijer, D. K. F., 207, *218*
Mellberg, J., 398, *405*
Mellema, J., 196, *213*
Melsen, B., 395, *403*
Melton, J. L., 33, 34, *45*
Mendieta, C., 366, 371, *376*
Menger, N., 271, *281*, 329, 330, 331, *354*
Menges, G., 226, *238*
Menon, G. K., 34, *46*
Merckel, A. H. J., 360, *373*
Meredith, M. P., 364, *375*
Merkle, H. P., 67, *80*, 70, 72, *81* 106, 109, *118,* 123, *150,* 123, *153,* 233, *239,* 242, 247, 260, *275,* 261, *276,* 261, 263, *280,* 274, *284,* 287, 297, *313,* 312, *314,* 311, *315, 316, 317*
Merlet, J. P., 272, *282*
Merrill, A. H., 32, *44*
Meyer, G., 166, 181, *187*
Meyer, J. M., 2, *19*, 206, *218,* 244, *275,* 292, *314*
Meyer, W., 134, *155*, 253, *278,* 342, *355*
Miani Jr., A., 163, *186*
Michaels, A. S., 30, *42*
Michaels, S. E., 394, *403*
Michalowicz, C., 372, *379*
Michotte, Y., 206, *218*
Miethke, M. C., 37, *48*
Mihailova, D., 253, *276*
Miki, Y., 368, *377*
Miles, T. S., 123, *151*
Miller, S. A., 56, *61,* 86, 93, *98,* 255, *279*
Miller, A. J., 360, *373*
Mills, G. D., 104, *117*
Mima, H., 76, *82*

Min, B. M., 106, *117*
Minabe, M., 369, *378*
Mirth, D. B., 111, *119,* 396, 397, *404*
Mitchelsen, J. J., 32, *44*
Mitomi, M., 76, *82*
Mitropoulos, C. M., 176, *188*
Mix, D., 312, *316*
Miyamoto, M., 361, *374*
Mizobe, M., 130, 131, *153*
Mock, D., 104, *116*
Moe, D., 103, *115*
Moffat, A. C., 57, *61, 62,* 134, *153,* 134, *154,* 253, *276*
Mok, Y. C., 351, *357*
Molema, G., 207, *218*
Moll, R., 103, *116*
Møller, I. J., 394, *403*
Møller, N., 324, 325, 326, 339, *353*
Møller-Sonnergaard, J., 329, 331, *354*
Monaghan, P., 104, *117*
Montenegro, L., 348, *356*
Moolenaar, W. H., 58, *63*
Moran, J., 367, *377*
More, F. G., 345, *356*
Moreno, E. C., 195, *213,* 203, 208, *216,* 387, *401*
Moreau, F., 272, *282*
Morgan, P. H., 134, *154,* 253, *277*
Morgan, P. R., 103, *115*
Morgan, R. A., 209, *220*
Morgan, S. N., 388, *401*
Morisaki, K., 368, *377*
Mortazavi, S. A., 225, *237*
Moss, D. E., 33, *45*
Moulin, A., 16, *24*
Moulin, D. E., 350, *357*
Mount, L. E., 18, *25*
Moyer, C. A., 31, *43*
Muhler, J. C., 323, 324, *353*
Mundy, G. R., 347, *356*
Munzer, J., 70, 72, *81*, 123, *150,* 297, 312, *314*
Muranushi, N., 59, *63*
Muranishi, S., 59, *63*
Murayama, Y., 361, *374*
Murphy, S. E., 104, 111, *116*
Murrah, A., 12, *22*
Murray, J. J., 391, 392, 394, *402*
Murray, G. R., 270, *281*
Murray, P. A., 203, 208, *216*
Murrell, W., 51, *60,* 85, *97*
Murty, V. L., 198, *215*
Myers, R. N., 32, *44*
Myhill, J., 144, *156*

N

Nacht, S., 86, *97*
Nagai, A., 361, *374*
Nagai, T., 16, *24, 25,* 68, 69, 72, 74, *80*, 70, 72, *81*, 123, *150, 151, 152,* 227, 228, 231, 232, 233, *238,* 265, *280,* 273, *283,* 286, *313,* 297, *14,* 312, *315*
Nagelkerke, J. F., 108, *118*
Nair, J., 104, 111, 112, 113, *117*
Nakada, Y., 123, *152*
Nakae, H., 203, *216*
Nakagaki, H., 159, 161, 162, 163, 166, 178, 184, *186,* 168, *187,* 170, 173, *188*
Nakajima, Y., 59, *63*
Nakamichi, C., 69, 74, *81*, 123, *152*
Nakamura, H., 170, 173, *188*
Nakayama, T., 16, *24, 25,* 68, 69, 70, 72, 76, 79, *81*, 123, *151,* 126, *152,* 135, 149, *156,* 273, *283*

Nambu, N., 16, *25,* 68, 72, *80*, 123, *150, 151,* 123, *152,* 227, 231, *238*
Nancollas, G. H., 194, 195, *212, 213*
Nanny, D., 11, *22,* 244, 245, *275*
Naruchi, T., 265, *280*
Nascimento, A., 273, *283*
Natte, R., 58, *62*, 123, 127, 128, *151*
Nattress, B. R., 159, 161, 162, 163, 166, 178, 184, *186,* 164, *187,* 167, 171, 173, 183, 185, *188,* 179, *189*
Navas, E., 103, *116*
Navazesh, M., 204, *217*
Neal, P. J., 10, *22*
Neary, E. R., 329, 345, *354*
Neeser, J. R., 103, *115*
Neiders, M. E., 198, *215*
Nelson, S. L., 364, *375*
Nemanic, M. K., 29, *42*
Nemeth-Coslett, R., 328, *353,* 332, *354*
Newcombe, R., 367, *377*
Newman, H. N., 360, *373,* 366, 367, *376*
Newman, M. G., 371, *379*
Nguyen, V. C., 196, *214*
Nicholas, C. V., 205, *218*
Niederman, R., 366, 371, *376*
Nieuw Amerongen, A. V., 203, *216,* 204, *217*
Nigalaye, A., 232, *239,* 268, 273, *283*
Niibuchi, J. -J., 205, *218*
Nikiforuk, G., 384, 387, *401*
Nilsson, L., 103, 104, 113, *115*
Nimmerfall, F., 205, *217*
Nip, T. J., 350, *357*
Nishihata, T., 111, *119*
Nishijima, K., 369, *378*
Nishimura, H., 123, 126, *152*
Nishizuka, Y., 33, *44*
Nissen, S. S., 371, *378*
Niu, S., 58, *62*, 70, 79, *82*, 123, 127, 128, *151, 153*
Noach, A. B. J., 207, *218*
Noda, K., 130, 131, *153*
Noed, C. E., 247, *276*
Noguchi, T., 368, *377*
Norderyd, J., 371, *379*
Nordstrom, J. L., 32, *44*
Norling, T., 371, *378*
Nozaki, Y., 274, *284*
Nugteren, D. H., 35, *46*
Nummikoski, P., 393, *403*
Nuuja, T., 393, *403*
Nyman, A., 393, *403*

O

O' Kneeffe, M. K., 332, *354*
O' Neill, C. T., 123, *150*
O' Connell, A. C., 166, *187*
O' Connell, B., 209, *220*
O' Neill, C. T., 232, *239,* 272, 273, *282*
O' Sullivan, E. A., 164, *187*
Obernesser, M. N., 361, *374*
Oda, D., 103, *115*
Odle, B. M., 361, *374*
Odumosu, A., 134, *155*
Oemrawsingh, I., 198, *215*
Offenbacher, S., 33, *45* 361, *374,* 364, 365, 366, *375,* 366, 371, *376,* 371, *379*
Ofstead, R. F., 289, *314*
Ögaard, B., 388, 395, *401,* 39, *403, 404*
Oh, C. K., 16, *25,* 69, *81*, 123, 124, 125, *151*
Oh, V. M. S., 253, *277*

Ohashi, K., 134, *155,* 253, *277, 278*
Ohata, I., 76, *82*
Ohta, M., 274, *284*
Okabe, K., 265, *280*
Okada, H., 203, *216,* 368, *377*
Okada, Y., 123, *151*
Olanoff, L. S., 16, *25,* 58, *62,* 86, *98,* 135, 136, 138, *155,* 253, *278,* 297, *314*
Olejnik, O., 77, *83*
Oliveby, A., 345, *356,* 351, *357,* 390, *402*
Olsen, W. A., 79, *83*
Olsen, B. L., 350, *357*
Onken, H. D., 31, *43*
Oppenheim, F. G., 194, *212*
Orlando, R. C., 86, *97*
Orme, M. L 'E., 134, *154,* 253, *278*
Ormstad, K., 103, 104, 113, *115*
Örnerfeld, H. -O., 398, *405*
Orntoft, T. F., 103, *116*
Otero-Espinar, F. J., 272, 273, *283*
Ouhayoun, J. P., 102, 103, *114,* 103, *115*
Overberger, C. G., 226, *238*
Ovrebo, R., 398, *404*
Ozil, P., 272, *282*

P

Paalzow, L., 66, *80*
Pace, N. L., 123, 127, 128, *151*
Pack, A. G., 336, *354*
Page, R. C., 359, *373,* 361, *374,* 363, *375*
Palcanis, K. G., 361, *374*
Panders, A. K., 207, *219*
Pang, K. M., 351, *357*
Pappas, N. A., 296, *314*
Paranchych, W., 203, *216*
Park, H., 222, 223, *236,* 224, *237,* 292, *314*
Park, N. H., 106, *117*
Parker, R. B., 361, *374*
Parnes, S. M., 104, *116*
Paronen, P., 76, *82*
Paronen, P., 108, *118*
Parsons, D. F., 104, *116*
Past, T., 134, *155*
Patanapiradez, V., 385, *400*
Patashnick, S. R., 359, *373*
Patel, R. M., 95, *100*
Paterson, J. W., 134, *154*
Paterson, R., 227, *238,*
Paul, P., 32, *44*
Paunio, K., 371, *379*
Pavirani, A., 209, *219,* 209, *220*
Peach, J., 270, *281*
Pearson, J. P., 224, *237*
Pearson, S. K., 166, *187*
Pechersky, J. L., 8, *21*
Pedersen, M., 106, 108, *118*
Pedersen, A., 176, 177, 178, *189,* 390, *402*
Pedersen, M., 332, 333, 338, 339, *354,* 340, 341, 346, *355*
Pedrazzoli, V., 371, *379*
Pendrys, D. G., 392, 393, *403*
Peppas, N. A., 206, *218,* 222, 223, *236,* 226, 228, 229, *238,* 272, 273, *282,* 292, 296, *314*
Perkins, B. H., 368, *378*
Perricaudet, M., 209, *219,* 209, *220*
Person, P., 88, 95, *99*
Persson, R., 361, *374*
Peschier, L. J. C., 76, *82*
Peters, A., 6, *20*
Petersen, J. K., 207, *219*
Petersson, L. G., 395, 396, *403*
Pfeiffer, C. C., 345, *356*
Phillips, R. W., 398, *404*

Pickup, M. E., 134, *154*, 253, *276*
Pihlstrom, B., 372, *379*
Pikal, M. J., 268, 274, *284*
Pimlott, S. J., 135, *155*
Piotrowski, J., 103, *115*
Pitcher, G. R., 360, *373*
Pochi, P. E., 40, *48*
Polverini, P. J., 104, 105, 110, 111, 112, 113, *117*
Polymeropoulos, M. H., 196, *214*
Ponchel, G., 206, *218,* 223, *236,* 264, *280,* 272, 273, *282,* 272, *282,* 287, 312, *313*
Ponec, M., 32, *44*, 78, *83*, 86, 88, *98,* 256, *280*
Porchet, N., 196, 197, *214*
Potter, R. H., 351, *357*
Potts, R. O., 10, *22,* 40, *48*, 76, *82*
Poulsen, S., 395, *403*
Povey, S., 106, *118*
Prakobphol, A., 192, 198, 199, 200, 202, *212,* 198, 200, *215,* 203, 208, *216*
Preston-Martin, S., 14, *23*
Prevo, M., 27, *41*
Price, J. C, 104, *116*
Primosch, R. E., 167, 174, 178, 181, 182, *188*, 387, 390, *401*
Prostak, L., 361, *374*
Prottey, C., 33, 34, *45*, 35, *46*, 40, *48*
Prunerias, M., 10, *21*
Purkis, P. E., 103, *115*
Purves, R. D., 140, *156,* 258, *280*
Putt, M. S., 323, 324, *353*

Q

Qi, H., 111, *119*
Quadros, E., 16, 18, *25,* 123, 124, *150,* 234, *239,* 297, 302, *315*
Quinn, J., 34, *46*
Qvist, C., 176, *188*

R

Raadal, M., 398, *404*
Raehs, S., 311, *315*
Raj, P. A., 194, 195, *212*
Ralph, J. P., 164, 165, 166, 167, 168, 169, 170, 173, 176, 178, 174, 181, 183, 184, *187,* 387, 390, *401*
Ramasubbu, N., 194, 195, *212, 213,* 200, *215,* 204, 205, *217*
Randhawa, M. A., 134, *155*
Ranga Rao, K. V., 272, *282*
Ranney, R. R., 361, *374*
Ranta, R., 393, *403*
Rao, G. S., 95, *99*
Rapley, J. W., 364, *375*
Rashidbaigi, Z. A., 86, 87, 90, *98*
Rasmussen, S. N., 123, *152,* 271, *281,* 347, *356,* 349, 350, 351, *357*
Rassing, M. R., 106, 108, *118,* 271, *281,* 268, 274, *284,* 312, *316,* 328, 329, 331, 332, 333, 334, 336, 337, 338, 339, 343, *354,* 340, 341, 342, 346, *355,* 347, *356,* 349, 351, *357*
Rathbone, M. J., 76, *82*, 135, 136, 137, 138, 144, *155,* 146, *156,* 158, 183, *186,* 176, 177, 178, *189,* 242, 244, 245, 247, *274,* 260, 265, 266, *275,* 253, *277,* 254, *279,* 286, 287, *313,* 312, *316*
Ratner, B. D., 226, *237*
Raub, T. J., 106, 107, *118*
Raubertas, R. F., 176, 177, 178, *189,* 390, *402*
Raul, V. A., 312, *316*

Raw, M., 271, *281*
Rawle, L., 367, *376*
Rawlins, D. A., 123, *153*
Readling, R. D., 86, *97*
Record, D. W., 328, *353,* 342, *355*
Reddy, M. S., 192, *211,* 193, 198, 199, 200, 202, *212,* 198, 200, 202, *215,* 203, 208, *216,* 223, *236*
Reed, H. W., 176, *188*
Reeh, E. S., 194, 195, *212,* 202, *215*
Rees, T. D., 362, *375*
Regnier, M., 10, *21*
Rehfeld, S. J., 31, *43*
Reibel, J., 103, *115*
Reichard, G. A., 32, *44*
Reidenberg B., 350, *357*
Reilly, S., 104, *117*
Rein, H., 28, *41*
Reinerston, R. P., 31, *43*
Reinling-Zappa, M., 361, *373*
Rekosh, D., 203, *217*
Remon, J. P., 123, *150,* 206, *218,* 223, *236,* 232, *238,* 397, *404*
Rennert, O. M., 198, *215*
Repta, A. J., 57, *62,* 86, 88, *98,* 95, *99*
Rhodes, A. R., 40, *48*
Rhodes, M., 204, *217*
Riber, E., 13, *23,* 40, *49*
Rice, R. H., 6, 13, *19, 20,* 35, *47*
Richardson, C. F., 194, 195, *213*
Richardson, D., 12, *22*
Ridall, A. L., 193, *212*
Rider, J. N., 326, 327, 329, *353*
Rider, P. H., 326, 327, 329, *353*
Rindum, J., 338, 346, *355*
Ring, J., 40, *48*
Ringler, M. B., 104, *116*
Ripa, L. W., 395, *403*
Risemberg, H., 104, *116*
Ritschel, G. B., 69, *81*, 123, 124, 125, *150*
Ritschel, W. A., 16, *25*, 69, *81,* 123, 124, 125, *150, 151,* 297, *314*
Robb, R., 16, *24*
Robertson, A. M., 196, *214*
Robinson, C., 158, 159, 161, 162, 163, 166, 178, 183, 184, *186,* 164, 165, 167, 168, 169, 170, 173, 174, 176, 178, 181, 183, 184, *187,* 171, 185, *188,* 179, *189,* 387, 390, *401*
Robinson, J. R., 16, *25,* 51, 52, 56, 58, *60,* 70, 77, 79, *82*, 86, 87, 89, 90, 93, 95, 96, *97,* 88, *99,* 109, *118,* 129, *153,* 206, *218,* 222, 223, *236,* 224, *237,* 233, *239,* 244, 245, 247, 256, 260, *275,* 268, 274, *284,* 285, 286, 287, 288, 292, *313, 314,* 312, *317*
Robinson, N. L., 328, *353*
Rodda, J. C., 385, *400*
Rodrigues, A. L., 398, *404*
Rodu, B., 268, 273, *283*
Rodwell, V. W., 32, *44*
Rogers, C. E., 235, *239*
Rogers, N. J., 16, *24,* 68, 71, 77, 78, *80*, 69, 74, *81*, 76, *82*, 123, *152, 153,* 308, *315*
Rojanasakul, Y., 66, *80*
Rolla, G., 14, *24,* 360, *373,* 364, *375,* 344, *356,* 388, *401,* 394, 395, *403,* 395, *404*
Romanowski, A. R., 8, *21*
Rompen, E., 370, 372, *378*
Rooney, L., 9, *21,* 29, *42*, 52, 56, *60,* 87, 96, *99,* 254, *279*
Rordorf-Adam, C., 361
Rose, M. C., 196, *214,*

Rosenfeld, M. A., 209, *220*
Rosenthal, E. R., 209, *220,*
Rosenthaler, J., 205, *217*
Rosenzweig, K. A., 87, *98,* 123, 124, *150, 151*
Ross, J. W., 389, *402*
Rossomando, E. F., 361, *374*
Roth, G., 12, *22*
Rothman, S., 28, *41*
Roukema, P. A., 198, 203, *215, 216*
Roussel, P., 199, *215*
Rowlands, C., 224, *237*
Rowland, M., 228, 234, *238,* 273, *283*
Rowlatt, C., 106, *118*
Rubright, W. C., 14, *24*
Rudney, J. D., 202, *215*
Rugg-Gunn, A. J., 385, *400,* 391, 392, 394, *402*
Rummelt, A., 70, 72, *81,* 123, *150,* 297, 312, *314*
Rupniak, H. T., 106, *118*
Russel, A. L., 381, *400*
Russell, C. M., 268, 273, *283*
Russel, M. A. H., 271, *281*
Russell, R. J., 368, *378*
Rynar, J., 361, *374*
Rytting, J. H., 76, *82,* 108, *118,* 111, *119*

S

Sabatier, M., 272, *282*
Sachs, D. P. L., 349, *357*
Sacks, P. G., 104, *116*
Sakaguchi, R. L., 202, *215*
Saleeby, D. E., *238*
Samaranayake, L. P., 312, *316*
Samejima, M., 130, 131, *153*
Sandow, J., 312, *316,* 312, *317*
Sandow, R. J., 123, *153*
Sarosiek, J., 205, *218*
Savanapridi, C., 271, *281,* 332, 351, *354*
Sawaf, M. H., 102, 103, *114, 115*
Saxegaard, E., 395, *403*
Saxen, U. P., 360, *373*
Scaletta, S., 88, *99*
Scannapieco, F. A., 194, 195, *213,* 203, 208, *216,* 204, 205, *217*
Schachtele, C. F., 385, *400*
Schaeffer, A., 103, *116*
Schaub, R. M. H., 207, *219*
Schenk, P., 7, *20*
Schenkels, L. C. P. M., 203, *216*
Scherrer, R. A., 291, 292, *314*
Schesmer, K. R., 134, *154,* 253, *278*
Scheuplein, R. J., 28, *41,* 29, *42*
Schiffman, S. S., 16, *24*
Schiller, D. L., 103, *114*
Schiller, G., 207, *219*
Schimmele, R. G., 323, 324, *353*
Schlesinger, D. H., 194, 195, *212, 213*
Schluckebier, S. K., 195, *213*
Schluger, S., 359, *373*
Schmid, H. H. O., 31, *44*
Schmid, P. C., 31, *44*
Schneider, L., 40, *48*
Schoenberg, J. B., 14, *23*
Schoenholtz, D., 341, 342, *355*
Scholz, M. T., 291, 292, *314*
Schor, J. M., 232, *239,* 268, 273, *283*
Schreiner, E., 9, *21,* 29, *42*
Schreiner, V. J., 86, *97*
Schroeder, H. E., 4, 6, 8, 9, 16, *20, 21,* 363, *375*
Schürmann, W., 134, *154, 155,* 253, *277*
Schurr, W., 67, *80,* 123, *153,* 135, *155,* 312, *316, 317*

Schuster, G. S., 103, 105, 108, *115,* 104, *116*
Schut, H. A. I., 104, 111, *117*
Schwartz, I. L., 210, *220*
Schwartz, J., 361, *374*
Scott, D. B., 381, *400*
Sedman, A. J., 253, *277*
Seitz, H. K., 14, *23*
Sela, M. N., 367, 372, *377,* 369, *378*
Semba, I., 12, *22*
Semple, W. F., 320, *353*
Senel, S., 56, *61,* 108, *118*
Seremet, T., 104, 110, 111, 113, *116*
Serra, M. C., 398, *404*
Sezaki, H., 59, *63*
Sforza, C., 163, *186*
Shaaya, A. N., 297, *314*
Shabana, A. H. M., 102, 103, *114, 115*
Shade, W. B., 10, *22*
Shanley, D. B., 123, *150*
Shannon, I. L., 192, *211,* 207, *219,* 389, 390, *402*
Shapira, L., 361, *374*
Shariati, M., 386, *401*
Sharma, S. C., 342, *355*
Shaw, J. E., 27, *41*, 30, *42*
Shefter, E., 16, *24*, 68, 71, 77, 78, *80*, 76, *82*, 86, *98,* 123, *152,* 274, *284,* 297, *315*
Shepherd, M. G., 382, *400*
Shern, R. J., 111, *119*
Shey, J., 398, *405*
Shields, C. P., 386, *401,* 390, *402*
Shim, Y. S., *400*
Shimabukuro, Y., 368, *377*
Shonik, J. A., 32, *44*
Shotton, D. M., 56, *61*
Shriner, D., 31, *43*
Siddiki, B., 196, 197, *214*
Siegel, I. A., 14, 16, *24, 25,* 27, 29, *41*, 57, *62,* 68, 72, 79, *80*, 86, 87, 93, *97,* 90, 93, *99,* 123, *151, 152,* 254, 255, 256, *279,* 261, 263, *280*
Siegmund, C., 361, *374*
Simon, M., 6, *20*
Simon, S. A., 16, *24*
Simonsen, K., 271, *281,* 347, *356*
Sindet-Pederson, S., 111, *118*
Singer, L., 389, *401*
Singh, B. B., 104, *116*
Skartveit, L., 398, *404*
Skutches, C. L., 32, *44*
Slaga, T. J., 104, *117*
Slivka, S. R., 103, 104, 108, 109, *114*
Slomiany, A., 198, *215,* 205, *218*
Slomiany, B. L., 103, *115,* 198, *215,* 205, *218*
Slop, D., 206, *218,* 397, *404*
Slots, J., 362, *374*
Smalley, J. W., 13, *23*
Smart, J. D., 225, *237,* 233, *239,* 272, *282,* 291, 292, *314*
Smith, D. C., 14, *24,* 158, *186*
Snell, E. E., 32, *44*
Snipes, W., 123, *153,* 268, 272, *281*
Sobrero, A., 266, 268, *280*
Socransky, S. S., 361, *374*
Soder, P. O., 247, *276,* 95, *100*
Söderholm, S., 393, *403*
Soei, Y. L., 78, *83*
Sojar, H. T., 203, *216*
Solt, D. B., 104, 105, 110, 111, 112, 113, *117*
Somogyi A., 348, *356*
Song, J. H., 342, *355,* 343, *355*
Soni, S. -D., 194, 195, *212,* 200, *215*
Sonies, B. C., 207, *219*

Sorenson, H., 103, *116*
Soskolne, W. A., 367, 372, *377*, 369, *378*, *379*
Southam, J. C., 111, *118*
Speight, P. M., 4, *19*, 40, *48*, 86, 93, *98*
Spies, F., 56, *61*
Sprake, S. A., 253, *278*
Sprecher, H. W., 33, *45*
Squier, C. A., 2, 4, *19*, 7, 9, *20*, 8, 10, *21*, 11, 12, *22*, 12, *23*, 14, *24*, 16, 18, *25*, 5, 18, *26*, 27, *41*, 29, 36, *42*, 31, 32, 34, 36, 38, *43*, 40, *44*, 34, *46*, 35, *47*, *48*, 51, 52, 55, 56, *60*, *61*, 59, *63*, 76, *82*, 86, 93, 95, *97*, *98*, 87, 88, *99*, 96, *100*, 103, 108, *115*, 104, 111, *116*, 204, *217*, 242, 247, 260, *274*, 244, 245, *275*, 254, *279*, 285, 286, 287, *313*
Sreebny, L. M., 195, *213*
Stabholz, A., 367, 372, *377*
Stafford, R. G., 16, 18, *25*, 86, 93, *98*
Stamm, J. W., 382, *400*
Stanley, T. H., 58, *62*, 70, 79, *82* 123, 127, *150*, 128, *153*, 269, *280*
Stannard, J. G., 382, *400*
Starcke, E. N., 207, *219*
Stashenko, P., 361, *374*
Steele, J. G., 106, *118*
Steinberg, D., 369, *378*
Steinert, P. M., 6, *19*, 6, *20*
Stellfeld, M., 364, 371, *375*
Steward, A., 70, 72, *82*, 207, *219*
Stier, L. E., 209, *220*
Stinson, M. L., 361, *374*
Stinson, M. W., 192, 198, *212*, 223, *236*
Stolinski, C., 6, *19*
Stoltze, K., 103, *115*, 338, 346, *355*, 364, 371, *375*, *378*, *379*
Stoner, G. D., 104, 111, *117*
Stookey, G. K., 176, *188*, 350, *357*
Strachan, D. S., 345, *356*
Strahan, J. D., 360, *373*, 366, *376*
Strang, A. M., 199, *215*
Stratford, R. E., 95, *99*
Stratford-Perricaudet, L. D., 209, *219*, *220*
Strauss, J. S., 37, 40, *48*
Strecker, G., 199, *215*
Streisand, J. B., 58, *62*, 123, 127, 128, *151*
Strong, M., 159, 161, 162, 163, 166, 178, 184, *186*, 164, *187*, 168, 169, 170, 173, 176, 184, *187*, 167, 174, 178, 181, 182, *188*, 387, 390, 390, *401*, 389, 394, *402*
Strous, G. J., 196, 200, *213*, 197, *214*
Sturzenberg, O. P., 360, *373*
Sugimoto, I., 69, 74, *81*, 123, *152*
Sullivan, A., 167, 176, 184, *187*
Summerly, R., 31, 32, 34, *43*
Sundin, Y., 366, *376*
Sundqvist, K., 103, 104, 105, 106, 110, 111, 113, *115*, 112, *117*
Sutherland, J. M., 134, *154*, 253, *278*
Suzuki, T., 130, 131, *15*
Suzuki, Y., 368, *377*, 265, *280*
Svanberg, M., 398, *404*, *405*
Swallow, D. M., 196, *214*
Swartz, M. L., 398, *404*
Swartzendruber, D. C., 6, *19*, 7, *20*, 10, *21*, *22*, 31, 32, *43*, 33, 34, *45*, 34, 35, *46*, 36, 38, *47*, *48*, 76, *82*, 285, 286, *313*
Sweeney, T. M., 31, *43*

Sweetana, S. A., 90, *99*
Synosky, S. P., 321, *353*

T

Tabak, L. A., 96, *100,* 192, *211,* 198, *212,* 200, 202, *215,* 203, 208, *216,* 204, *217,* 207, *219,* 223, 224, *236,* 246, 247, *275*
Taggart, E. J., 366, 371, *376*
Taichman, L., 104, *117*
Takagi, A., 205, *218*
Takahashi, K., 361, *374*
Takashiba, S., 361, *374*
Takatori, T., 69, *81*, 123, 126, *152,* 273, *283*
Takeuchi, K., 369, *378*
Takigawa, M., 361
Tamura, E., 369, *378*
Tamura, T., 369, *378*
Tan, S. C., 247, *276*
Tanaka, M., 16, *24,* 123, *152*
Tanner, A., 366, *376*
Tanquaery, A., 396, *404*
Tanzer, J. M., 123, 132, 133, *150*
Tapsonyi, Zs., 134, *155*
Tartaglia, G., 163, *186*
Tarwater, O., 396, *404*
Tatevossian, A., 388, *401*
Tavakoli-Saberi, M. R., 104, 105, 107, 108, 109, 110, 112, 113, *117, 118,* 111, *119*
Taves, D. R., 389, *402*
Taylor, M. J., 182, *189*
Teboul, M., 369, *378*
Temple, D. J., 134, *154, 155,* 253, *278*
Ten Cate, J. M., 176, *189,* 386, *400*
Tenovuo, J. O., 246, *275*
Tfelt-Hansen, P., 66, *80*
Thakkar, N. S., 207, *219*
Thaysen, J. H., 210, *220*
Thesleff, I., 393, *403*
Thomas, N. W., 78, *83*
Thompson, L., 209, *220*
Thomsen, M. E., 336, *354*
Thorburn, D. N., 312, *316*
Thorn, N. A., 210, *220*
Thornqvist, E., 174, *188*
Thylsrup, A., 176, *188,* 176, *189,* 345, *356,* 384, *400, 401,* 389, *402,* 393, *403*
Timmins, P., 123, 126, 127, *151,* 226, 234, *237,* 234, 235, *239,* 268, 273, *283*
Tipnis, V., 302, *315*
Tirendi, S., 348, *356*
Tjalve, H., 104, 105, 106, 110, 111, 113, *117*
Tobey, N. A., 86, *97*
Toda, H., 368, *377*
Toftgard, R., 103, 104, 113, *115*
Tolo, K., 8, 16, *21,* 10, 16, *22*, 56, *61,* 86, *97,* 86, *98,* 256, *279, 280*
Tomlinson, E., 134, *154,* 253, *276*
Tomomatsu, E., 369, *378*
Tomomatsu, T., 369, *378*
Tonetti, M., 366, 371, *376*
Tong, G. L., 253, *277*
Toon, S., 228, 234, *238,* 273, *283*
Topp, E. M., 95, *99*
Toribara, N. W., 196, 197, *214*
Torres, G. I., 203, 208, *216*
Totdal, B., 398, *404*
Touchard, F., 206, *218*, 272, 273, *282*
Toumba, K. J., 167, *187,* 397, *404*
Traczyk, T. N., 34, 35, *45*, 34, *46*
Trapnell, B. C., 209, *220*
Treagar, R. T., 31, *43*
Trejdosiewicz, L. K., 106, *118*
Triggs, E. J., 57, *62,* 134, *153,* 253, *276*

Trushin, N., 104, 111, *116*
Tsai, H., 196, 200, 202, *214,* 207, *219*
Tsamtsouris, A., 382, *400*
Tseng, C. -C., 194, *213*
Tsuchiya, S., 205, *218*
Tucker, I. G., 76, *82*, 129, *153,* 134, *154,* 176, 177, 178, *189,* 242, 245, 247, 260, 265, 266, 254, *279,* 286, 287, *313,* 312, *316,* 368, *378*
Turner, P., 58, *62,* 134, *154,* *155*, 253, *277, 278*
Turunen, T. M., 76, *82*, 108, *118*
Tuyns, A. J., 14, *23*
Tveit, A. B., 398, *404*
Tyrer, J. H., 134, *154*, 253, *278*

U

Uematso, A., 369, *378*
Ullbro, C., 395, *403*
Umemoto, T., 369, *378*
Urtti, A., 76, *82*, 108, *118*
Ussing, H. H., 90, *99*

V

Vadgama, P., 205, *218*
Valdez, I. H., 195, 204, *213*
Valentijn-Benz, M., 203, *216,* 204, *217*
van den Brink, I., 56, *61*
van der Ven, P. F., 207, *219*
van Dyke, T. E., 361, *374*
van Halbeek, H., 199, *215*
van Harten, J., 66, *80*
van Lennep, E. W., 210, *220*
van Loveren, C., 386, *401*
van Muijen, G. N. P., 103, *115*
van Palastein Helderman, W. H., 360, *373*
van Rijn, L. J., 207, *219*
van Steenbergen, T. M. J., 362, *375*, 370, 372, *378*
van Winkelhoff, A. J., 362, *375*
van-Seuningen, I., 197, *214*
Vandelli, M. A., 228, *238*
Vandenhoven, G., 370, 372, *378*
Vanderfaeillie, A., 370, 372, *378*
Varboncoeur, A. P., 361, *374*
Varonne, R., 369, *378*
Veall, N., 328, 329, 333, 336, 337, 345, *354*
Vedtofte, P., 103, *115, 116*
Veerman, E. C. I., 203, *216,* 204, *217*
Veillard, M. M., 16, *25,* 70, 72, *81* 129, *153,* 224, *237,* 233, *239,* 268, 274, *284,* 312, *317*
Venegas, M., 103, *116*
Verain, A., 272, *282*
Verhoef, J. C., 51, *60,* 56, *61,* 86, 88, *98,* 108, *118,* 221, *236,* 242, 245, 246, 247, 261, *274,* 256, *280,* 296, 297, *314*
Verma, M., 196, 210, *213*
Vermeer, B. J., 32, *44*
Vermey, A., 207, *219*
Vermey, T., 207, *219*
Viaje, A., 104, *117*
Vigne, P., 58, *63*
Visch, L. L., 207, *219*
Vissink, A., 207, *219*
Vlachou, A., 382, *400*
von der Fehr, F. R., 394, *403*
von Heijne, G., 197, *214*
von Unruh, G. E., 348, *356*
Voorhees, J. J., 33, *45*
Voorspoels, J., 123, *150*
Vora, K. R. M., 253, *278*
Vos, H. L., 196, *214*
Vyas, S. P., 265, 268, *280*

W

Wade, W., 367, *377*
Wadsworth, J., 134, *155,* 253, *278*
Waerhaug, G., 360, *373*
Waerhaug, J., 344, *356*, 363, *375*
Wagner, J. G., 253, *277*
Wakshull, E., 10, *22*
Walgreen-Weterings, E., 203, *216*
Walker, J. A., 14, *24*
Walker, L. A., 326, 327, 329, *353*
Walker, M., 77, *83*
Wallenstein, S., 350, *357*
Walters, K. A., 77, *83*
Walton, R. P., 66, 67, *80*
Wamer, T. M., 14, *23*
Wan Yusof, W. Z. A., 366, *376*
Wang, E., 32, *44*
Wang, L. -Y., 66, *80*
Ward, S. A., 134, *154,* 253, *278*
Warm, R., 67, *80*
Warren, S. J., 123, 126, 127, *151,* 226, 234, *237,* 235, *239,* 268, 273, *283*
Warren, C., 336, *354*
Washington, N., 270, *281,* 271, *282*
Watanabe, S., 158, *186,* 173, *188,* 366, *376*
Waterman, H. A., 196, *213*
Watson, E., 57, *62,* 86, 87, 93, *97,* 254, *279*
Watt, F. M., 6, *20*
Wayne, J. P., 336, *354*
Weatherell, J. A., 159, 158, 161, 162, 163, 166, 178, 184, *186,* 164, 165, 167, 168, 169, 170, 173, 174, 176, 178, 181, 183, 184, *187,* 171, 182, 185, *188,* 179, *189*, 387, 390, *401,* 398, *404*
Weaver, M. L., 123, 132, 133, *150*
Weaver, W., 14, *24*
Webb, J., 207, *219*
Wechter, W. J., 360, *373*
Weder, H. J., 134, *154*, 253, *277*
Weetman, D. A., 158, *186*
Wehmeyer, K. R., 364, *375*
Wei, S. H. Y., 395, *404*
Weiffenbach, J. M., 207, *219*
Weinberg, D. S., 350, *357*
Weinstein, G. D., 40, *48*
Weissbach, R., 67, *80*
Wenander, A., 366
Wennemark, J. R., 134, *154*, 253, *277*
Wermerskirchen, A., 261, 263, *280,* 311, *315*
Wersall, J., 7, *20*
Wertz, P. W., 6, *19,* 7, *20,* 10, *21,* 12, *22,* 18, *26,* 31, 32, 34, 35, 36, 38, *43,* 40, *44,* 33, 37, *45, 46, 47,* 37, *48, 49,* 51, *60,* 76, *82,* 103, 108, *115,* 244, *275,* 285, 286, 287, *313*
Wettstein-Knowles, P., 33, *45*
Wheatley, V. R., 31, *43*
Wheeler, K. P., 77, *83*
White, R. J., 35, *46*
Whitmore, D. A., 77, *83*
Wiedermann, W., 361, *374*
Wieriks, J., 123, *151*
Wieruszeski, J. M., 199, *215*
Wiesenfeld, D., 207, *219*
Wikman, A., 205, *217*
Wikstrom, M., 362, *374*
Wildnauer, R., 40, *48*
Williams, A., 110, *118*
Williams, D. M., 4, *19,* 12, *22,* 40, *48,* 86, 93, *98*
Williams, D. R., 364, *375*
Williams, M. L., 31, *43*
Williams, P., 207, *218*
Williams, R. C., 360, *373*
Williamson, M. P., 197, *214*

Wilson, C. G., 182, *189*, 270, *281*, 271, *282*
Wilson, C. W. M., 134, *155*
Wilson, I. B., 197, *214*
Winer, R. A., 95, *100*, 247, *276*
Winkelmann, R. K. J., 1, *18*
Winn, D. M., 14, *23, 24*
Winrow, M. J., 364, *375*
Winsor, T., 28, 31, *41*
Winter, S., 103, *115*
Wintraub, B. U., 34, 35, *46*
Winzler, R. J., 198, *215*
Wisniewski, N., 296, *314*
Witzel, F., 336, *354*, 341, 342, *355*
Wojciechowski, N. J., 134, *154*, 253, *277*
Wolany, G. J. M., 70, 72, *81*, 106, 109, *118*, 123, *150*, 242, 247, 260, *275*, 261, *276*, 274, *284*, 297, 312, *314*, 311, *315*, *317*
Wolff, K., 9, *21*, 10, *22*, 29, *42*, 34, *46*
Woltz, A., 103, *115*
Woodford, W., 320, 329, 348, *353*
Woodley, D., 10, *21*
Woodley, J. F., 206, *218*
Worthington, H. E. C., 233, *239*, 291, 292, *314*
Worthington, H. V., 176, *188*
Wotman, S., 192, *211*, 246, 247, *275*
Wouessidjewe, D., 272, 273, *282*
Wright, I. S., 67, *80*
Wright, J. T., 164, *187*
Wu, A. M., 202, *215*
Wyandt, C. M., 326, 327, 329, *353*
Wynder, E. L., 14, *23*

Y

Yamahara, H., 130, 131, *153*, 286, 287, *313*
Yamamoto, A., 58, *63*, 88, 95, *99*
Yamamoto, M., 265, *280*
Yamashita, S., 70, 72, *81*
Yanagibashi, N., 16, *24*, 123, *152*
Yang, B., 273, *283*
Yang, K. Y., 342, *355*
Yano, K., 135, 149, *156*
Yardley, H. J., 31, 32, 34, *43*
Yashiki, T., 76, *82*
Yeung, F. I. S., 367, *376*
Yiu, C. K. Y., 395, *404*
Yoneyama, K., 209, *220*
Yoshimura, K., 209, *220*
Young, D. Y., 207, *219*
Young, J. A., 210, *220*
Young, J. M., 351, *357*
Young, W. W., 103, *116*
Yukimatsu, K., 274, *284*
Yum, S. I., 27, *41*
Yuodelis, R., 359, *373*

Z

Zaki, S. A., 324, 329, 330, *353*
Zambon, J. J., 362, *374*
Zappa, U., 361
Zawacki, S., 204, 205, *217*
Zeigler, F., 103, 104, 108, 109, *114*
Zero, D. T., 176, 177, 178, *189*, 390, *402*
Zhang, H., 58, *62*
Zhang, J, 58, *62*, 70, 79, *82*, 123, 127, *150*, 128, *151*, *153*
Zheng, H., 112, 113, *119*
Zibell, S. E., 323, *353*
Ziboh, A., 33, *45*
Ziegler, R., 67, *80*, 135, *155*
Zielenski, J., 198, *215*
Zimber, M. P., 103, 104, 108, 109, *114*

Subject Index

A

Advantages as a site, 15, 66, 242, 286
Apthous ulceration, 14
Artificial salivas, 207
Autoradiography, 55-56

B

Basal lamina, 10
Buccal mucosa
- blood flow, 286
- thickness, 245, 286

C

Cellular composition, keratinized, 6
Cellular composition, nonkeratinized, 7
Cellular differentiation, 6-7
Chewing gum
- advantages, 319-320, 346
- clinical applications, 319, 346, 352

[Chewing gum]
- composition, 320-321
- cultural aspects, 320-321
- definition, 320
- factors affecting release, 328-342
- formulation, 322, 335-336
- history, 320
- in vitro release assessment, 323-340
- manufacture, 322-323
- safety aspects, 351-359

Classification of oral mucosal drug delivery systems, 263-265
Comparison with other routes, 242
Confocal laser scanning, 55-57

D

Dental caries, 383
Dental enamel, 383-384
Dento-gingival junction, 7-9
Disadvantages as a site, 85
Dosage forms, systemic, 266-274
Drug candidate selection criteria, 248-256

E

Epithelial cell and tissue cultures
advantages, 102
application in drug delivery, 107-113
cell lines, 105-106
disadvantages, 102
dissociated cell cultures, 104-105
explants, 104

F

Fluoride
definition, 382
sources, 382
Fluoride delivery systems, 391-398, 345-346

G

Gingivitis
definition, 359
Glycomimetics, 208-209

H

Hydrogels, 225-235
drug release from hydrogels, 227-230
ideal properties, 235
mechanism of release, prehydrated hydrogels, 228
mechanism of release, swelling hydrogels, 228

I

In vitro methods
advantages, 85-86
animal models, 86-87
design, 89-90
tissue viability and integrity, 89
uses, 86, 96-97
In vivo methods
absorption cells, 123-129
animals, 123-132
buccal absorption test, 134
disc methods, 135-148
dosage forms, 123
perfusion cells, animal, 129-132
perfusion cells, human, 135-148
Insulin, 68-72

L

Lamina propria, 10-11
Lichen planus, 14

M

Mechanism of absorption, 29
Membrane coating granules, 6-7, 9, 34-36
Metabolic barrier, 95-96
MG1, 191, 198-199
MG2, 192-193, 200-202
Mouth - see oral cavity
Mucin composition, 196, 198
Mucins, 196, 198-202
function, 202-204
properties, 202-203

[Mucins]
role in barrier function, 205-206
role in drug delivery, 206-207
Mucoadhesive delivery systems, 231-235
Mucoadhesives
definition, 222
mechanisms, 222
physicochemical features, 222
role in drug delivery, 227-228, 231
testing, 224
Mucus
barrier function, 95-96
components, 191
composition, 192-195
function, 191-195
properties, 191
structure, 192, 223

O

Oral cavity
function, 244
physical description, 243-244
Oral mucosa
blood flow, 11, 245
composition, 31-39, 244-245
organization, 2
regional variation, 2, 4, 52
structure, animals, 15-18
structure, human, 2-4, 52
thickness, 244-245
tissue turnover time, 4, 6
vascular drainage, 11

P

Paracellular route, 53-54
Patch delivery systems
adhesion, 290-293
bioavailability, 298-299
characteristics of drug release, 294-295
comfort, 300
composition, 290
design, 287-290, 306, 312
dimensions, 306
in vivo adhesion, 300-302, 304
load, 289
manufacture, 289, 296, 306
oral mucosal versus transdermal route, 288
pharmacokinetics, 304-311
placement sites, 300, 304
preclinical evaluation, 297
shape, 289
size, 287
thickness, 306
tolerance, 297-298
toleration, 300-302, 304
Pathways - see routes of drug transport
Periodontal delivery systems, 365-371
Periodontal disease
definition 360-361
etiology, 359
pathogenesis, 361
treatment, 360
types, 361-362
Periodontal pocket
anatomy, 362
biopharmaceutics, 364
Permeability
animal models, 15-18
effect of aging, 12
effect of dentures, 41

[Permeability]
effect of extrinsic factors, 13-14
effect of inflammation, 12-13
effect of mucosal disease, 14-15
individual variation, 40
regional variation, 40
role of blood flow, 96
Permeability barrier, 28-29, 38, 52
Permeability coefficient, 91-93
Permeation enhancers
characteristics, 73-74
mechanisms, 76-77
structure/effect relationships, 74, 76
structures, 75
toxicity, 78-79
Proteins and Peptides, 67, 73, 95, 308-312

R

Routes of drug transport, 29-30, 53-54, 58

S

Saliva
composition, 246
direction of flow, 164-166
[Saliva]
film thickness, 159-160, 224, 247
function, 245-246
location of major glands, 245-246
location of minor glands, 224-225
movement of substances, 166-168
pH, 247, 286
role, 385
volume, 158, 160, 162, 246
Salivary proteins, 193
Surface area of oral mucosa, 4, 159, 245

T

Teeth, 243
Transcellular route, 53-54

V

Vesiculo-bullous lesion, 15
Visualization techniques, 55-56

X

Xerostomia, 195, 204